the complete book of
hairstyling

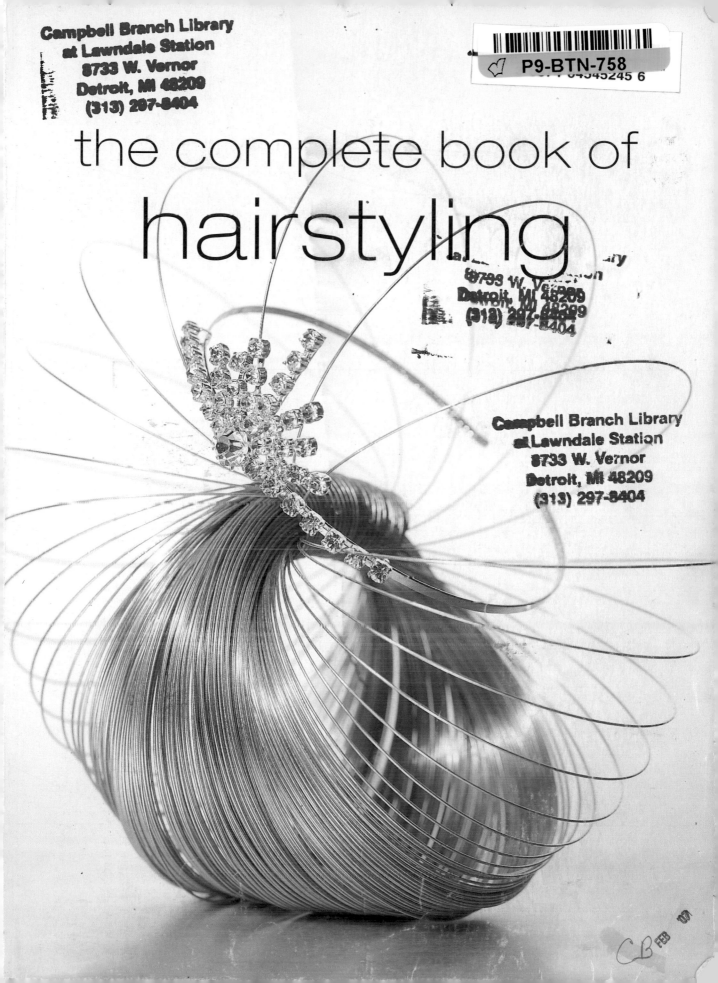

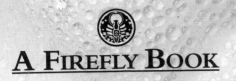

A FIREFLY BOOK

Published by Firefly Books Ltd., 2002

Third printing, 2005

National Library of Canada Cataloguing in Publication Data

Worthington, Charles
    The complete book of hairstyling
includes index.
ISBN 1-55297-576-2
    1. Hairdressing. 2. Hair—Care and hygiene. I. Title.
TT972.W65 2002   646.7'24   C2001-902196-8

Publisher Cataloging-in-Publication Data (U.S.)

Worthington, Charles.
    The complete book of hairstyling / Charles Worthington. — 1st ed.
[304] p. : col. ill. : photos. ; cm.
Includes index.
Summary: Hairstyling ideas and instructions, professional secrets, emergency quick fixes and hair care for women.
ISBN 1-55297-576-2 (pbk.)
1. Hairstyling. 2. Hairdressing. I. Title.
646.724   21   CIP   TT972.W67   2002

Published in Canada by
Firefly Books Ltd.
66 Leek Crescent
Richmond Hill, Ontario L4B 1H1

Published in the United States by
Firefly Books (U.S.) Inc.
P.O. Box 1338, Ellicott Station
Buffalo, New York 14205

Text: Carmel Allen (City Hair), Karen Wheeler (Big Date Hair), Emma Craven (Vacation Hair) and Lisa Helmanis (Big Day Hair)
Photography: Hugh Arnold (model), Patrice de Villiers (still life)
Illustrations: Jason Brooks
Stylists: Sophie Kenningham and Rachel Davis
Make-up: Chase Aston and Maggie Hunt
Editorial Manager: Venetia Penfold
Art Director: Penny Stock
Project Editor: Zia Mattocks

Printed and bound in Dubai

the complete book of
hairstyling

Charles Worthington

FIREFLY BOOKS

contents

foreword

I defy anyone to underestimate the power of hair and its ability to transform the way you look and feel! Your hair is your most important fashion accessory and the first thing that people notice about you. It speaks volumes about your personality, lifestyle, look and, most of all, what sort of mood you're in: casual and laid-back, minimal and understated, glamorous and sexy, sleek and neat or wild and va-va-voom. What's important to me, as a hairdresser who has witnessed and enjoyed the buzz that people get from a great cut or a new style, is to make fabulous hair accessible to everyone every day of the year. The aim is to make sure you can enjoy hair that is in peak condition and fulfilling its maximum potential whether you're at home, away on vacation, preparing for a change of image or planning your wedding. Most of all, though, I think hair should be fun – it should be about enjoying your individuality and finding a hairstyle that suits you and your lifestyle.

Charles Worthington

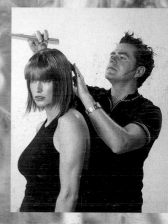

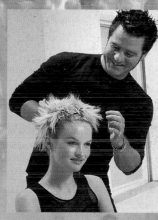

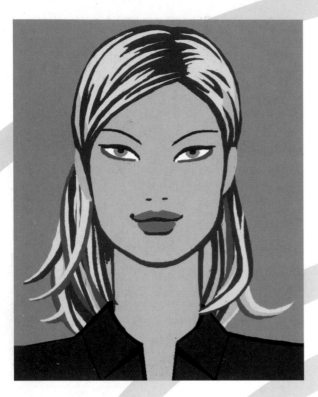

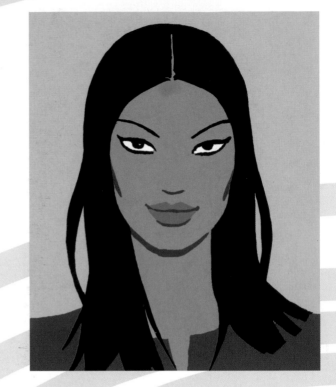

polly

jaz

Polly is a career babe — traditional, yes, but she's got a twist. Her A's in math means she can add up her buying splurges as fast as the computers at Visa. She always looks immaculate and only her closest friends know that her sleek blonde hair is the result of painstaking styling to iron out its natural wave. Polly's money-crazy boyfriend Harry is inclined to insensitivity and it's beginning to get her down. She needs something — or someone — to inject a bit of excitement into her life. Everyone thinks she's as straight as her hair, but she's about to show them a new side to her character.

Jaz (short for Jasmine) is your regular club bunny. She loves all things hip, cool and girlie. Her earliest memory is of dressing up in the contents of her mother's overstuffed wardrobe — and clothes are still her greatest passion. She can't remember the last time she took off her make-up before going to bed but, with her long, thick, shiny black hair, she always looks stunning nevertheless. Always the party girl, Jaz will try anything once and dreams of landing herself a high-glamour job in fashion. She's not fussy, as long as it fuels her passion for fashion, fun and trying out new hairstyles.

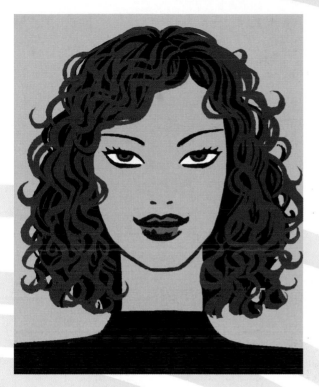

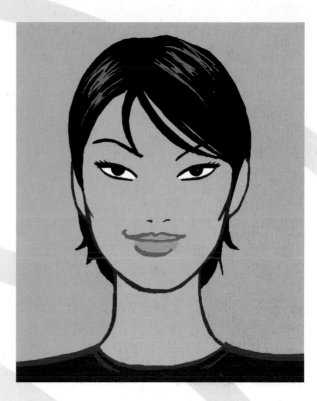

kate

laura

Kate looks like a pre-Raphaelite painting: unruly curly red hair, milky complexion and rosy cheeks. She works as a personal assistant to the marketing director of Crunch Cookies — not a good career choice when you have a sweet tooth and are prone to overindulgence. Kate is a hopeless romantic with an insatiable crush on her boss. But spending hours daydreaming of weekends away with him in exotic destinations isn't getting her anywhere. It's time to make some changes, and it's not just her looks and love life that are in need of a revamp, her career needs something of a kick-start, too.

Laura is a tomboy: lean and androgynous with a short crop. Her uniform is urban cool — more combat boots and running shoes than pencil skirts and high heels. She wouldn't be seen dead in anything glittery. Laura loves to work out but is fiercely competitive and intimidates most of her fellow gym-goers. A struggling TV researcher who wants to make gritty documentaries and dreams of winning an Emmy, Laura's recognized the benefits of networking. She's also trying to attract the attention of a certain assistant producer and decides that a redefined image — still tomboy but with a feminine twist — just might be the answer.

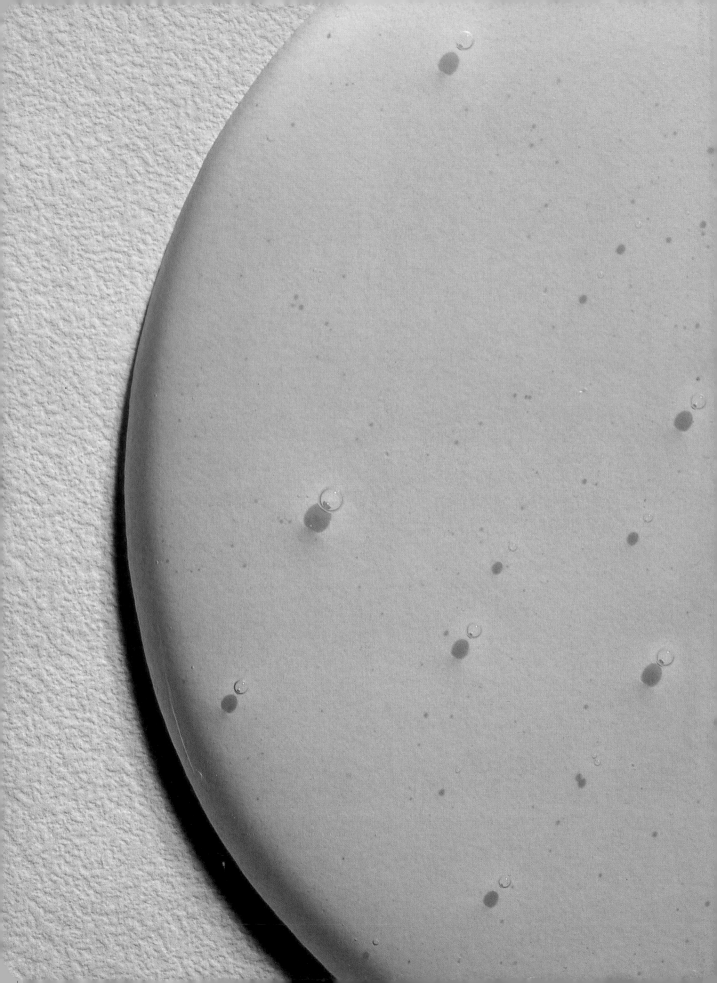

city hair

Discover the **perfect** haircare routine to suit your particular **needs**, cuts to enhance your face shape, colors to **complement** your **skin tone** and just-left-the-salon **styling** techniques to help you achieve and **maintain** salon-style hair every day of the week. City Hair **answers** your everyday hair needs, whether it's **redefining** your **image** to help you get **ahead** at work, coping with "stressed" **hair** or getting caught with a **last-minute** after-work **party** invitation.

hair basics

home, sweet home

"Oh, Polly," moaned Kate, tossing back her unruly red curls and flinging herself down perilously on Polly's new white couch, glass of red wine in hand. "I can't believe you've agreed to let Chrissie come and stay for a month — what a nightmare." Polly did indeed know that Chrissie could be high-maintenance (to say the least), but then so, too, could Kate. She grimaced as a drop of wine from Kate's glass splashed onto her candy-striped pyjamas, but at least it didn't hit the couch.

With the help of her parents (rich) and her first city bonus, Perfect Polly — as the others called her in their more green-eyed moments — had bought a loft in Tribeca, chosen largely for its proximity to fashionable, but much more expensive, Soho. Polly had proceeded to install her BFs: Laura, her best friend from NYU and her two oldest friends from highschool, fashion-mad Jaz and, of course, Kate. Playing the part of landlady to what seemed at times like a bunch of teenagers was enough to make Polly's cool blonde locks curl at the ends even more than they were prone to do naturally.

"Oh, come on, Kate. Don't you remember what fun Chrissie was at school?" said Jaz, who was looking forward to having someone to swap the latest make-up tips with. Jaz was also eager to update her long curtain of thick black hair inherited from her Indian mother, and Chrissie, a beauty therapist on Virtual Airlines, would be able to fill her in on all the latest looks in Paris.

"She'll hog the bathroom and leave her make-up and clothes all over the place," said Kate grumpily. "And she'll steal everyone's boyfriend."

"Polly's the only one among us who's got a boyfriend," said Laura, looking up from her book on the mating habits of otters. Laura, a TV researcher on a wildlife program, could always be relied upon to be blunt (rather like her boyish crop). But having never actually met the infamous Chrissie, she had no strong views on her imminent arrival. Instead, she asked, "Why is she coming to stay, Pol? I thought she was based in Los Angeles now."

"Something to do with a record producer she met on one of her flights," said Polly. "Apparently he's promised to get her an audition with a new girl band."

"Oh, for God's sake," said Kate, who, if the truth be told, was more than a little jealous of Chrissie's thin thighs and exciting life. Her own thighs were not so svelte (thanks to her sweet tooth), while her job as a PA at Crunch Cookies couldn't be more boring.

Polly, meanwhile, was looking forward to a little distraction (her boyfriend Harry certainly wasn't providing it) and Chrissie was bound to liven things up…

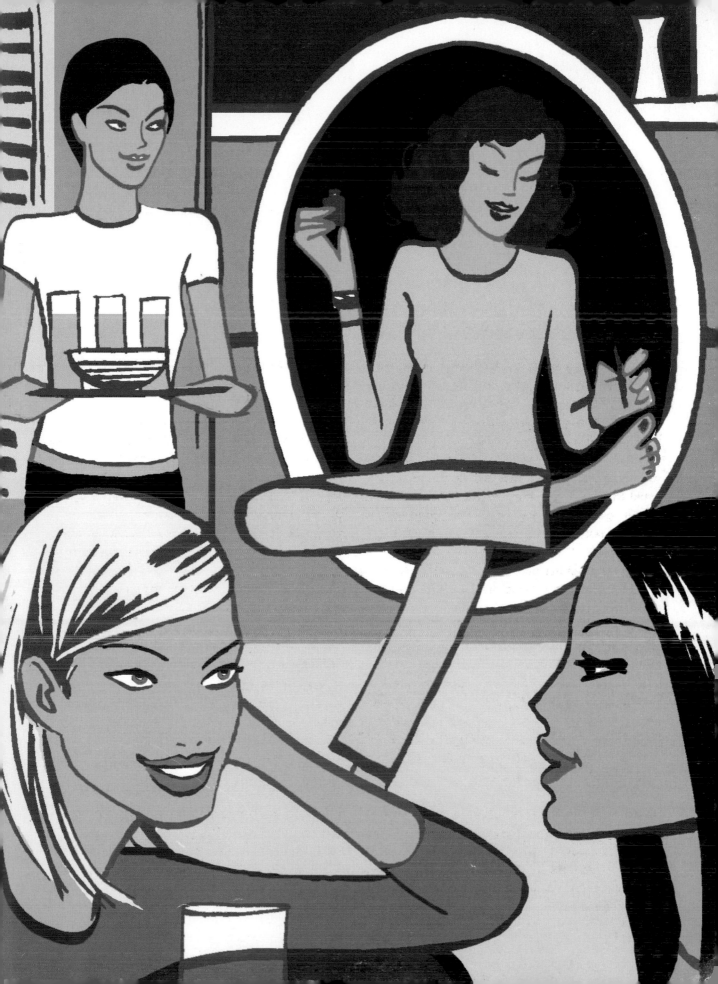

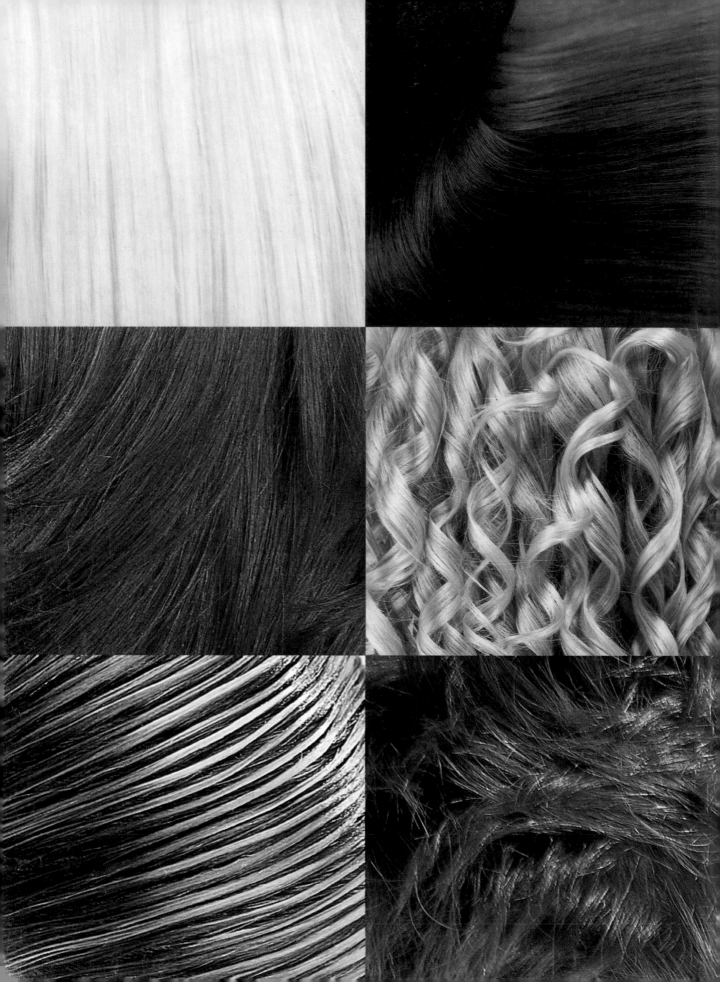

head start

Nothing reflects inner health, vitality and wellbeing quite like a clear complexion, sparkling eyes and — your crowning glory — glossy hair. Beauty comes from within, and if you have an unhealthy diet and lifestyle, your hair — like your skin — will suffer. Fatigue and stress will also wreak havoc on your hair, so modern haircare must be holistic and take into account all aspects of your lifestyle. When you are tense, your scalp tightens and the blood capillaries contract, reducing the amount of oxygen and nutrients that reach the hair follicles; the production of sweat increases, causing a greasy scalp; and, over prolonged periods of time, stress may even lead to hair loss. A good, relaxing scalp massage can help maintain a healthy head of hair, relieving tension and increasing blood flow, which will, in turn, nourish the root and hair follicle (see page 26 for how to do it).

Clean, shiny hair is a joy to have and head-turning to watch. Yet how often have we been told that our hair is dead, that it is just a build-up of deceased protein cells, strands of keratin which feel no pain when they're cut? This much is true. But hair is also organic in the same way as leather or wood is organic. Just think of how a favorite pair of shoes responds to a good polish, or how a wooden surface shines after a little elbow grease and beeswax. Nourish and condition them and they will shine, "breathe" and last for years. With the same love and attention, so will your hair. Taking care of your locks is a three-step affair: providing nourishment, treating it with care and using the right products. The simple routines, tips and advice that follow will ensure that you have great salon-style hair every day.

food for thought

The bottom line is that you can't expect to have healthy hair if you eat unhealthily. Whatever products you put onto your tresses, the only real solution is a long-term one that comes from within — a varied diet full of essential vitamins, minerals and other nutrients. Your scalp — where the root and follicle are formed and where "live" hair grows and develops — forms part of your skin, the largest organ of the body but the last in line to receive nourishment from the food we eat (hence the number of skin creams that deliver vitamins and minerals topically). A poor diet means impoverished skin and scalp. If you know your diet is not balanced and you don't want to compromise the health of your hair, then supplement it with a vitamin B complex, antioxidants (including vitamins C, E and beta-carotene), gamma-linolenic acid (GLA), fish oil, linseed oil and the minerals selenium and zinc (see page 28 for more on this). Many pharmacies sell a good all-round hair and skin supplement.

gently does it

We wouldn't dream of tugging our favorite little black dress on over our head without undoing the zipper, or putting our new silk panties in the dryer for 30 minutes on a high heat setting. So why do we think nothing of committing similar crimes to our hair? Imagine your hair to be as precious as a cashmere sweater set; treat it accordingly and you will reap the rewards. Your tools are all-important: poor-quality brushes and combs will scratch the scalp and damage the hair shaft, so don't stint on these (see page 24). Hair is elastic to some extent, but too much pulling will overstretch and ultimately snap it, causing split ends.

no products, no style

Using the right products on your hair could make bad-hair days a thing of the past. The plethora on sale in any pharmacy, supermarket or salon makes choosing the ones appropriate for your hair type confusing. Slick advertising and packaging makes it even more difficult to get it right. Do you want to go herbal, organic, scientific, fruity or unscented? Will it make your hair bigger, softer, fuller, blonder or seal your split ends? The claims can often be overwhelming — and you just want your hair to look great. The first thing to do is to determine your hair type; once you've got that right, then you can think about the extras. Read on to find out how...

hair types

Most people tend to wash their hair every day so they probably do not know exactly what hair type they have.

Your hair type is a combination of three factors:

1 The condition of your scalp — is it dry, oily or flaky?

2 The characteristics of your hair — is it fine, frizzy, coarse, curly, wavy, straight or color-treated?

3 Your environment — do you live in the country or the city? Is your office air-conditioned? Is the climate hot and humid, wet and windy or dry and hot?

normal hair

If your hair is neither prone to oiliness or dryness, you are one of the lucky few to have normal hair. Look after it well with products that keep it clean, conditioned and protected from environmental damage.

combination hair

Five to six hours after washing, hair begins to show signs of oiliness around the roots and yet the ends of the hair remain dry. Oiliness can be caused by overuse of conditioners and styling products, as well as by humidity and pollution.

oily hair

The hair will look oily, dull and "dirty" along the length of the hair shaft. If you suspect oily hair, part it and gently rub your forefinger along your scalp, then rub your thumb and forefinger together. If it feels slippery, you have an oily scalp and overactive sebum glands.

HAIR SNIP

TO CHECK WHICH HAIR TYPE YOU HAVE, WASH YOUR HAIR AS NORMAL AND LET IT DRY NATURALLY. THE NEXT MORNING, BEFORE WASHING YOUR HAIR AGAIN, CHECK FOR SIGNS OF DRYNESS OR OILINESS. YOUR HAIR TYPE WILL CHANGE IF IT CANNOT ADJUST NATURALLY TO CHANGES IN YOUR ENVIRONMENT. IT WILL ALSO PROBABLY CHANGE (BOTH SCALP AND HAIR SHAFT BECOMING DRIER) IF IT IS CHEMICALLY COLORED OR PERMED.

dry hair

Dry hair will look dull, lifeless and parched; at its worst, it may look fuzzy and straw-like. If you suspect your scalp is dry, look at the white flakes on your shoulders before brushing them away. Small, powdery flakes are often the result of stress, too much alcohol and fatigue. If they are larger, translucent and moist, then it is a case of dandruff, due to an overproduction of sebum in the hair follicles, rather than a dry scalp.

hair textures

curly hair

Often the cuticles (the overlapping keratin cells that form hair) do not lie flat on curly hair because of the curved nature of the shaft. This can lead to dull-looking hair and frizz. Overcome this with leave-in conditioners, shine enhancers and conditioning sprays.

black hair

Black hair is usually dry, brittle and fine. Hydrate the hair with conditioning products and massage the scalp gently to promote healthy growth and the production of sebum, the body's natural hair conditioner.

straight hair

The shaft of the hair is straight and, if the hair is in good condition and the cuticles are lying flat (the use of styling lotion can encourage this), straight hair can look super-shiny. In less than ideal conditions, split ends and breakages may be noticeable.

coarse hair

This type of hair can look fuzzy and wiry after shampooing. Use a serum or leave-in conditioner to close and smooth the cuticle and do regular deep-conditioning treatments.

fine hair

Often this type of hair can look lank and lifeless soon after washing. Overconditioning will weigh the hair down, so only use those types of products sparingly. Always use volumizing products specially formulated for fine hair.

chemically treated hair

Although coloring processes are more gentle than ever, some still change the make up of your hair permanently. Give colored hair extra support by using rehydrating shampoos and conditioners that have been specifically designed for this hair type. Also, check that they contain sunscreen to protect your hair from damage caused by ultraviolet light and keep your color looking fresh for longer.

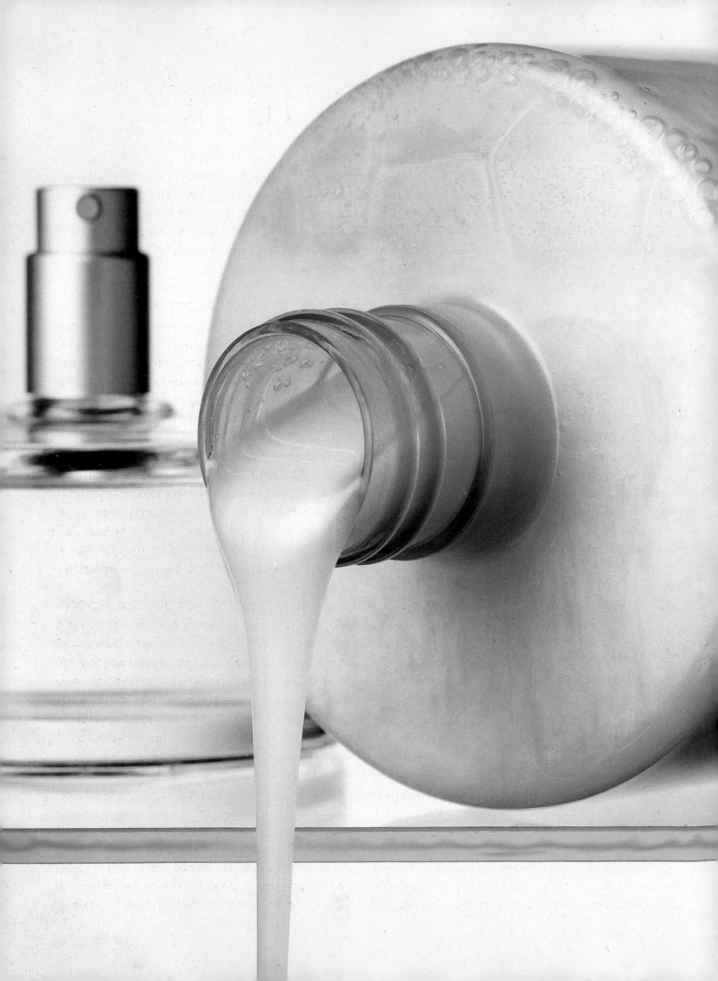

dream routine

Compare your haircare regime to your skincare regime: face — cleanse, tone, moisturize and protect, apply make-up; hair — shampoo, condition and protect, style, finish. A shampoo will gently but effectively cleanse the hair shaft, while a conditioner will moisturize your hair like a good face cream moisturizes your skin. Appropriate styling and finishing products will protect it from heat and oxidation from ultraviolet light and pollution which create dangerous free radicals. There are more benefits to be had by following a four-step haircare regime — shampoo, condition, style, finish — than by relying on a shampoo alone.

Few women skip a step in their skincare routine (are there still women who just use soap and water?) because modern products are designed to work together. The same is true of haircare products. Have you noticed how wonderful your hair looks when you have just been to the hairdressers and had the full treatment of shampoos, conditioners, styling products and finishing spray? Use them all regularly and your hair will become stronger, more flexible and resistant to damage. It's a cumulative effect.

shampoos

Beauty skeptics love to disparage the relative merits of so-called designer shampoos. "There's no difference between them and dishwashing liquid," is their collective cry. Well, they are wrong. Here's why: There is no denying that a bubble bath might share similar ingredients to a shampoo. But, as with humans whose bodies are made up of 90 percent water and yet each one is unique, it is the other 10 percent that makes all the difference. There are many special ingredients added to shampoos that can make hair look and behave as you would like, so experiment to find one that performs best for your hair type. Most modern shampoos are gentle enough to use every day and, in many cases, will actually improve the condition of hair. It is not necessary to scrub your hair like you might your clothes because the surfactant properties of the key ingredients in shampoos allow grime, dust, oil and dirt to lift away from the hair shaft, leaving your hair clean and porous for conditioning.

pH-balanced shampoos

Using a shampoo that is not pH-balanced could damage your hair, so make sure you choose products carefully. Be extremely cautious of baby shampoos as some of these are not pH-balanced and are formulated for scalp care rather than for nourishing and cleansing the hair.

dandruff shampoos

Dandruff shampoos have changed dramatically in the past few years. Coal tar, the traditional dandruff remedy, has been replaced by new wonder ingredients such as piroctone olamine. The shampoo acts as an exfoliant to help shed the surplus cells. The best anti-dandruff shampoos include tea tree oil, a natural antiseptic that will not overdry the scalp or damage hair

frequently asked questions

Q Is shampooing regularly bad for your hair and will it fade color?

A No, as long as you use good products that are pH-balanced and contain conditioning agents to seal the cuticle and lock in color.

Q Why does my hair feel greasy and my scalp dry after shampooing?

A This comes from not rinsing out products thoroughly. Always rinse the hair until it feels "squeaky clean" to the touch.

Q Do shampoos, conditioners and styling products cause build-up and if so, what can be done?

A Some products' ingredients can cause a build-up or intolerance. This can be prevented by using a detoxifying shampoo every two weeks, which will also cleanse the hair from outside pollution.

the five-step shampoo

1 Thoroughly drench hair for 30 to 60 seconds before you apply shampoo — you'll need less product and washing will be easier on the hair. Rub a little shampoo between the palms of your hands before smoothing it over the surface of the hair.

2 Gently massage the head, but do not rough up the hair or pull long hair up onto the scalp — it causes tangles. Long hair will be cleansed as the shampoo washes out with the water.

3 When massaging, use the tips of your fingers, not the palms of your hands. This helps stimulate the scalp and stops you from roughing up the cuticle.

4 Rinse, rinse and rinse again. Poor rinsing results in dull hair and a flaky scalp, caused by dry soap flakes. Finish with an ice-cold rinse. It will close the cuticle and stimulate the scalp, ensuring healthy growth and extra shine.

5 To towel-dry, squeeze and pat hair dry. Do not rub it too vigorously with the towel as it will rub the hair cuticle the wrong way.

conditioners

There is much more to conditioners than just their moisturizing ingredients: laws of physics come into play each time you apply one. The positively charged polymers of small and large cationic molecules in the conditioning agents are attracted to and attach themselves to the negatively charged, damaged areas of your hair. In this way, each strand of hair is coated with protective binding and moisturizing ingredients, so conditioners can actually help repair weakened hair. As skincare formulations have become more advanced, so, too, have haircare products, enabling the ingredients to penetrate much deeper, leaving hair better conditioned and feeling lighter.

hair masks

Deep conditioning treatments and hair masks work on the same principle as everyday conditioners, but because they are left on the hair longer, they have more time to penetrate the hair shaft. The ingredients are easily absorbed by the hair, so there is no need to leave the treatment on longer than the recommended time. Use an intensive conditioner or hair mask once a week for super-shiny hair, especially if your tresses are prone to dryness.

leave-in conditioners

These are designed to condition and add shine but do not leave the hair limp which makes them ideal for people with fine, flyaway or difficult-to-manage hair. They are best applied away from the roots.

conditioning tips

Identify your requirements when choosing a conditioner to suit your hair and scalp type, but remember its limitations. No conditioner can replace essential nutrients that are lacking in your diet.

Always read the manufacturer's notes. These provide much more information than ever before, so you are less apt to make the wrong choice.

Once you have applied a hair mask, cover your hair, either with aluminum foil or plastic wrap, both of which lock in the heat and enable the product to penetrate deeper (heat will open the cuticle wider).

Alternatively, soak a towel with hot water and wrap it around your head — you have the bonus of extra heat and the steam will stop the hair from drying.

When you rinse out conditioner, finish with a cold blast of water which will close the cuticle, leaving hair glossy and shiny. It will also stimulate blood flow to the scalp, encouraging healthy hair growth.

Key ingredients to look out for in your miracle in a bottle: wheatgerm oil, a natural moisturizer; green tea extract, which helps to retain moisture; and provitamin B_5, which enhances shine.

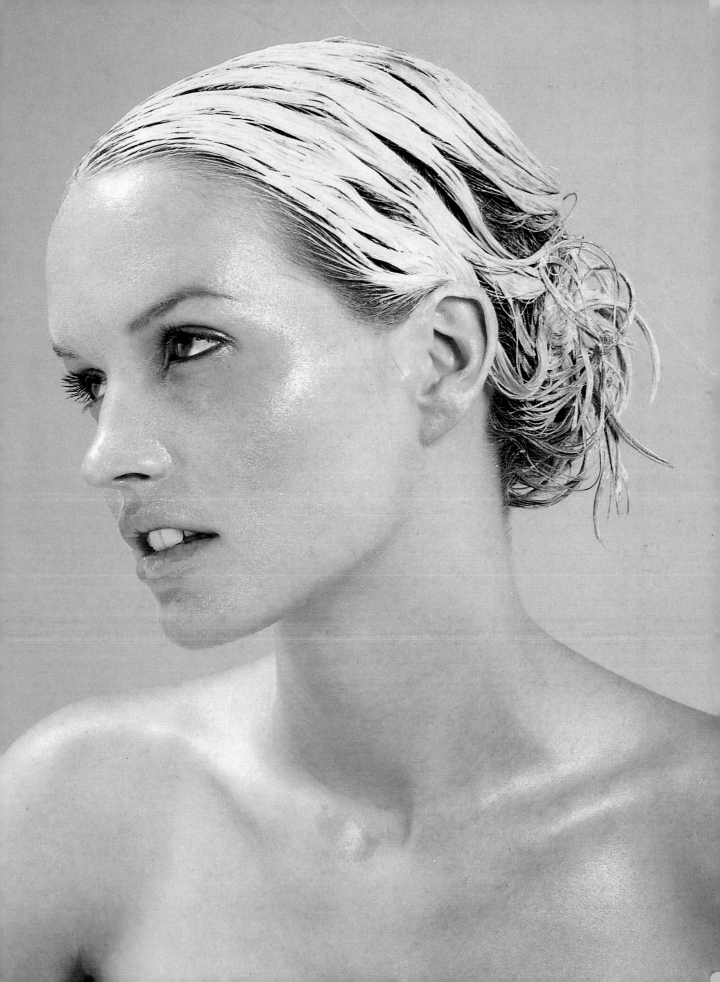

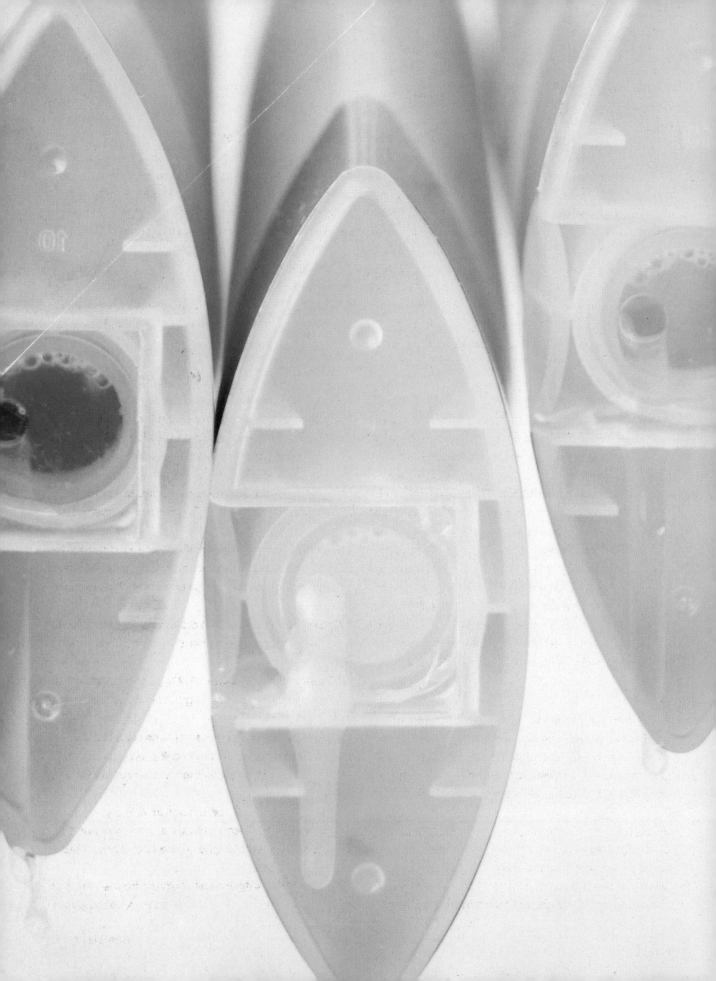

product power

Hair without styling product is like a sandwich without filling; it's the best way to get the most out of your locks. To maintain tip-top condition, use products that are specially formulated for your hair type and that correspond with your shampoo and conditioner. Avoid sticky products, as these tend to create build-up and can ruin the condition and health of your hair. Also, don't overload your hair — it may lose volume and look limp. Forget old myths about styling products; they have improved dramatically in recent years to give added manageability and the control you need to create certain looks. Try out as many products as you can to see which you like, and ask your stylist for advice.

mousse
The light, airy consistency of mousse makes it easy to distribute evenly. The hold factor depends on the resin content — more resins means more lift and hold.

thickening and volumizing sprays
Like mousses, styling sprays use flexible resins to add body and volume. They give even coverage and tend to be softer and lighter than mousse; the spray application means it can be directed to specific areas, such as bangs or the roots. Both sprays and mousses help combat static. Styling spray is ideal to use on wet hair or as an instant pick-me-up between shampoos to give great shape and renewed shine and bounce. It leaves hair looking natural and protects it from heat-styling damage.

gels
These are used to sculpt a style and contain water-soluble resins and silicones that provide a firm hold. Depending on the ratio of water to oil in the formula, gels can vary in consistency from ones that set hard after application to those that keep a wet look.

wax
Originally used in Black haircare, waxes (or pomades) became the hair gels of the 1990s. Used sparingly, waxes (which contain petroleum jelly) give shine and hold down wandering strands by virtue of their adhesive consistency.

shine enhancers
The latest hair styling innovation is a volatile silicone which imparts brilliant shine to hair with none of the heaviness of wax. It must be used very sparingly, otherwise hair looks oily. The spray versions tend to be heavier and can't be controlled as well as serums in a pump bottle.

straighteners
These temporarily close down the cuticle to achieve a smooth, sleek finish. Use one in conjunction with a straightening blow-dry (see page 63) and Jennifer Aniston's look could be yours.

always read the label
There are key ingredients to watch for when choosing the right products for your hair type. There is no need to be blinded by science for a moment longer — all will be revealed:

Amino acids act as humectants, drawing moisture into the hair.

Cationic ingredients are positively charged molecules (usually polymers) that are attracted to damaged areas of the hair shaft and lock on to smooth and repair.

Green tea extract is an antioxidant that combats free radical damage and improves hair health.

Panthenol or Provitamin B_5 penetrates the hair shaft to improve strength, moisture and shine.

Polymers give bounce and manageability. Water-soluble silicones and dimethicones coat the hair to smooth the cuticle and add shine.

Vitamin E, or tocopherol, is a protective antioxidant that slows down oxidation caused by pollution, smoking, chlorine and UV exposure.

Wheatgerm oil moisturizes the hair and also decreases static.

working with brushes

It seems like such a simple and obvious thing — using the right tool for the job — and yet few people do it. The choice of brush can affect how fast your hair dries, how smooth it is and how much volume you can create. Good-quality bristles protect hair from splitting and stretching, making styling and combing easier and painless, while poor-quality brushes and combs will scratch the scalp and damage the hair shaft. When choosing a brush, always check that the teeth and bristles are smooth.

paddle brush

Broad and rectangular, it smooths hair and works best on long, straight styles. The rubber cushioning on the paddle ensures extra-smooth, static-free hair.

roller and curling brushes

Used with a hairdryer, roller and curling brushes become mobile curlers and achieve volume. Some have a metal barrel that conducts heat from the dryer to reduce drying time. These can be detached from the handle to form a roller, which is ideal for creating long-lasting volume. If your hair has a tendency to be static, then lightly spray the metal barrel with hairspray.

volumizing brushes

These are the ones with an "open" head and fewer bristles or teeth than most other brushes. The holes work like air vents to circulate warm air from a hairdryer and increase volume and bounce.

smoothing brushes

An essential day-to-day brush that often has a rubber cushion holding the bristles, helping to counter static electricity. It is good to have a mix of natural and nylon bristles — nylon ones will grip, while natural will smooth.

tail combs

Used for sectioning hair when blow-drying or setting, they are the only way to create a perfect part.

pick combs

These "open" up curls and separate kinky, wavy hair.

fine and medium combs

Both of these are used for backcombing and delicate detangling, but are best used by a hairstylist.

wide-tooth combs

Use these to comb conditioner through wet hair.

brushstrokes

Hair is elastic to some extent, but harsh brushing will overstretch and ultimately break the hair.

1 Always brush your hair before shampooing to massage the scalp, help loosen dead skin cells and detangle any knots (the hair becomes more fragile and thus more difficult to detangle when wet).

2 Always brush from the tips up, not from the roots down. This is the best way to detangle hair.

3 To remove a tangle, comb from the base of the tangle to hair tips, working upwards slowly.

4 Once hair is tangle-free, brush from the roots to the tips to distribute sebum along the hair shaft and increase its natural shine.

5 Ignore the "100 brushstrokes a day" credo. Too much brushing will overstimulate sebum production and increase the chances of oily hair, breakage and split ends. In Victorian times when this old-wives' tale was coined, 100 strokes a day was a good way of preventing hair lice from multiplying because it destroyed the eggs and damaged the insects. Yuck! Times have changed and now so should our grooming habits. Rapunzel had more time on her hands than you.

6 Keep brushes and combs clean and free from stray hairs and product build-up. Add a little shampoo to lukewarm water and soak them for about five minutes, then leave to dry naturally.

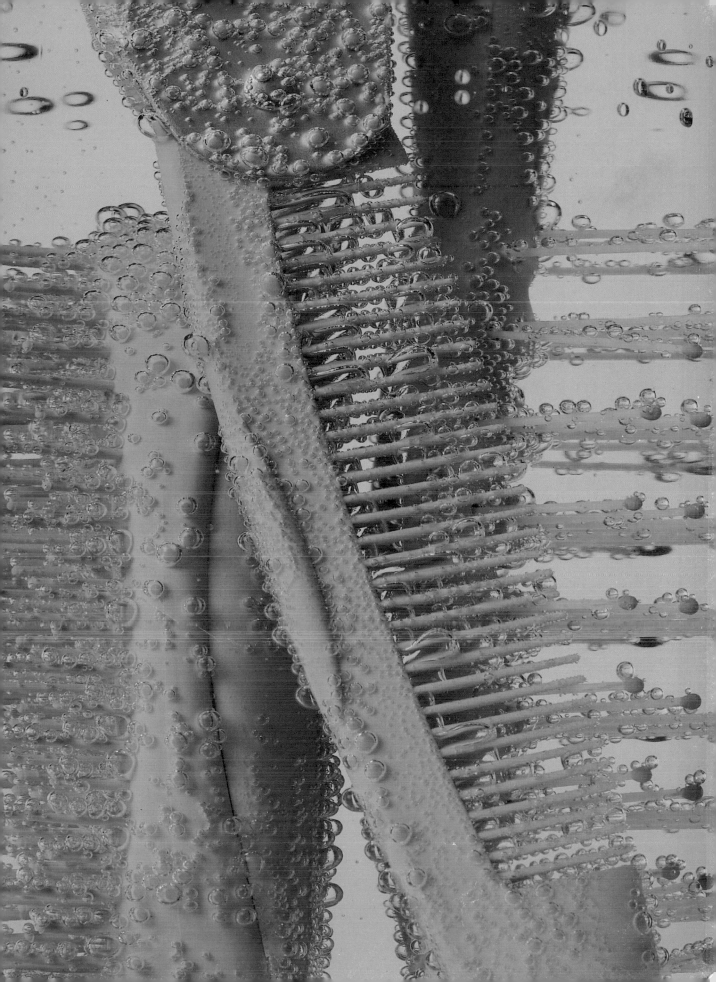

inside, outside

In a perfect world we would all be calm, collected and look the picture of health. Unfortunately, though, all too often we are subject to stress, but how we deal with it determines how well we cope and, ultimately, how good we look. Taking supplements, exercising and allowing time to eat well, sleep well and relax will not make your life go more smoothly, but it will give your inner resources an extra boost that will help you manage stress and still have enough energy left to keep your inner light shining brightly.

expect the unexpected

From relatively minor disruptions like the washing machine flooding to more serious problems of health and demands from your work and family, life is full of situations beyond our control. Inevitably, this means we often have to change the best-laid plans at the last moment and adapt accordingly. When we are fit and healthy we are more able to deal with problems and to respond more effectively to them.

don't be too harsh on yourself

Good habits are easy to break and no one is immune to temptation. If your willpower isn't as strong as you'd like, maybe you are expecting too much of yourself. Reconsider your goals. Few people manage to eat a perfectly balanced diet or keep up an exercise routine all of the time.

learn to compromise

We all lead busy, busy lives and free time has become a luxury. If a few microwave meals are a way of spending precious time with your family, then so be it. But you don't have time to relax? You don't have to be in a yoga class to practice slow, deep breathing — do it while driving home in your car or while sitting on the bus.

get as much help as you can

Develop a support system of your favorite products, dietary supplements and pampering treats that you can use to nurture your sense of wellbeing. Keep a list of the numbers of good health, beauty and alternative therapists on hand so that booking a reflexology appointment becomes as easy as phoning for takeout.

stressed hair

When you are worried and stressed, the first part of your body to become tense is the shoulders. When the neck and shoulders are constricted, the supply of oxygen and blood to the scalp is inhibited. Inevitably, your hair becomes stressed, too, and the signs are a flaky scalp, dull hair and, eventually, hair loss. When you are stressed, your nails and hair are the first to be ignored by your body's natural vitamin distribution process — and this is also true for pregnant women. It is absolutely essential to replace lost minerals and vitamins, both internally and externally.

1 Massage the scalp and learn to relax. It relieves tension and increases blood flow which nourishes roots and hair follicles. Gently work your fingers around your head, massaging all the time. Start at the perimeter of the head and work inwards, making sure your fingers never leave the scalp.

2 A flaky scalp can be due to dehydration — especially after too much alcohol — so take a bath to unwind, rather than reaching for the wine bottle. Always drink at least eight large glasses of water every day.

3 Think about supplementing your diet with vitamins and minerals.

4 Eat your greens. Green vegetables have a high iron content that will encourage the growth of healthy hair.

5 Eat oily fish like salmon. The oils encourage the flow of sebum, giving flexibility to the hair.

6 Essential oils are good for wellbeing and can also benefit the scalp and hair when a few drops are diluted in vegetable oil or warm water. Rose absolut is moisturizing; tea tree and eucalyptus oils have antiseptic properties which are soothing for a dry, tight scalp; and lavender is supremely relaxing.

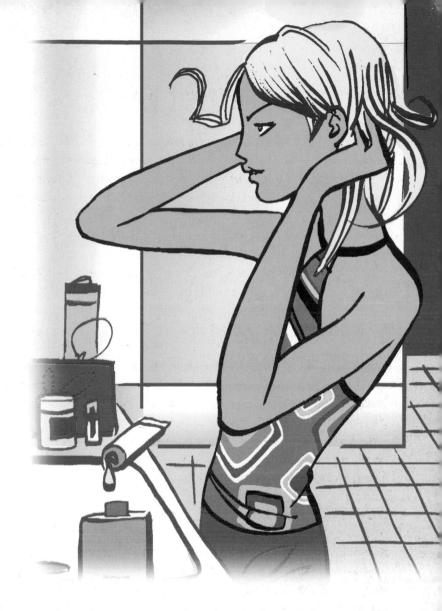

Having spent the night on a mattress on Polly's floor, Chrissie feels overwhelmed, jet-lagged and out of sorts. She didn't get the red-carpet treatment she'd been expecting — her sleeping arrangements left a lot to be desired and where was she meant to hang up her (extensive) wardrobe? Standing in the bathroom under the glare of a very unflattering light, she realizes that she is experiencing the mother of all bad-hair days. Chrissie's fine flyaway locks are

...chrissie's frazzled-hair crisis

looking fluffy, fuzzy and lank. Her job as beauty therapist on Virtual Airlines has caused big problems on the static front. All those long, carpeted corridors at the airport, the nylon upholstery and the stylish beret she's forced to wear ensure that sparks fly every time she brushes her hair. It's no wonder she's failed to pull the handsome dot.com entrepreneur who commutes to San Francisco every week; each time she gives him a back massage he complains of static shocks. And now this. She looks like a cross between an aging rock star and Cousin Itt from *The Addams Family*. Working frantically through the contents of the bathroom cabinet, she experiments with every hair product she can lay her hands on in an attempt to groom her sorry, straggling strands — but to no avail. It

finally dawns on Chrissie that no amount of styling lotion is going to solve her hair crisis. What her stressed-out mane really needs is some back-to-basic haircare — the magic H_2O (at least eight glasses a day) and some dietary supplements like vitamins B and C (a balanced diet is not one of Chrissie's strong points).

fringe benefits

The debate about whether or not to take supplements is on-going. Many doctors and dieticians believe that a balanced diet, containing plenty of fresh fruit and vegetables, should provide all the nutrients the body needs to function efficiently and at its optimum. However, the lifestyle that many of us lead means that we are frequently under stress and exposed to toxins — from an intake of caffeine, nicotine, alcohol and overprocessed food, and also from ultraviolet rays, pollution and radiation from office equipment — which can deplete the body's supply of essential nutrients.

supplements for hair, skin and nails

Beta-carotene is an antioxidant that is converted in the body to form vitamin A.

Omega-3 provides essential fatty acids.

Starflower oil is a rich source of an essential fatty acid, gamma linolenic acid (GLA), which acts as a building block for healthy skin and hormone balance.

Selenium is a mineral needed for the action of many antioxidant enzymes.

Vitamin B complex promotes healthy hair and skin and supports the central nervous system.

Vitamin C is an antioxidant that destroys harmful free radicals caused by pollution.

Zinc is a mineral that is essential for the proper functioning of over 100 enzymes.

warning

Most supplements are virtually non-toxic but you must be careful. A good all-in-one multivitamin, multimineral and an antioxidant formula is ideal, but if in doubt, ask a doctor, dietician or pharmacist for advice and **always** follow the manufacturer's dosage instructions. If you are experiencing any serious problems with your hair, consult a doctor for advice.

supplements for stress

Beta-carotene, selenium and **vitamins C** and **E** with **zinc** work together as antioxidants to disarm damaging free radicals caused by stress.

Bilberry helps prevent the premature death of body cells.

Calcium and **magnesium** deficiencies are common in highly stressed individuals and can result in anxiety, fear and even hallucinations.

Dong quai supports the kidneys, central nervous system and the adrenal glands, which are among the most susceptible organs to stress.

Gamma-aminobutric acid (GABA) acts as a tranquilizer and is important for proper brain function.

Gingko biloba aids brain function and circulation.

Hops help to ease nervousness, restlessness and stress.

Kava kava relaxes the mind as well as the body.

L-Tyrosine is an effective sleeping aid.

Valerian is another powerful sleeping aid when taken at bedtime and it also helps ease stress-related headaches.

Vitamin B complex, plus extra **vitamin B_6 (pyridoxine)**, **B_{12}** and **B_5 (panothenic acid)** are necessary for health and the proper functioning of the nervous system; B_5, in particular, is an anti-stress vitamin needed by the thymus gland.

Vitamin C with bioflavonoids is essential for the functioning of the adrenal gland, which produces anti-stress hormones.

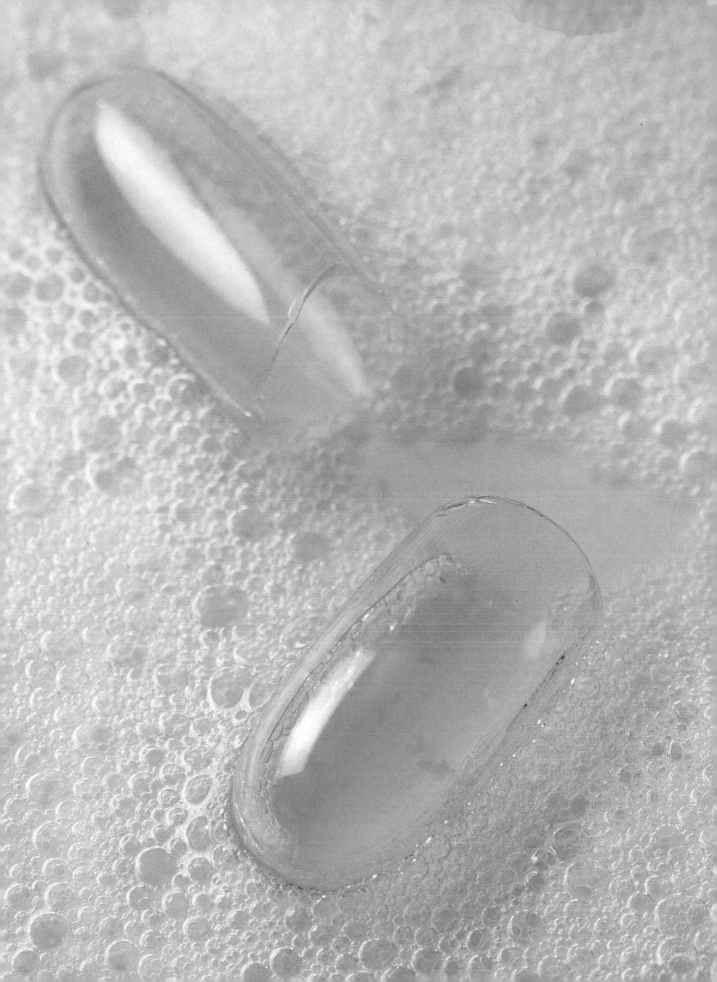

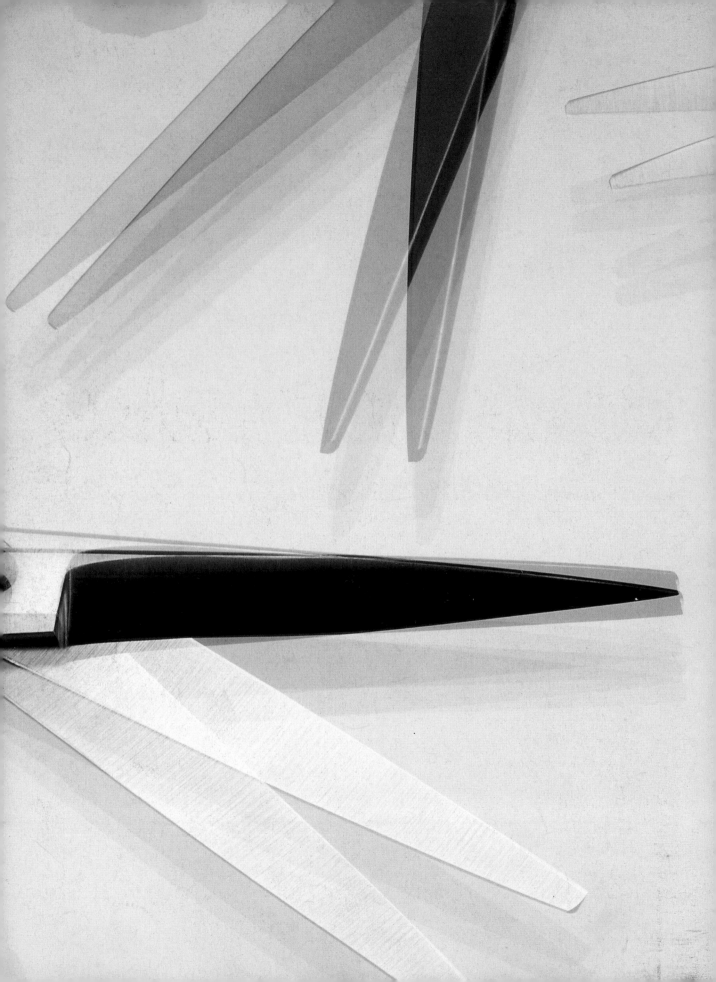

your hair talks

chrissie comes to town

"I can't tell you how thrilled I am to be here," said Chrissie, gliding elegantly into the sitting room, bare-footed and bare-legged, save for a silver chain around her ankle that jangled as she moved. The girls were lined up on the (once) white couch, marveling at how glamorous their new house guest looked. Despite the fact that it was Sunday morning, Chrissie was wearing full make-up, artfully contrived to look as if she was wearing none at all.

"So I've brought each of you a little present from L.A.," she was saying, dipping into a big honey-colored leather bag that Jaz instantly recognized as a designer label that you had to join a 12-month waiting-list to own. "For Polly, my gracious hostess ... something sexy to go under all those deathly boring navy-blue suits that you have to wear to work." Chrissie handed over a little parcel of shell-pink tissue paper containing a scarlet silk camisole with black lace trim. "I thought it might spice things up a little with Harry," she added. Polly blushed the same color as the camisole. It would take more than this to spice things up with Harry, her boyfriend since college. He was a nice enough guy, but these days he seemed to get more turned on by share prices than by Polly's choice of lingerie. Their relationship had gone a little flat, to say the least. It was a good job that she had flirtatious e-mails from her colleague in Miami to look forward to. At least "cyber-Simon", as she called him, was adding a little fizz to her life. "And for you, Kate... a new cellulite cream," Chrissie was saying. "I've heard from girlfriends who have cellulite that it really works." Kate glowered as Chrissie handed over the tube of Fat-busting Miracle Lotion. Jaz, meanwhile, was thrilled with her set of brain-boosting nail polishes containing ginkgo biloba — "absorbed through the nail bed to improve brain function" — and oblivious to the implied insult. "And Laura, I think this scent is just the ticket for you. It smells... well, very feminine," said Chrissie, in what was clearly a dig at Laura's tomboy style. Laura, who never wore perfume, stifled the urge to laugh as she eyed the blurb on the label: "Fatal: The scent that spells instant attraction." Love her or loathe her — and Laura hadn't made her mind up yet — there was no denying that Chrissie was a blast.

"Now girls, the good news is that Steve, the record producer I told you about, has invited me to the opening of Shaft, a new bar in Soho, on Saturday night," Chrissie continued, "and I've managed to get you all on the guest list."

"Thanks, but no thanks. I've already got plans," lied Kate, who would rather boil in oil than spend an evening with Chrissie.

"Count me in," declared Jaz enthusiastically (she was already painting her toenails orange).

"I'm game," said Laura. "What about you, Pol?"

"I'd love to, but I'm flying to South Beach on Saturday afternoon for business and I'll be away for the rest of the week," replied Polly, who could hardly contain her excitement at the prospect of finally meeting Simon, her sexy (she hoped) cyber-suitor.

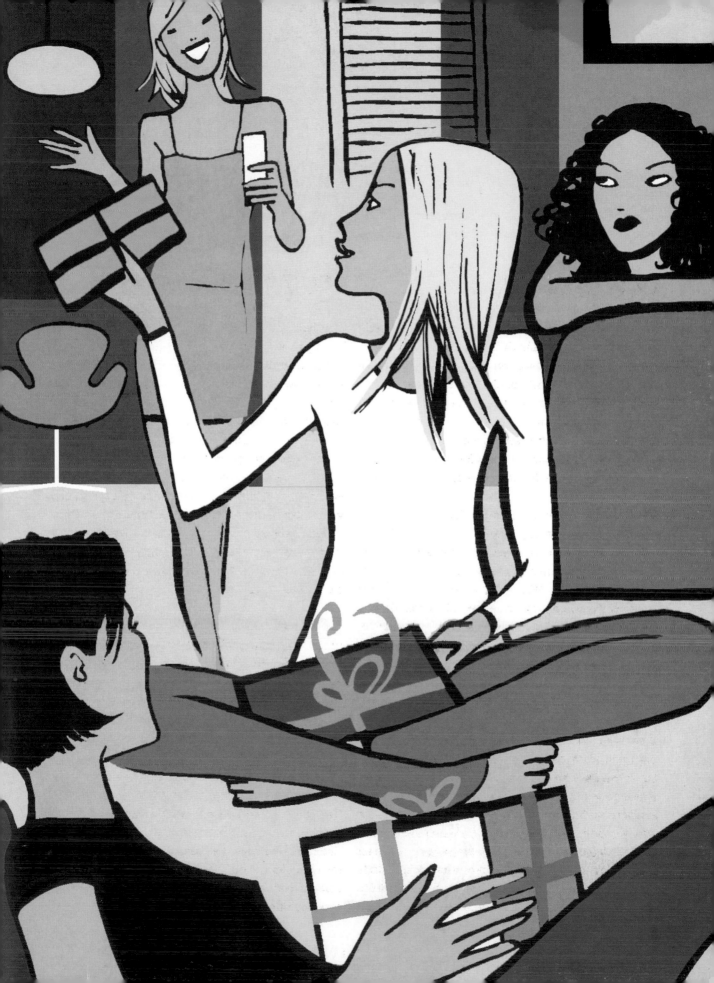

cut it

There are no limitations to your choice of style or cut. Modern fashion and beauty tells us that anything goes: all that matters is that you feel happy and confident with your look. If you have a long, sloping jaw, traditional thinking would tell you to avoid a short gamine cut, but if you like it and have the confidence to wear it, the chances are you will pull it off beautifully. Just look at all those quirky models who don't fit the perfectly proportioned, blonde-hair, blue-eyed aesthetic. But if you don't feel brave enough to throw caution to the wind, here are few guidelines that will guarantee that a cut suits your face and flatters your features in a more classical manner.

face shape

The best way to determine your face shape is by doing the mirror trick (see page 36). Alternatively, get a photo taken or rely on your hairdresser to define your profile. Certain features can be minimized or emphasized by a hairstyle. A prominent nose or chin can be countered by bangs. An angular jawbone means you can wear gamine Audrey Hepburn cuts and crops, while a long, sloping jawbone doesn't always work with short hair.

Remember that your face shape changes with age. Your jaw will inevitably grow less defined and your complexion less radiant and smooth as you grow older. The good news is that a clever cut and color can make you look younger and feel better. Don't get stuck in a rut, repeating the same hairstyle time and time again. Keep moving with the times. After all, what suits you at 18 is unlikely to look good when you are 30. Nothing dates you faster than make-up and a haircut, and yet nothing is quite so simple to change as these.

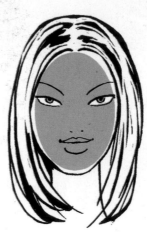

oval face

This classic shape suits any look. With this in mind, use your hairstyle to create an illusion of the perfect oval by balancing the proportions.

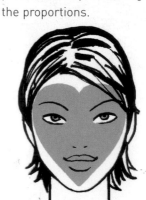

heart-shaped

The narrowing of the face can be countered with the extra volume of a layered bob, which flicks outwards at chin level.

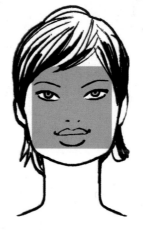

square face

Soften up the edges with a style that breaks up the symmetry. Play with off-center parts, graduated layers and soft curls.

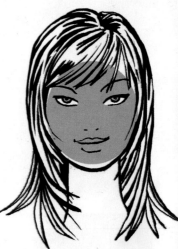

round face

Soft, feathered cuts with layers coming forward onto the face look stylish and sophisticated and also slim down a fuller face.

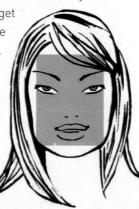

long face

Bangs disguise a long forehead, while a chin- or shoulder- length style adds volume and broadens the face.

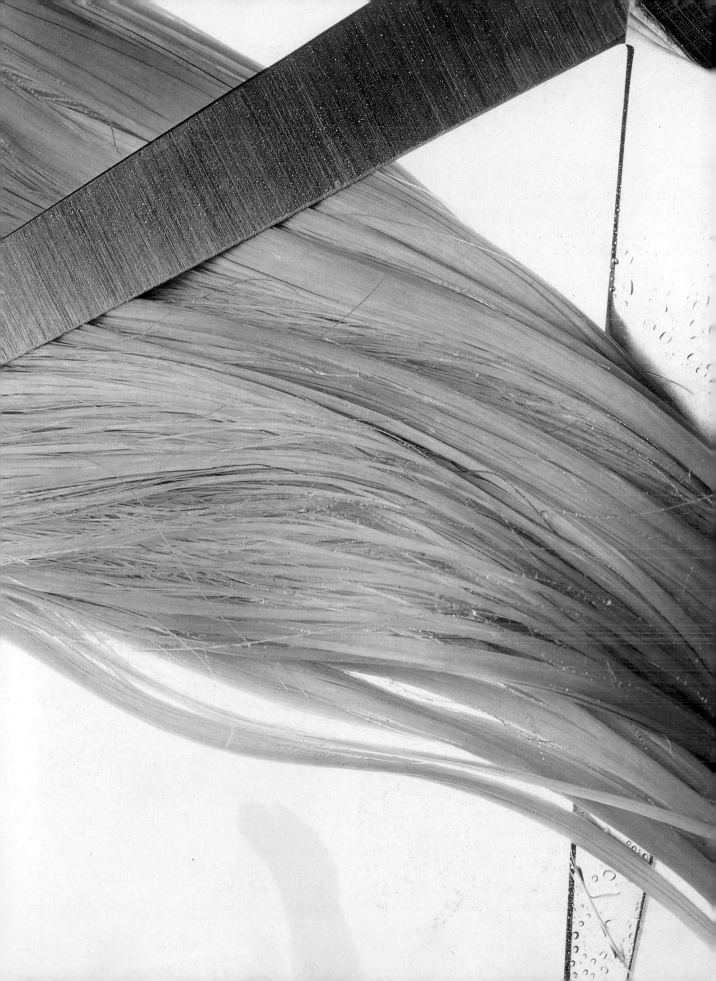

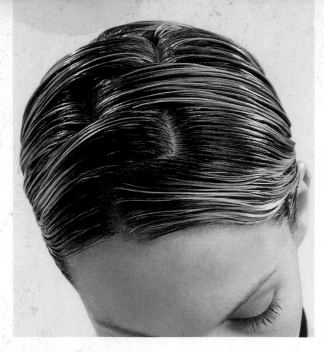

body proportion

As well as considering your hair type and face shape, a good hairdresser will also take into account your body shape, proportions and size when consulting you about a restyle. This is why it is important that he or she sees you to discuss your ideas before you are sitting in a chair, shrouded in a gown and with your hair wrapped up in a towel.

Very long, flowing hair on a short body frame will shorten the body even more; conversely, a short, gamine crop will not work well on a body that is broad-framed and tall. Big-volume, curly shoulder-length hair on a short, plump torso will just accentuate width; while a short, spiky cut on a tall person can be intimidating.

how to determine face shape

1 Stand in front of your mirror.

2 Using your hands, pull all your hair away from your face.

3 Take a lipstick (not your favorite) and, at arm's length, draw an outline of your face on the mirror.

4 Like it or not, what you are left with is your face shape.

parting company

Creating a new part is the quickest and cheapest way to update a style and change your look and face shape. Each season, one type of part dominates the fashion shows — from the zigzag to the deep, side parting just above the ear. For a long time only center parts would do. Use a tail comb to experiment. Hold it by the teeth at a low angle and use the handle to part the hair. Keep the tip in contact with the scalp to get the most control.

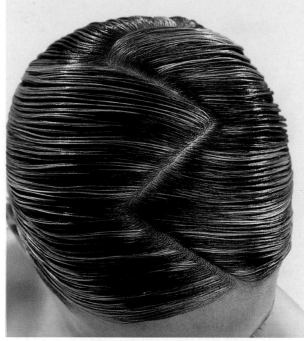

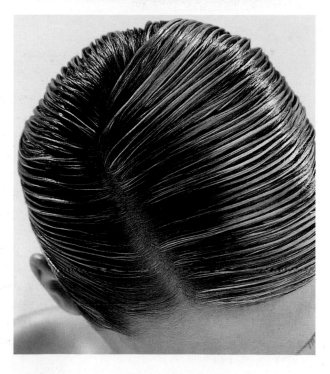

Laura is quite the antithesis
of Jaz. That's not to say she
doesn't care about her image —
she always manages to look
effortlessly cool — she just can't
be doing with Jaz's overwhelming
"girliness". Listening to her and

...laura's restyle

Chrissie prattle on last night
about the best pink nail polish
and where to buy the prettiest
handkerchief tops had almost
driven her to commit a violent
act. Laura has a much more
pragmatic approach to beauty.
She loves to work out and has
had the same boyish crop —
quick to wash and dry after her
gym sessions — since she
started college over five years
ago. She knows that it's
definitely time for a restyle

(her mind was well and truly
made up when she heard
someone refer to her as "him"
— she did have her back
turned, but nevertheless it was
not a moment she ever wants
to revisit). Laura books up an
appointment with her hairstylist
who, after a lengthy discussion
— enthusiastically cuts and
restyles her hair. The end
result gives her more height on
the crown, soft, wispy bangs
on her forehead and light curls

on the nape of her neck. The
crowning glory, however, is that
this new style disguises her
large forehead and shortens
her long face (not that she
would ever admit to caring
about these features) —
amazing how a cut can change
the shape of your face. Laura
strides out of the salon with
a spring in her step, secretly
hoping that the assistant
producer in Current Affairs
will sit up and take notice.

the cutting edge

A good haircut should make you feel fantastic. It should increase your confidence, make you feel sexy, taller, slimmer, more powerful, and, most importantly, it should reflect your personality. Styled in the right way, a haircut can even act as an instant "facelift," helping to detract attention from areas of the face that show signs of ageing and, instead, highlight your most flattering features, perhaps great bone structure or beautiful eyes. A good cut will give your entire look a new lease on life — while a little color on your tresses will make it look thicker and shinier, too (see page 44). Hair is usually the first thing to be changed when a woman is making a major life change — perhaps a new career direction or at the beginning (or end) of a relationship. A visit to the hairdresser's for a bit of pampering or reinvention is also a sure-fire way to lift a bad mood. Once you've found the right hairstyle, everything else falls into place. Whatever the reason and whatever the style, always have a trim every six weeks to avoid split ends and to help maintain condition and manageability.

cutting considerations

There are three essential points to consider before embarking on any change of image:

1 Be realistic. How much time do you really want to spend on your hair every day? Also, how much time have you got realistically? If you choose a style that requires too much time, you will never get the look you want.

2 Straight, curly, dark or blonde, wavy or wispy, make the most of what you've got. Hair always looks its best when it is in fabulous condition and has a fantastic cut.

3 Use your ammunition! Products are essential daily tools for achieving shine, body and manageability on all hair types. Experiment a little and learn which products suit your hair best and how to use them.

the long and the short of it

Long, romantic, tumbling tresses remain a classic look and a favorite with the opposite sex. To counter the hippie "curtain" effect and make your hair seem less heavy, as well as keep locks in excellent condition, choose a layered cut. This will add shape around your face to give a defined and confident style. With well-shaped layers, hair will not fall too heavily across the face. But be warned: there's nothing worse than straggly, uncared-for, hair snaking down your back, so don't bother growing it if you don't want to spend time brushing, washing, drying and styling it.

With its mix of modernity and femininity, short hair can be extremely sexy. It is a great option for women who want a strong, feminine image, a personal signature, yet a low-maintenance style. Short, sassy, sexy styles are on the rise — think Meg Ryan, Gwyneth Paltrow and Cameron Diaz. Casual or glamorous, layers help to define texture and volume, giving the hair greater depth and making styling simple.

going for the chop

Ultimately, whether you opt for a long or short style, determining your face shape, hair type and texture will help you to find the most flattering cut. Once you have this basic information to work with, you can then adapt catwalk styles or ideas from the pages of beauty magazines to create an individual look. The key thing to remember is that face shape should trigger off the hairstyle. In the same way as a beautiful frame enhances a picture, if you've got the right hairstyle for your face shape, then your whole face will look prettier and fresher and your eyes will stand out. Your good features will be emphasized. Enjoy your hair's own unique style and, with the advice of your hairdresser, select a style to enhance what you've already got. If you try to change your natural hair too much, you may end up compromising on its condition and become a slave to a high-maintenance look in the process.

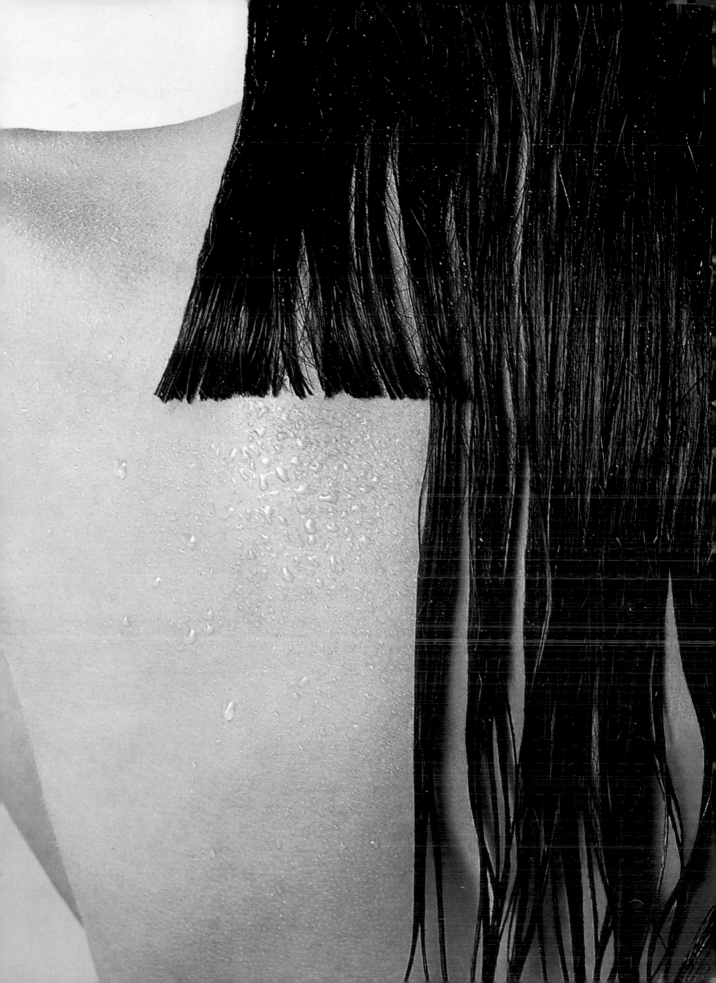

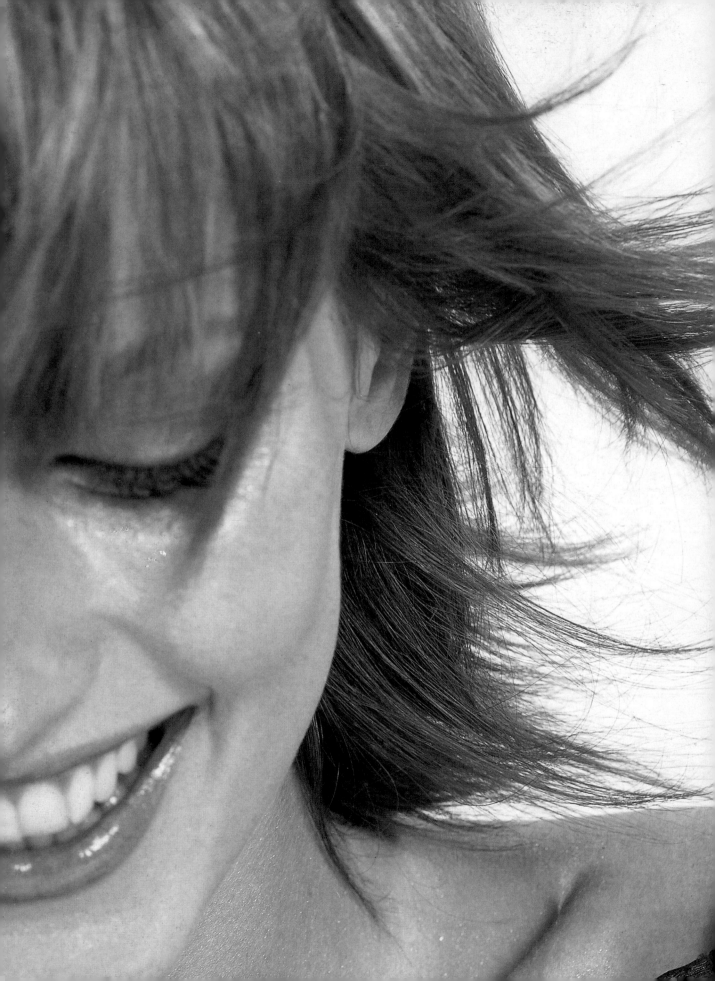

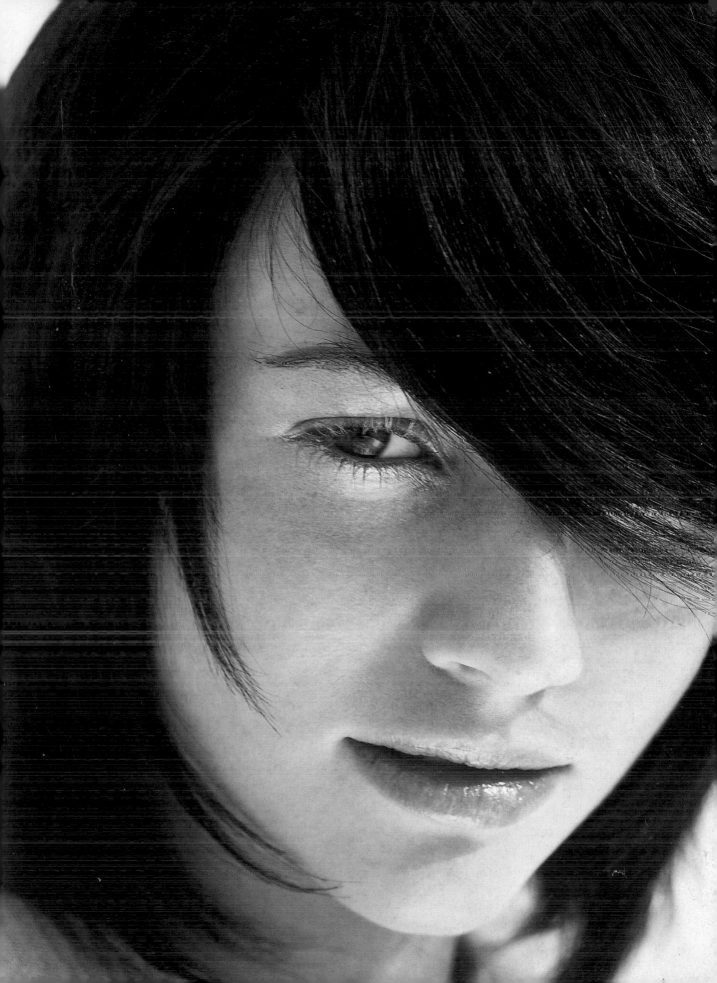

your hairdresser

Finding a hairstylist with whom you "click" is like any other relationship — although it's unlikely you'd ask a friend to make you look and feel like a groovier version of your favorite actress. You need chemistry, you need trust and you need to be able to convey your ideas in such a way that they can be easily interpreted. If you are considering a radical cut but don't have a hairdresser you trust, make appointments for a few blow-drys at different salons. Mention your ideas to the stylist looking after you and decide with whom you feel most at ease. All good salons offer a free consultation, but having a blow-dry will allow you to experience how a stylist works, rather than just listen to their suggestions. Above all, visiting a salon should be a pleasurable experience. You want to feel pampered and relaxed, confident in the knowledge that when you walk out you are going to look and feel like a million dollars, not nervous and edgy, wishing you'd brought a paper bag with you.

Recommendations from friends are a good way of finding a reputable stylist, but we are all subjective in our choices, and one person's dream stylist could be another's idea of hell. If you see someone with a haircut you like, ask them who did it. After all, you wouldn't hesitate to question where someone got their stunning high heels that you liked, now would you?

the consultation

Taking along a picture of a cut or color you like is a good starting point and avoids confusion. Compile a "look book" — a scrapbook or folder where you keep magazine tear sheets of styles you like, as well as photographs of yourself when you had a particularly good cut or color. It's also useful to show your stylist pictures of looks that you really dislike. A picture is a good way of understanding one another's vocabulary — for you, titian may mean coppery golden highlights; for your stylist it may mean gingery red tones. However, do not expect to look like the person in the picture. Sadly for us, there is only one Rachel, one Meg and one Gwyneth.

reworkings and rewards

If you don't like a cut or style, be honest and tell your stylist. They would much prefer to rework it and sort it out for you, rather than have you leave disappointed. Conversely, if you really like a cut or receive a lot of compliments on a style, give the stylist that feedback. Everyone responds to praise and likes to know when a cut or style performs well.

If you are happy with the stylist's work, then tip, but don't feel uneasy if you can't afford to tip generously. Ask any hairdresser and they are thrilled if they receive a thank-you card or see a customer leave the salon looking genuinely happy. Equally, if you buy a bottle of the shampoo, conditioner or styling product that your stylist has used, this indicates that you want to re-create the look at home.

hairdressers' translation service

Choppy This is the result when hair has been cut using a texturizing method — for example, razor-cutting to give a "choppy finish."

Feathering Using a razor to cut hair instead of scissors. This creates a much more random finish, leaving the hair more disheveled and creating that lived-in look.

Flick-outs This involves blow-drying the hair so that it flicks outwards at the ends to create volume and width, instead of blow-drying the hair under, which is a more traditional look.

Texturizing A method of cutting using tools such as a razor, clippers or texturizing scissors. These are like ordinary cutting scissors, but one blade is serrated, enabling the stylist to reduce weight evenly throughout the cut.

Volume To build hair and add life, volume can be temporary or permanent.

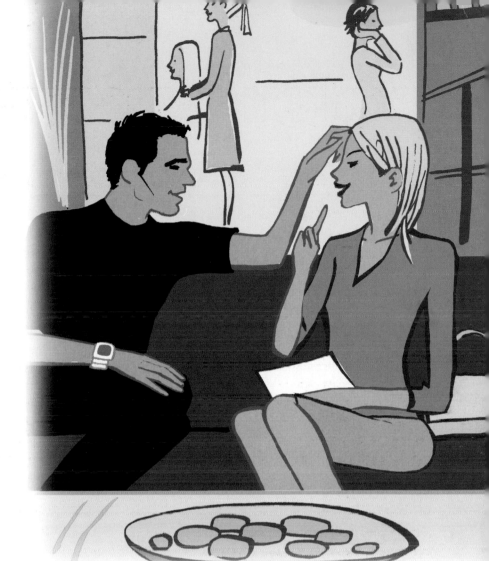

...polly's hair therapy

Chrissie's arrival at the house has precipitated a bit of a *crisis* in Polly's life. She takes one look at Chrissie's suitcase — the contents of which are now strewn across her bedroom floor — and can't help but compare her own black, grey and navy blue power suits and boring black and white basics with Chrissie's endless supply of skimpy tops in every shade of pink and purple, bead-fringed capri pants and flirty, diaphanous skirts. And

was that a rhinestone, heart-shaped body jewel stuck to her sensible beige carpet? Polly decides there is nothing else for it but to book a day at her favorite hair and beauty spa for a bit of head-to-toe pampering. She's been "seeing" Charles for years — he always has a knack of understanding exactly what she wants, and has a chair-side manner to die for — not to mention the great haircuts. After plenty of hair chat (so

much better than therapy), Polly decides to have her shoulder-length blonde hair lightly layered, which will soften her face and groove up her look. Best of all, it can be souped up with products for that hip rock-chick look — although the latter probably won't go down too well with the suits on the top floor at work! Polly feels fantastic. Harry won't recognize her — on second thoughts, he probably won't even notice.

color coding

Color adds sheen, texture, thickness, depth and life to your hair and can be used either to enhance your natural hair color or to explore a different side of your personality and change your image. Never be afraid to experiment, especially when you have a trusted stylist with whom you feel safe enough to be a little more daring. A good colorist will work with your skin tone and personality to create an effect that suits your style and boosts your confidence.

HAIR SNIP

MODERN HAIR COLORANTS ARE ENRICHED WITH CONDITIONING INGREDIENTS, SO YOU CAN ENHANCE YOUR NATURAL COLOR WITHOUT DAMAGING THE HEALTH OF YOUR TRESSES. HOWEVER, ANY CHEMICAL TREATMENT MEANS THAT THE HAIR WILL REQUIRE GENTLE HANDLING. USE EXTRA-NOURISHING CONDITIONERS AND APPLY A HYDRATING MASK ONCE A WEEK TO REPLENISH MOISTURE. AVOID HOT-OIL TREATMENTS AS THEY TEND TO STRIP OUT COLOR.

hue are you?

An experienced colorist is able to determine quickly whether you are a "whisper," "talk" or "scream" type of customer — in other words, whether you would be more comfortable with a few lowlights in your mousey brown hair or whether you are an extrovert who will feel perfectly at ease with a platinum-blonde crop. Often a customer profile questionnaire is used as part of a two-way discussion between stylist and customer to establish which colors will go best with your personality, as well as which will suit your complexion.

natural mixes

The color of your hair should be from the same family (warm or cool) as your skin tone. If you have very pale skin, any color will look good; if you have pink skin, avoid reds and warm golds; if your skin has yellow tones, favor deep reds and avoid golds; those with black or olive skin should stay dark, adding richness and depth with lowlights. Use the following guide to help determine what hair color will best suit your complexion and coloring, or try on wigs or hairpieces.

the home color zone

Use the color chart on pages 48—9 to work out whether you are a "warm" or "cool" customer. This will help you determine which hair colors will best enhance your skin tone (see right).

1 Stand in front of a mirror in good (preferably natural) light, holding the color chart just underneath your chin.

2 Slowly move it from left to right and back again and observe which color tones are the most flattering to your complexion.

3 Repeat the process a few times and ask the opinion of a friend.

warm

Eyes: brown, hazel, green or dark brown.

Skin: freckles, golden beige, bronze or golden brown.

Hair: golden or strawberry blonde, golden brown or auburn, chestnut or dark brown.

cool

Eyes: gray-blue, gray-brown or rose-brown.

Skin: beige, rose-brown or cocoa.

Hair: ash blonde, ash brown, beige blonde, black, burgundy or plum.

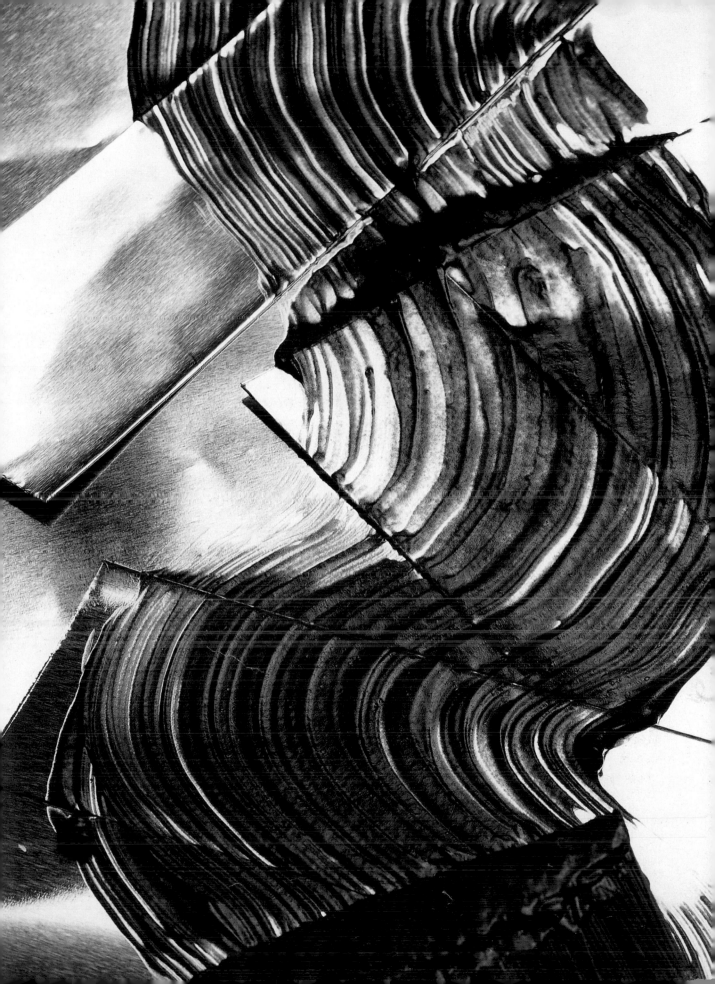

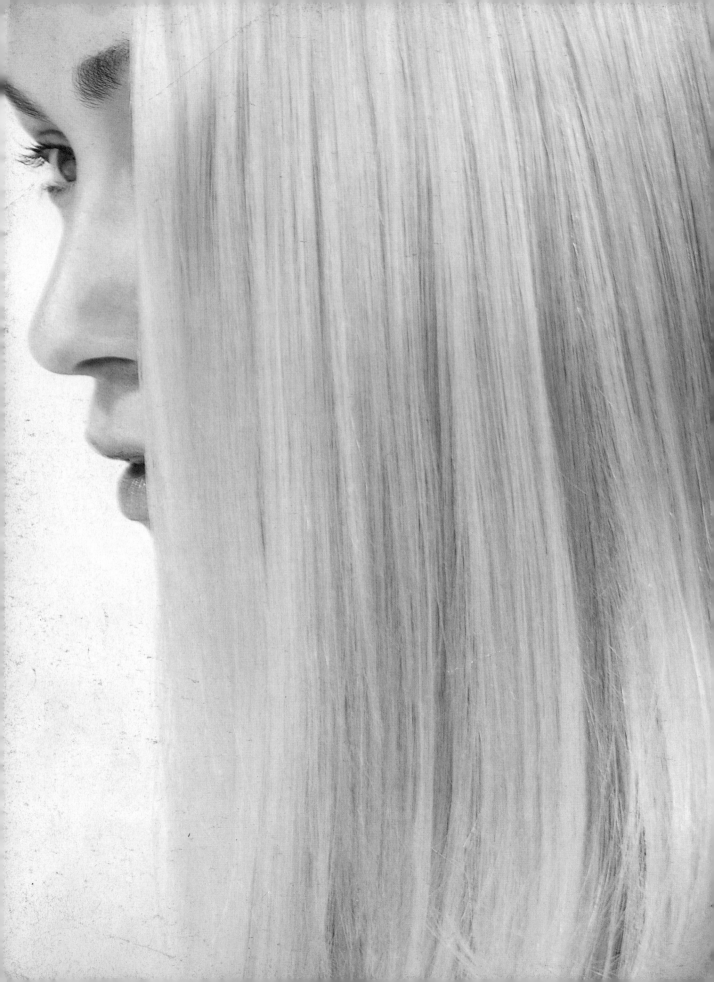

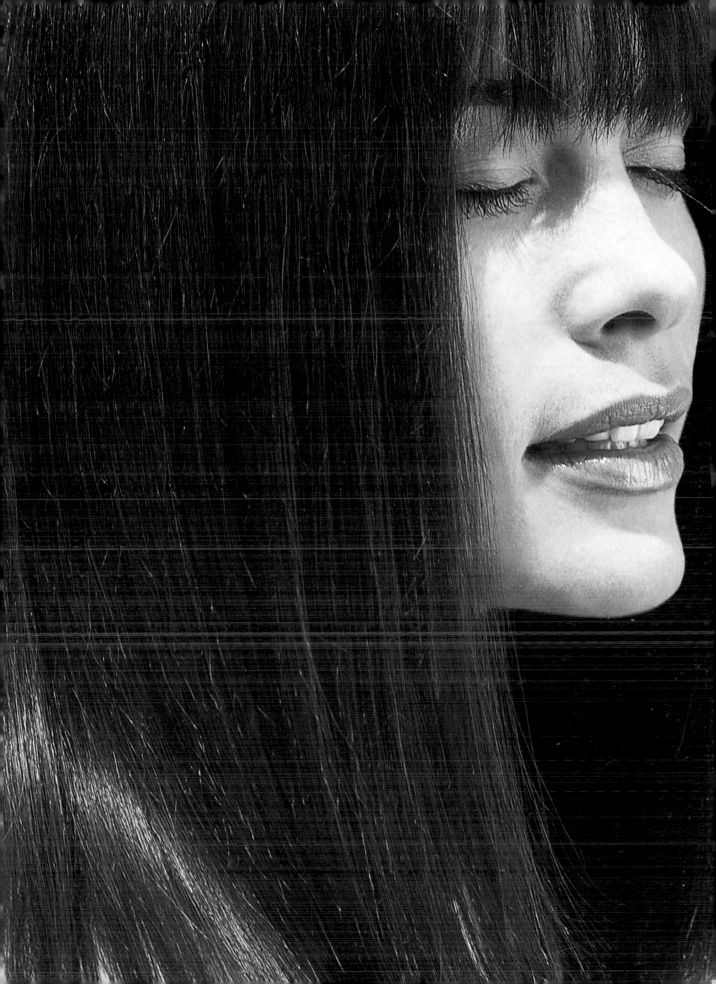

ool

semi-permanent color
These colors are made by a... dyes that penetrate slightly into the hair... then simply wash away. They last for ... and can make hair... and only darker or warmer ...

highlights
With highlights, strands of hair are placed in foils and dyed a lighter shade than your natural color. Bold ... a dramatic fashion effect, while fine pieces give ... natural look. As the dye is permanent, the roots ... reappear also band when the highlights grow out.

permanent color
... improve the condition of the hair while ... make hair lighter, darker or change the ... does not appear artificial, ... tone. This process can be ... as small sections of color.

lowlights
With lowlights, strands of hair are placed in foils and dyed a darker shade than your natural hair color. The dye is permanent. This is a very good method of adding depth and tone to dull hair — you can be as subtle or as bright as you want.

color wash
Change your look for the weekend with a color wash. This temporary color is available as a colored mousse or setting lotion and will last for just one wash. Also known as vegetable colors, these are excellent for refreshing faded color and can be used as a conditioning treatment.

tone on tone

This technique adds tone and shine. It will not lighten hair, but gives it sheen and life. Tone-on-tone lasts between four and six weeks. This can also be used within creative-color techniques to give subtle, even depth.

shading

Two or three shades of color are applied to each "slice" of hair. Semi-permanent color can be used for a subtle look; tone-on-tone for visible color; and permanent color for a dramatic effect. This is a good technique for thickening fine hair, as the multicolor shading gives depth.

chunky lights

Normally applied on the top of the head and around the face, color is added to wide-woven pieces of hair. Softer or stronger colors can be used to create different effects. This technique is best when slightly contrasting colors are used, as it will make the color stand out.

bleaching

This technique is used to lighten hair or to create results that cannot be achieved with high-lift color. Bleaching agents lighten the pigments of the hair and rinsing stops the process at the required shade. It's a job best left to the experts, as toning is a major part of this process.

duo/trio color

A creative technique using tone-on-tone color, which can be semi-permanent or permanent. Color is applied in two sections to cover the entire head and can be subtle or dramatically different. Duo color means two colors only; trio is three colors only.

waxes and pomades

Color waxes or pomades are a totally temporary coloring method, ideal for those who like to go wild at the weekend but have to look professional during the week. It is applied after the hair has been dried and styled to give a dramatic look. If you have very blonde or bleached hair, do a test strand to make sure it doesn't stain the hair and will wash out.

tonal blast

The tips of the hair are first lightened and then tone-on-tone color is applied. The lightened pieces of hair will show the tone more dramatically. This color adds definition to shorter haircuts and works best when stronger colors, such as reds and coppers, are used.

warm

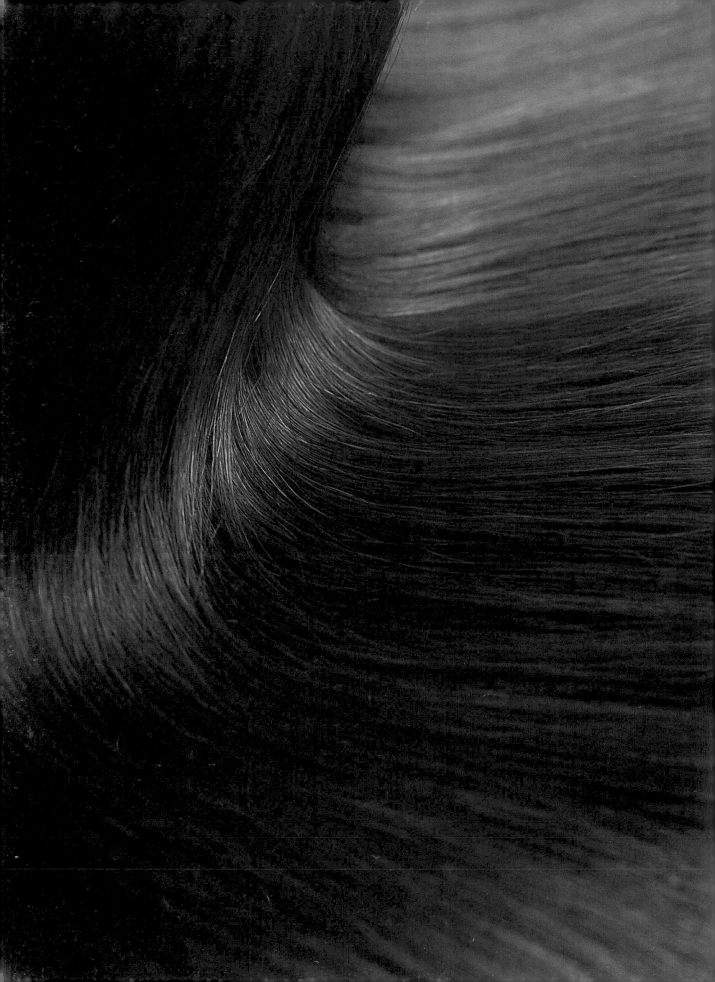

...jaz's creative-color experience

Jaz's girlfriend, Vicci, whose passion for fashion equals Jaz's, has a younger sister who's a junior stylist at a top salon. She's told them they're looking for models for creative coloring and, since Jaz has such great hair, would she be up for it? Stupid question! Jaz is there as quickly as you can say highlights. She's been chosen for tie-dyeing — cool. What amazing timing with this party coming up at Shaft with Chrissie and the girls. She really wants to look hot — apparently it's going to be packed with movers and shakers from the media and the fashion crowd. Jaz can hardly contain her excitement, which is not quite so cool, she realizes. While the hairstylist divides her hair into sections, she pictures herself working the room at Shaft and holding court, with a hip designer hanging on to her every word. These happy thoughts are interrupted by a serious style issue. What shade of nail polish will look best with her fuchsia-pink, bias-cut slip dress? Before she knows it (amazing how absorbing such matters can be), her hair has been sectioned with hair bands, scrunched up, colored, washed and blow-dried. And — hey presto — her dark black, glossy locks are now mottled with variegated shades of red. Fab — it's just like the skirt she bought last weekend. Love it!

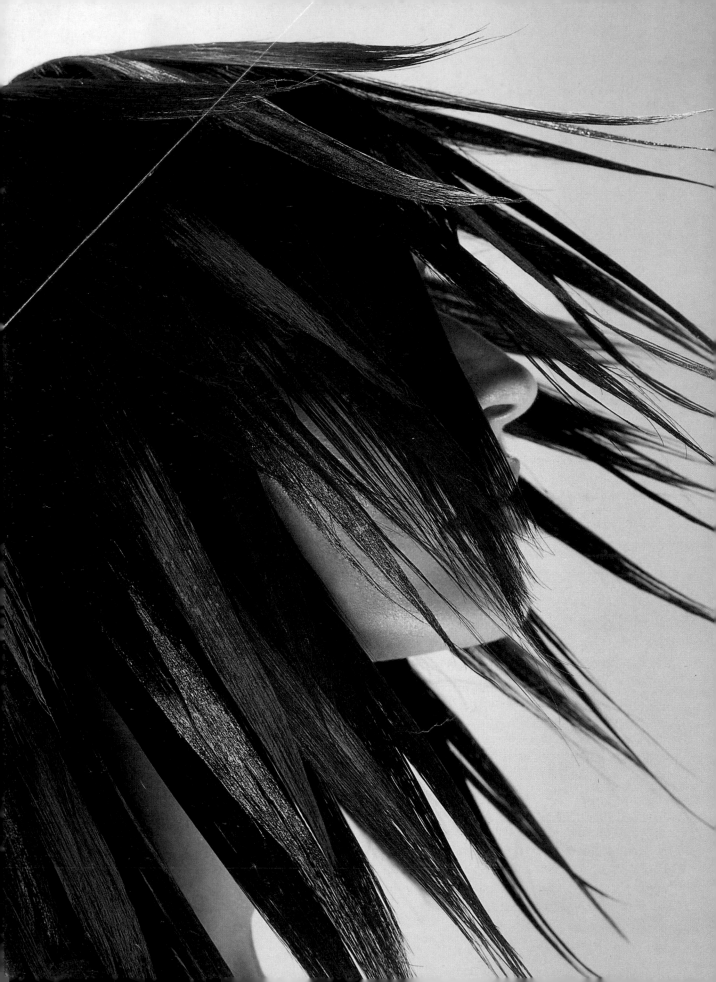

coloring tips

lighten up, but **not** at home

Attempting to lighten your hair yourself, using home-made preparations, lemon juice or — horror — bleach, is an extremely precarious business. Do without that must-have pair of feathered mules if need be, but leave your highlighting to the professionals. If you don't, you'll probably end up having to visit the salon anyway for a rescue job.

troubleshooting

If your hair has been colored in a salon and you are unhappy with the end result, talk to your hairdresser. There are several things they can do. Color can be masked or returned to your natural shade. Brassy or yellow bleached hair can be toned down with silvery or ashy temporary color and a tint will also cover bleached hair. A color stripper or reducer can also be used by your hairdresser to remove permanent tints. Repeated shampooing will lift semi-permanent colors, but this damages the condition of the hair, so always apply a protein-restructuring mask afterwards.

refresh your tresses

To revive your hair color, use a color enhancing shampoo and conditioner once a week. Always follow the manufacturer's instructions and leave them on for the specified time. Minuscule amounts of color pigment are deposited on the hair shaft to revitalize and maintain the color. Vary this treatment with a shampoo and conditioner that has been specially formulated and designed to cope with the changes your hair has undergone.

shampoo/conditioner speak

Shampoos that have been specially formulated for color-treated hair are designed to condition and cleanse the hair, as well as prevent the color from fading. Conditioners formulated for color-treated hair leave a protective film around porous, damaged areas of the hair shaft, helping to lock in the color pigments and improve the condition of the hair, leaving it stronger and shinier.

don't be dull

If your hair has a tendency to look dull after it has been colored, a good, quick and very natural treatment is to crack a raw egg onto your head after shampooing and work it through the hair. Leave it for five minutes and then rinse it out thoroughly. Top tip: Use cold or lukewarm water; if the water is too hot you will find that the egg will scramble and it will be difficult to remove. The natural proteins in eggs will leave the hair shiny and full of body.

natural remedy

If you find yourself in a fix without professional products, you can resort to Mother Nature. If your colored hair has been in the sun and feels brittle and dry, mash up an avocado and work it into your hair after shampooing. Leave it on for at least five minutes to let the moisturizing oils penetrate the hair shaft, then rinse it off thoroughly.

fade out

If you find that your naturally brown hair starts to look dull and faded, steep three tea bags in a large jar of hot water, let it cool down and use it to rinse the hair. The natural dye in tea will even out and enhance the color of your hair. Similarly, if your naturally blonde hair starts to look dull, rinse it with a solution of camomile tea made as described above. The antioxidant ingredients in the tea will leave your hair fresh, bright and shiny.

chlorine alert

Swimming in chlorinated water can turn bleached or blonde-tinted hair an unsightly shade of green. To prevent this, use products that have been specially designed to protect the hair in chlorinated water, and always rinse your hair immediately after swimming. To restore natural and enhanced blonde hair to its former glory, massage tomato juice into the hair after shampooing; leave for a few minutes and then rinse it out thoroughly. The active ingredients in the tomato juice will neutralize the green color.

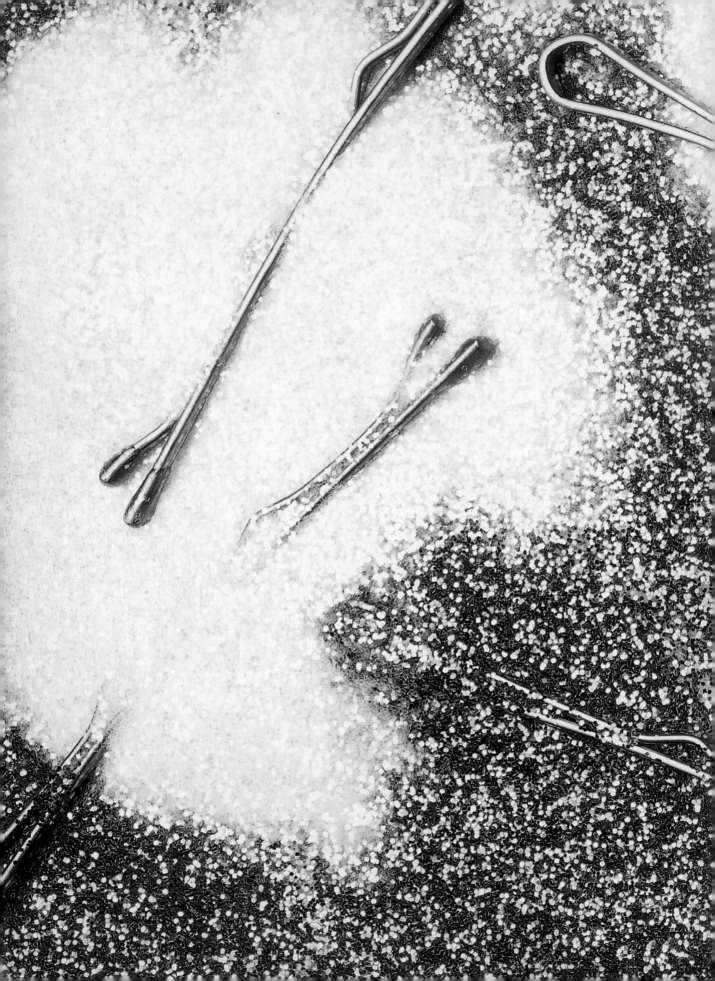

hair to wear

party prep in Tribeca

Saturday afternoon and very loud disco music was pumping out of the stereo over the non-stop whir of a hairdryer. There was definite excitement in the air. Chrissie was blow-drying Jaz's hair in the kitchen, Laura had just returned from her Fab Abs class at the gym and Polly was in her bedroom, packing for her trip to Miami. In less than 12 hours, she would finally meet cyber-suitor Simon. His last e-mail had been especially flirtatious: "Don't forget to bring your dancing shoes," he had written. It usually took Polly 20 minutes tops to pack for a business trip, but today she had dithered for several hours and instead of her usual organized approach, clothes and shoes were strewn Chrissie-style across the bed. Dizzy with excitement, she finally tossed the scarlet camisole, a pair of high heels and a bias-cut slip dress into her case, along with the sensible navy business suits, of course. She jumped guiltily when Kate poked her head around the door to say goodbye, "I'm off to the hairdressers. Have fun in Miami, Pol."

Kate was glad that she had a hair appointment to go to. Not only was the pounding music driving her mad, but the sight of their house guest running around in an endless selection of tight-fitting clothes — all flat stomach, long legs and sleek blonde hair — really was just too much. Still, it had increased Kate's resolve. After years of flowing, pre-Raphaelite locks and long floral dresses, the time had come to sharpen up her image and start climbing up that career ladder. She was even going to attend a Color Me Beautiful session at a girlfriend's house that night. Matthew — her handsome boss, the marketing director — wouldn't recognize her on Monday.

At 6 pm Polly's cab arrived. "Bye girls, I'm off now. Have a great time at the party," she yelled above the music. Laura was trying to watch a political discussion on television while she waited for Jaz and Chrissie to make their grand entrances. She had been ready for hours, having showered and scrunched some mousse through her hair at the gym. She was pleased with her new, slightly wispier crop, although it'd seemed to have escaped the notice of the assistant producer in Current Affairs. She had no idea what this party would be like, but she'd pushed out the boat and had swapped her uniform of jeans and running shoes for a slim-fitting skirt and — hell, it was worth a try — a spritz of "Fatal".

Jaz, meanwhile, had pulled out all the stops. She was desperate to wave goodbye to her job as a retail consultant at The Flag and land a plum position with a top designer. This party was the perfect opportunity for career enhancement, since it would be packed with fashionistas. Her new tie-dyed hair and matching red-and-black dip-dyed skirt ought to be enough to get her noticed.

Chrissie was also planning on having a little career advancement of her own. Determined to secure an audition — and a date — with Steve the producer, she had opted for "result wear."

Laura and Jaz gasped as she panthered into the living room. Her skin-tight black shell top was practically transparent, her heels as high as the Empire State Building and her fine, flyaway hair looked "Big" with a capital "B", thanks to some deft work with her hairdryer and some styling product. "Let's go, girls," she cried.

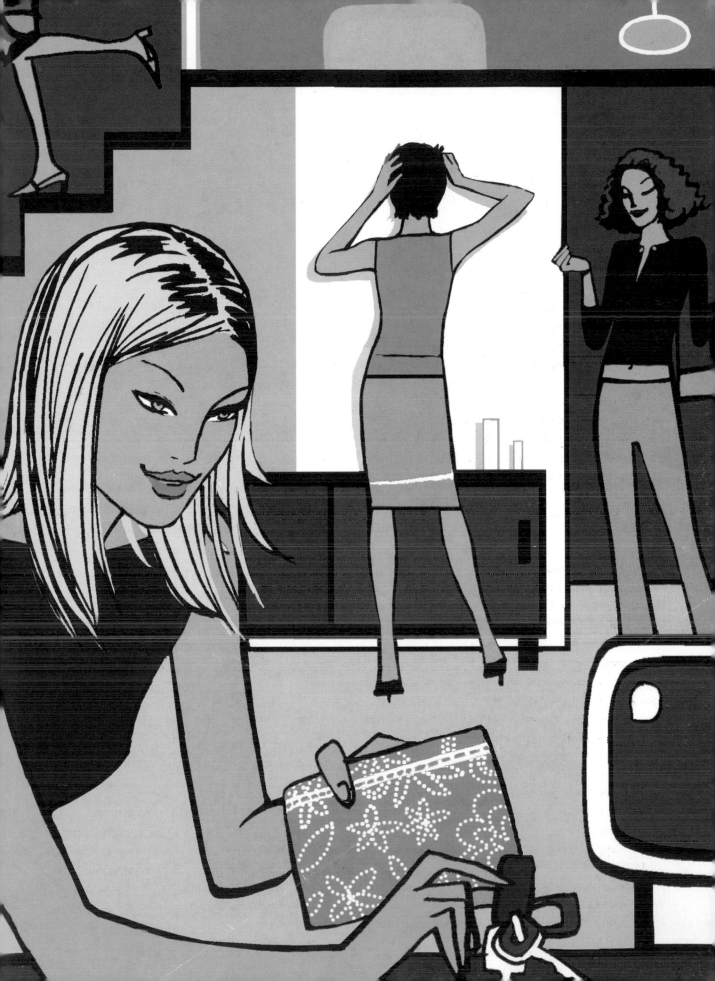

hair-styling

With a few good products and a little practice, anyone should be able to turn a bad-hair day into a good one. Learning how to use styling products effectively and achieving a good blow-dry at home are the first lessons. The critical point is the "damp to dry" stage when hair has a style "memory." If you overdry your hair, spritz it with a little water from a plant mister.

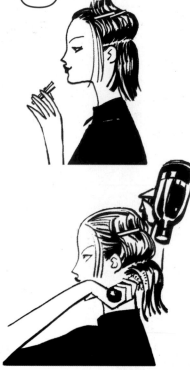

basic blow-dry

1 Gently pat as much moisture away from wet hair as possible using a towel. Rubbing the hair will ruffle the cuticles and cause tangles.

2 Hair loses one-quarter of its elasticity when it is wet, so gently comb it from the tips.

3 Tip your head upside-down and rough-dry your hair with the dryer on medium heat until it is 70 percent dry. Lift and separate the hair at the roots and through the length with your fingers to create volume.

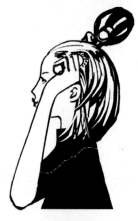

4 When the hair is still slightly damp, apply the styling product. Then section the back, top, bangs and sides with big clips.

5 Starting at the back, unclip and style one section at a time. Use a brush to lift the hair at the roots, then pull away to dry the length. Spend most effort and time on the front and side sections — once the frame to the face looks good, the rest follows.

6 A fine blast of cool air on the hair, while still under brush control, sets the hair and closes the cuticles, giving extra shine.

7 For the finishing touch, add a bit of shine enhancer, a little pomade to get a choppy look or just a spritz of hairspray to set the style.

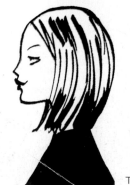

HAIR SNIP
ALWAYS RUN THE HAIRDRYER DOWN THE LENGTH OF THE HAIR SHAFT TO KEEP THE CUTICLES LYING FLAT.

TIP YOUR HEAD UPSIDE-DOWN AND SPRAY HAIRSPRAY AT THE ROOTS TO CREATE AMPLE VOLUME.

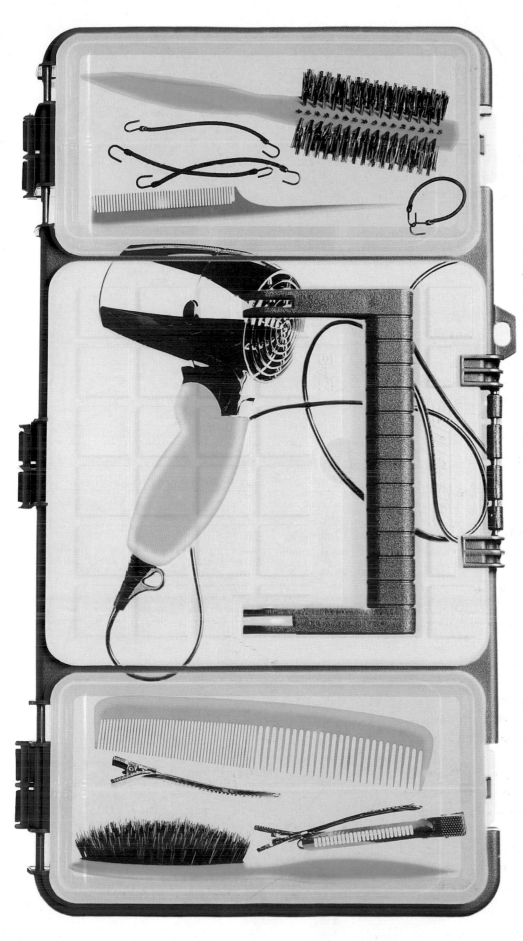

tool kit

brushes

Your hairstyle will probably require at least two different brushes, depending on the hair length. One should be a round brush for smoothing or curling and the other, a volumizing brush (see page 24).

hairdryer

Choose a hairdryer with a minimum strength of 1500 watts, several heat and speed settings and a cold button for finishing.

products

Have the appropriate mousse, gel, styling lotion or styling spray handy for your particular type of hair and style (see page 23).

comb

A comb is used for careful detangling, sectioning off hair for styling and for creating parts.

clips

These hold sections of hair out of the way while you are blow-drying and styling.

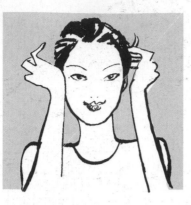

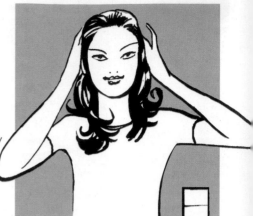

natural drying

1 Start by applying your chosen styling product, spreading it evenly through your hair using your fingers and finishing with a comb.

2 "Mold" your hair into the desired shape before drying it to ensure a perfect finish.

3 Start drying your hair, using your fingers as a brush. This gives maximum lift at the roots.

4 Dry all sections thoroughly and then finish using a light pomade.

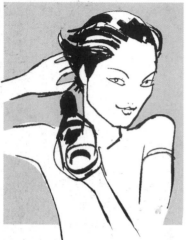

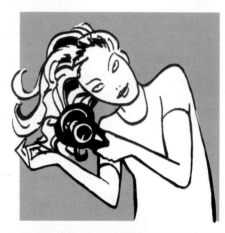

great curls

1 Apply a styling product that is suitable for your hair type — it is really important to start with a great foundation.

2 Tip your head to one side and, using the bowl of the diffuser, lift the hairdryer up and down into the hair with a gentle movement. Then tip your head to the other side and repeat.

3 When the hair is dry, tip your head forward and continue with a similar motion. If you find your hair is starting to go fluffy, spritz it with a shine spray.

4 When you have finished all the sections of the hair, gently run a gel evenly through it to create a more defined curl.

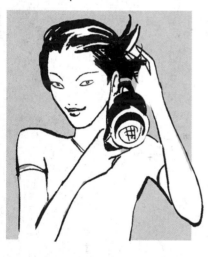

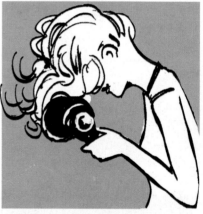

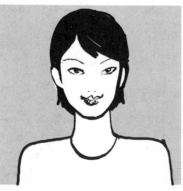

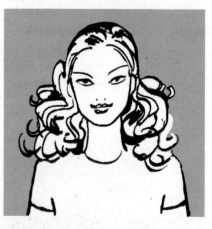

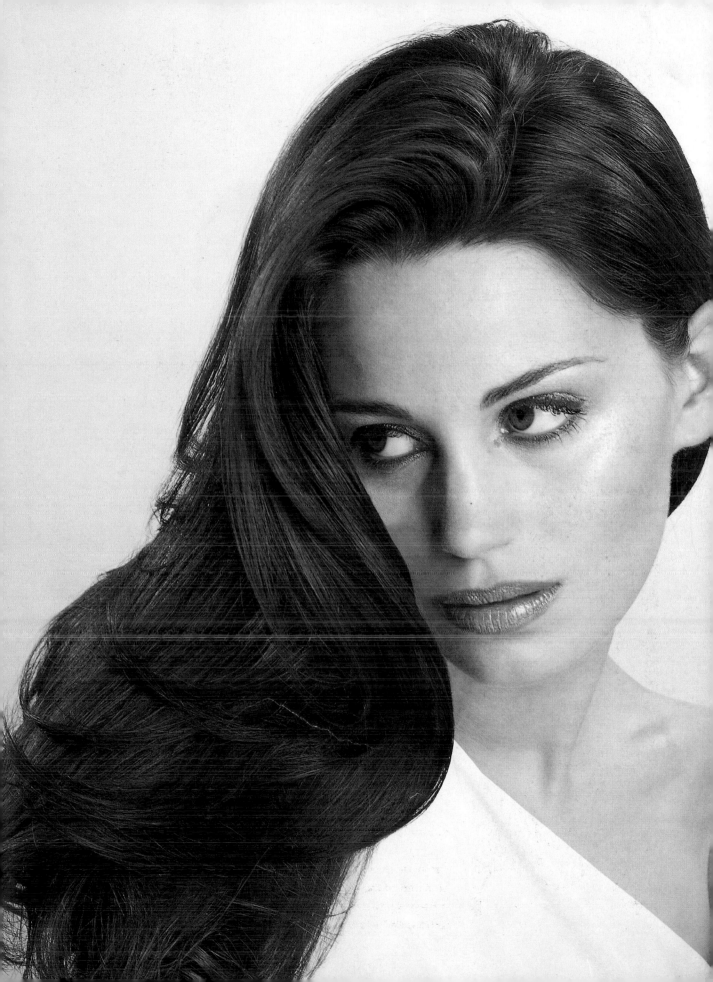

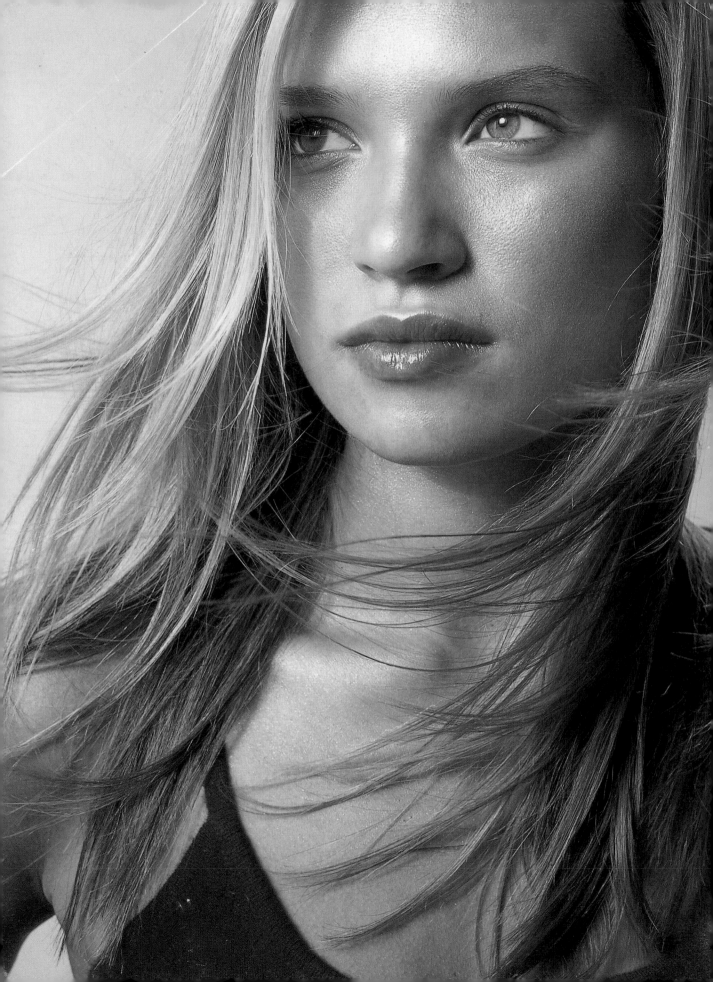

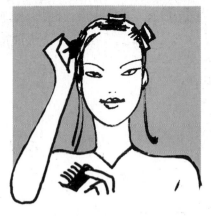

straightening

Here are some step-by-step tips for taming your tresses to create bone-straight sleek hair:

1 Start by applying your chosen product evenly through the hair — an anti-frizz serum is ideal.

2 Beginning at the back, use clips to section the hair. Avoid taking a section that is too big.

3 Using a paddle brush, dry each section in a downward motion. Start at the roots, taking the brush right through to the ends of the hair. To finish each section, give the hair a blast of cold air.

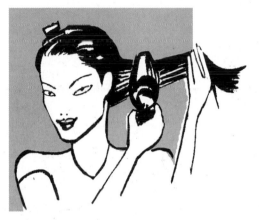

4 When all the sections of the hair are dry, lightly spray with hairspray to seal the cuticles.

5 Heat the straightening iron and, when it is very hot, run them section by section from the roots to the ends of the hair to ensure Cleopatra-style straight hair. This seals the cuticles of the hair, leaving it almost impossible for any moisture to penetrate the shaft.

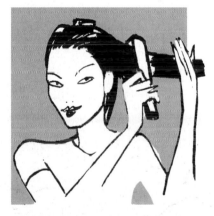

6 To complete the look, spray the hair with a light mist of shine spray.

HAIR SNIP

IF THERE IS A LOT OF MOISTURE IN THE AIR, OR IT IS VERY HUMID, USE AN ANTI-HUMIDITY SPRAY. THESE CONTAIN ANTI-HUMECTANTS WHICH SEAL THE HAIR AND BLOCK MOISTURE. A LEAVE-IN CONDITIONER WILL ALSO HELP PREVENT YOUR SLEEK LOCKS FROM BECOMING A FRIZZY MESS. ALTERNATIVELY, MIX TWO PARTS OF GEL WITH ONE PART OF STYLING LOTION AND APPLY IT TO WET HAIR.

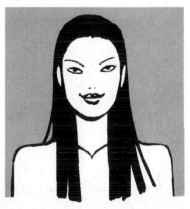

quick fixes

1 If your hair is short, try slicking it back into a sleek crop or just use pretty pins to decorate it.

2 If your hair is dirty, pin it up. Day-old hair is always easier to put up and will stay in place better than freshly washed hair. Turn unclean hair to your advantage by making a finger-combed ponytail on the crown of your head (avoid too much brushing as this increases the oiliness) and tie it with an elastic. Twist a length of hair around the elastic, fixing it with bobby pins as you go. Let locks of different lengths twist out if they want to; the more effortless the look, the higher the glam factor.

3 If your hair is curly, revitalize it by spritzing it with water and gently scrunching. If it has become frizzy, work a little styling lotion through each tendril, tackling it section by section.

4 If your hair is flat, try a little back-combing to give it lift. Start at the crown and work your way around to the sides. You don't need to backcomb all over, just enough to give a little lift.

5 Do not try to slick back dirty hair with copious amounts of wet-look gel. Although it looks good in magazines, in reality no one is fooled.

6 Never underestimate how long it takes to wash and dry your hair. Forfeit a shampoo for a bit of inventive yet speedy styling.

7 If you are not confident with bobby pins and combs (quick-fix 1), it is better to shower and leave with fresh, clean-smelling but perhaps damp hair than to get frustrated in front of a mirror.

8 Keep an emergency hair kit in the car or office that includes: a brush, a cordless straightener or curling iron, the nearly finished bottles of mousse and styling lotion from home, and a few pins and elastics that can save the day.

9 When you get given another hairdryer for Christmas, take one to the office. It is amazing how many times you get caught in the rain.

10 If your hair is really greasy and you have no time to wash it, apply some dry shampoo or talcum powder close to the roots. Massage it in gently to absorb the excess oil and then brush it out. Or, use a cotton pad to dab a little witch hazel onto the roots to absorb any grease.

style-and-go tips

1 To control static, flyaway hair, simply spray a comb with hairspray and gently run it through your locks.

2 Cheap shampoos containing strong detergents can strip your hair of its natural oils and make it seem dull, limp and lifeless.

3 If your hair is very tangled, work it through with a comb first before you begin to use your brush. This causes less damage.

4 Keep it cool. Using a hairdryer on a cool setting is good for the scalp, especially if you have greasy hair. Apply too much heat and the scalp will perspire for up to 15 minutes after you've finished drying, causing your hair to lose its shape. It will also activate the oil-producing glands. Whatever your hair type, avoid overdrying, too.

5 Sleep on a satin pillowcase to avoid "bed-head" hair. In the night your hair will slide gently across it, whereas cotton causes friction which can disrupt the hair cuticles.

6 If, on the other hand, you want to achieve "bed-head" hair, apply mousse to slightly damp hair before you go to bed. In the morning, simply arrange into place with pomade.

7 To keep the hair shaft healthy and prevent split ends, have a trim at least every six weeks.

8 Touch your hair as little as possible after styling it. Otherwise it will lose its shape and body and could become greasy.

9 Simple styles can be energized with temporary color. Try using hair mascara in bright blue or black for an extra-daring look.

10 To reduce the effects of static hair in the morning, wrap your hair loosely in a silk headscarf before going to bed. (Probably only worth trying if you sleep alone!)

11 To avoid flat hair, make sure your hair is totally dry when you go to bed. With slightly damp hair, you might wake up with a frizzy mop, and it's more likely to be flat against your scalp.

12 Two-in-one products can be a great timesaver, but avoid using those that are silicone-based. These build up a coating on the hair which makes styling difficult.

interview hair

Big hair with plenty lift at the roots was where stylish hair was at in the 1980s — think of the stars of *Dynasty* and *Dallas*. Thankfully, though, these days hair that means business is definitely sleek, easy and under control. Employers wonder if you can't keep your hair under control, how can you possibly be keeping your business under control either? Groomed hair is smart-and-together hair; a sleek ponytail, a smart, short crop or a bob are the perfect styles, and shiny, silky hair in tip-top condition is a must.

It is often quoted that employers decide in the first three minutes of an interview who they are going to employ. To make a good impression, ensure your hair is clean and shiny, as it is an obvious sign that you take care of yourself — the thinking being that if you don't take care of yourself, will you take care of your job? Make sure that your hair is not overly elaborate. If a style looks like it takes forever to create, you will be sending out signals that you will be wasting company time checking your reflection in mirrors. Leave elaborate hairstyles to ladies who lunch, who have nothing more important on their minds than their next Caesar salad. A ponytail can be elegant, but girly styles like braids are a no-no if you want to be taken seriously. Depending on the type of business, leave the pink bow and glitter hair clips for the evening. Your Hello Kitty hair accessories won't impress a bank or law firm.

updos

Sleek, chic and giving the appearance of being effortlessly elegant and well-groomed, long hair pinned up in a chignon always means business. Even simpler ponytails can work just as well on hair that is layered or growing out as on straight, one-length hair.

1 Tidy up growing-out layers and feathered-cuts by combing through some firm control mousse before tying back the hair.

2 Your hairdresser can show you how to attach a hairpiece in the same color as your own hair to add bulk to a thin ponytail.

3 Avoid tying your hair back towards the crown. Positioned too high, your chic updo will become a cheerleader's ponytail.

4 Keep a hairpiece for ponytails handy on business trips. That way, even if you don't have time to wash your hair, you can tie it back, slick it down and look super-stylish in a flash.

5 Wrap a small strand of hair around the elastic so that it can't be seen and fix it with a bobby pin on the underside. It finishes off the look better than a hair accessory. Alternatively, to make sure your ponytail is really secure, use wet string instead of an elastic to hold it. The string will contract as it dries, fixing the hair in place. As before, wrap a small section of hair around the string to hide it.

6 Slick down wispy bits with a little styling lotion and hairspray to keep the look sleek rather than sporty.

7 If your hair is fine and flyaway, wash it the day before so it's easier to handle and stays in place.

power bobs

The simple bob — with or without bangs; curled-up, curled-under or straight; short or long; blunt-cut or wispy — looks professional. There is a variation to suit everyone, so talk to your hairdresser about finding the one that suits you. It can be made sleeker or choppier with styling products, depending on your mood. It is the versatility of the bob that keeps it so fresh, even though it has been around since the 1920s.

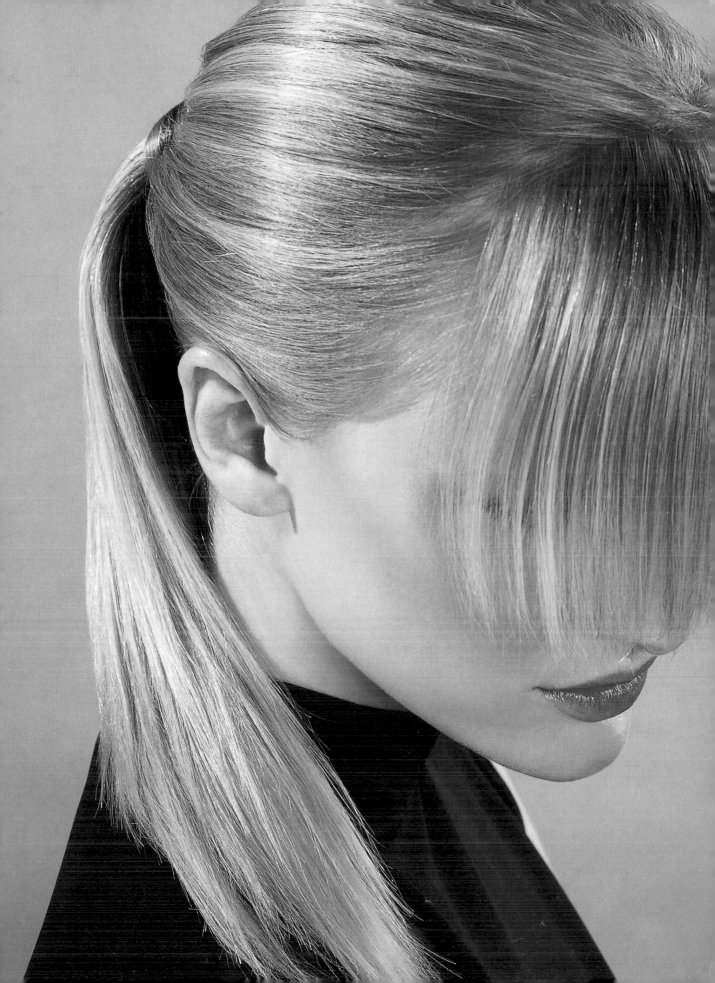

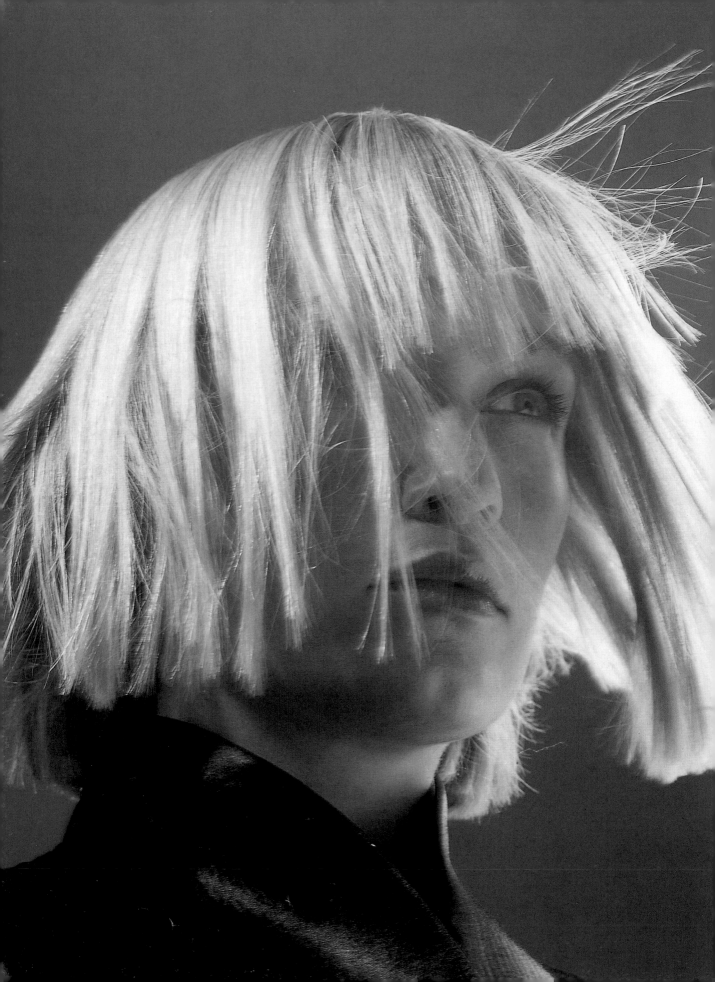

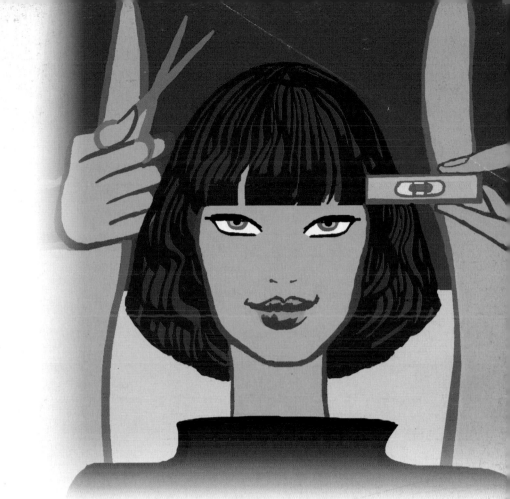

...kate's take on a power bob

Kate can't bear the thought of looking like a cross between a 1970s throwback from the easy-care perm days and Goldilocks for one minute longer. With her crush on Matthew the marketing director growing more intense by the week, Kate is increasingly interested in how she appears at work. While munching her way through a bag of the latest Crunch cookies (all in the name of research), she'd read a magazine article entitled confidently "How to Get Ahead at Work". Point number three, which was all about image and presentation, had made quite an impression. With new resolve — a woman with a mission — she hurtles to the hairdresser and demands a power bob (also advised in the very same article). Her patient stylist explains that a classic power bob is a no-no with her hair type; it was never going to look like Uma Thurman's poker-straight "do" in *Pulp Fiction*. What he can do, though, is a give her a sleeker, more groomed look, by taking off some length, adding some layers and generally tidying up her tresses into a bob shape. Kate starts feeling calmer and her breathing becomes more regulated as she watches herself being transformed into Miss Get Ahead at Work (and, more to the point, Miss How to Get Mr Marketing Director to Look Twice). Her stylist suggests blow-drying her hair straight (the closest she will ever get to a true power bob). Kate can't believe her eyes — she looks like Julia Roberts with sleek hair at the Oscars (sort of). Mr MD — wake up and smell the coffee! For the first time in her life, Kate can't wait to get to work on Monday.

work to play

The invite is for drinks at 7:30, or dinner at 8, yet you know you won't finish work until 6:30 at the earliest. Even if you do leave early, there is no way you can negotiate the cross-town, rush-hour traffic, get changed and get back in time. If you try (and everyone has done it once), you end up frazzled, in a foul mood and 30 minutes late. How much better, then, to make the work-to-play transition in the office or at a nearby gym?

One advantage of choosing a hairstylist near your office is that many salons now offer beauty treatments and have showering facilities available. Build a good relationship with your stylist and you will never have to change at work again. If an invite is sprung on you at the last moment and you have no change of clothes, it is amazing how a professional blow-dry can improve your spirits and your appearance. Your boring suit and white T-shirt suddenly look pared-down and Calvin Klein-ish with an expert coiff. If the salon option is out of the question, opt for one of these styles or try one of the quick fixes on page 64.

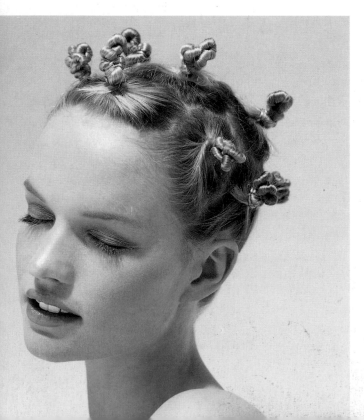

twisted sister

1 Start by dividing all of the hair into 2-in (5-cm) square sections. Use clips to hold them out of the way.

2 Starting at the nape, take each section individually and twist it tightly from the root through to the ends. As you work your way up each section, you'll find that it starts to twist down onto itself. Let this happen until it is sitting on your starting point, then secure it in place with a bobby pin.

3 Repeat this, working your way up the head to the crown, until you have twisted each section.

4 Finish by spritzing with a non-aerosol hairspray, to ensure a strong hold.

glam-hair updo

1 Loosely tie your hair back in a ponytail using a cloth-covered elastic to maintain a strong hold.

2 Lightly backcomb the ponytail section to create extra volume.

3 Fold sections of the ponytail into the middle of the head, securing them in place with bobby pins placed close to the elastic. This can be random — the beauty of the style is that it should look as if you've done it yourself.

4 When all of the hair is secured, lightly apply non-aerosol hairspray.

5 Choose an accessory to suit your outfit.

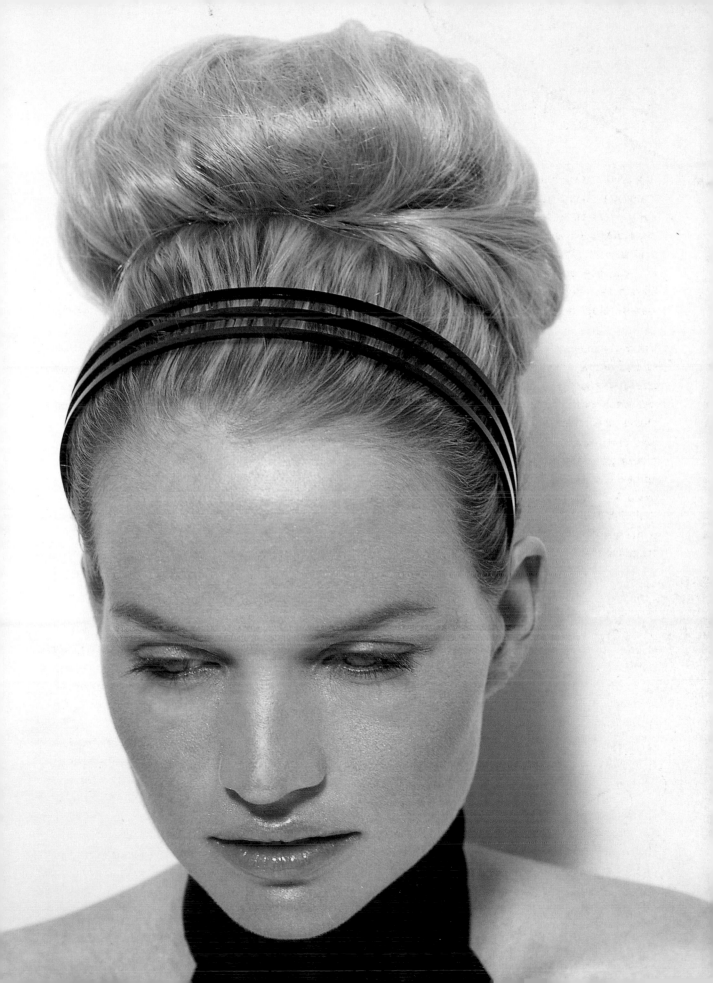

jet-set hair

Relatively inexpensive air travel has given most of us fast access to the "global village." Air travel was once strictly for the jet set, but now that it is no longer exclusive, no one pretends (not even the first-class passengers) that they feel glamorous after a 14-hour flight. Even though the in-flight wellbeing programs give tips on how to exercise (isn't sitting with your knees under your chin exercise?) and avoid dehydration, they never mention how to keep your hair looking as good on arrival as it did at departure.

dehydration

The air pressure in the cabin and the high altitude encourage dehydration, which leaves the skin and hair dull and lacking in radiance. This can only be prevented by drinking copious amounts of water and soft drinks, while avoiding tea, coffee and alcohol, all of which have a diuretic effect that will compound the problem. Drinking carrot and apple juice before a flight will also help to keep hair hydrated.

static

The dry, air-conditioned cabin atmosphere could not be better for static, nor worse for flyaway hair (the wispy rather than the jet-set sort). If you have ever tried brushing or combing your hair while sitting in your seat, you will know that you can hear the crackle of static over the noise of the engines. While there is nothing you can do to change the climate in the cabin, you can counter the static by fixing hair in place with firm control wax and gels, which give the hair weight. Resting a headscarf over the headrest will also help to reduce the friction between your hair and the back of the seat.

flaky scalp

Dehydration on board means an increased chance of developing a flaky scalp. If this happens to you, tie back your hair to avoid dandruff-like flakes on your shoulders. Once you are settled at your destination, a vigorous, but gentle, brushing will loosen any flakes.

Follow with a thorough scalp massage to increase the blood flow, and therefore nutrients and oxygen, to the scalp, as well as to release tension from the flight (see page 26). Finally, a shampoo and deep-conditioning treatment will remove any lingering flakes and restore moisture, bounce and shine.

Air-hair dos and don'ts

Don't fly with your hair weighed down with products or your face caked with heavy foundation. Fly with clean hair and a touch of lipstick, if you like.

Do spritz your face regularly with a hydrating mister to keep the skin soft and supple. Use it to refresh stale, dry hair, too.

Do drink plenty of uncarbonated mineral water.

Don't drink coffee, tea or alcohol.

Do always pack your skincare and haircare products in waterproof bags so there's no chance of them spilling their contents over your favorite silk dress.

Do tie your hair back to help prevent static building up. If you do get static hair, spray some hairspray onto your brush or comb and lightly run it through the hair.

Do pack a gentle, restorative shampoo and super-rich conditioner to revive your travel-stressed hair on arrival.

Do not despair. If you still look less-than-perfect on arrival — despite plenty of water and a first-class seat — simply act like a film star and wear a pair of dark "Jackie O" sunglasses, a smart hat, some red lipstick and a disenchanted air.

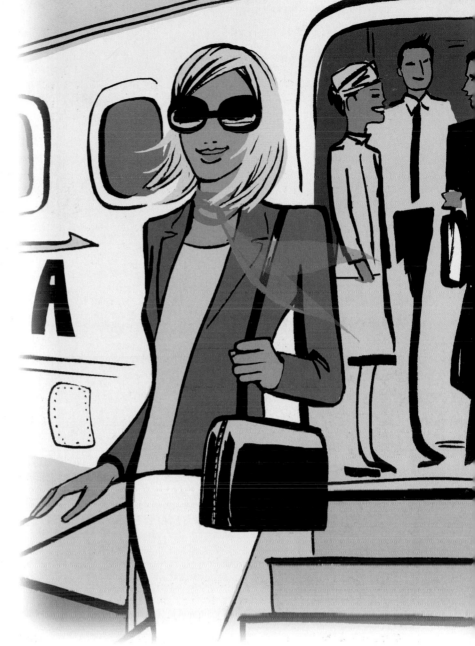

Never before has the prospect of a business trip to Miami seemed quite so exciting as it does now. Apart from the obvious retail opportunities, it's the anticipation of finally meeting cyber-suitor Simon, who has her heart fluttering like a teenager's. There is one problem, though — airplane hair — and she has to go straight out from the airport to a dinner meeting with no time for a hotel stop and hair overhaul. After a few hours of being subjected to the two demon hair enemies — static

…polly's air-hair dilemma

and dehydration — Polly's worried that she'll disembark with hair so frizzy and static that the only spark between her and Simon will be the electric shock she gives him when they shake hands for the first time. What to do? Hair in bun? Business-like but maybe too prim. Wear a headscarf? Ladylike-chic but a bit too prudish. A baseball cap? Not a good look with a suit. Polly hits a brick wall, but a quick phone call to her hair guru, Charles, solves the problem. Drink plenty of H_2O and carrot and apple juice before flying to combat dehydration. Another good tip, put a scarf on the headrest to prevent static from the nylon seat covers. Hah! She knew the scarf would come in handy. Armed with bottles of water and various fruit juice concoctions, her Hermès scarf knotted around her neck, Polly sashays down the corridors at La Guardia without a second thought for her boyfriend. Sorry, Harry.

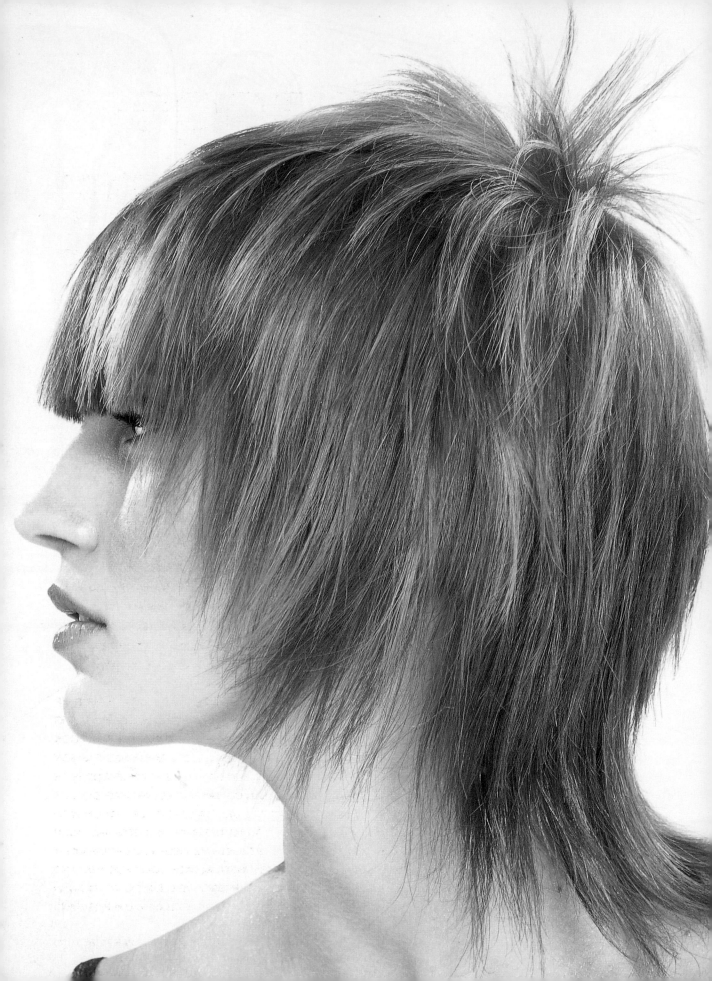

vive la change

We all know someone who has taken the plunge and had the big chop. It usually coincides with a big life change, invariably the end of a relationship. Cutting long hair short is a liberation and, when one considers how men prize long hair, it is a form of emancipation from their — his — ideals. There is bravery attached to a dramatic new look, too. A complete change of color or a cut — or both — can be tremendously energizing and rejuvenating. Some people thrive on change, whereas others need a gentle nudge to boost their courage.

considerations

Whether you're the sort of person who gets a real buzz from reinventing yourself or you take the cautious approach, don't do anything rash. Think carefully about your new look, consider all the options and ask advice from your stylist. The decision to chop off four years' worth of hair growth should not be taken lightly.

1 Think about why you want to have a dramatic change. Remember, a haircut won't bring a lover back or put the world right again, but it might restore your confidence, perk up your mood and give you a much-needed lift.

2 Are you prepared to change your wardrobe and make-up to accommodate a dramatic new hairstyle? For example, if you are naturally a brunette with long hair, having a short blonde crop will affect the coloring of your face and different clothes will suit you. Be prepared.

3 Copying someone else's style exactly never works successfully. Find a style or cut that inspires you, then, with the help of your hairstylist, make it your own.

4 A flexible hairstyle is the best one to have. You may love your spiky crop when it's just been done, but get bored with it after the initial impact has worn off.

5 Color, rather than cut, is the easiest way to effect a big change and yet still leave you with the option to reverse it. A cut is more permanent as it grows out slowly, at little more than half an inch a month.

6 If you are considering cutting long hair, try on a few short-styled wigs beforehand to make sure you like the way it looks.

7 If you are thinking of growing out a short haircut, use hairpieces to see if you like the feel of longer hair.

8 Make sure you're ready for a change and don't let anyone push you into doing anything you're not happy about.

9 Think of the upkeep. Will your new look be easy or an effort to style? Will it fit in with your lifestyle? How versatile do you need it to be? And how often will you need to revisit the hairdresser to keep it looking good?

HAIR SNIP
WHEN YOU'RE CONSIDERING GOING FOR A COMPLETE IMAGE-OVERHAUL, LOOK THROUGH PLENTY OF BEAUTY AND FASHION MAGAZINES TO FIND AS MANY PICTURES AS YOU CAN OF HAIRSTYLES AND HAIR COLORS THAT YOU LIKE. TAKE YOUR SELECTION WITH YOU TO THE HAIRDRESSER'S AND YOUR STYLIST WILL HELP YOU DECIDE WHAT ELEMENTS FROM EACH LOOK SUIT YOU AND YOUR HAIR TYPE. THAT WAY, YOU CAN CREATE A UNIQUE LOOK.

gently does it

If you like the idea of changing your image but just can't seem to get the courage to go for a complete reinvention, try a few subtle, temporary changes first. Ask your hairstylist to blow-dry your hair in a different way — if you are naturally curly, get them to blow-dry it completely straight; if you normally wear it forwards, framing your face, ask them to style it away from your face; or have it set in curlers to create gentle waves. If you always wear your hair loose, ask your hairdresser to show you a new way of pinning it up; or simply try parting it in a different way. You could even have a semi-permanent color rinse that will wash out in a few weeks. All of these devices can make you look and feel quite different without committing yourself to a radical change that may take years to reverse.

without bangs...

If you are flirting with the idea of having short hair, then think about moving towards that in stages rather than going for a crop in one fell swoop of the scissors. You could evolve from a one-length long cut to a layered Rachel cut, then a shoulder-length bob or a sexy layered "rock chick" style. You can then try a messed-up Meg Ryan cut and still have hair left to go even shorter. Gradual change is experimental and will give you time to play ideas out and find which styles and cuts suit your face and your personality best.

bangs or no bangs?

There are no hard and fast rules about hair type or face shape: some people simply do not suit bangs. It's a very personal thing. If you are thinking of having bangs but are not sure if they will suit you, or if you like bangs but don't want anything permanent which you will then have to grow out (a big bore), try faking it. It sounds unlikely but it does work!

How to do it: take a section of hair from the crown, comb it forwards over your forehead and arrange it as you would bangs. If you've got long hair, twist it to take away the length before taking it forwards. Adjust the width, length and density as required, then clip it securely just above the crown using a large clip. Alternatively, ask your hairstylist to attach a hairpiece. Leave your false bangs for 20 minutes to get used to them before deciding whether the look suits you.

moving on

Even the most dramatic changes lose their impact after a while, so the trick is to reinvent your look regularly to avoid getting stuck in a style rut. Think how differently Madonna looks at 40 compared with how she looked in her twenties. Many feel she looks younger now. True to type, she has grown her hair and left it long at the age when most women feel they have to go short. Luckily, hair does grow. So unlike that dolphin tattoo swimming across your buttock, even the most radical change of color and cut will grow out over time. Be brave and enjoy the positive power of transformation that a radical change can bring. (See overleaf — would you do it?)

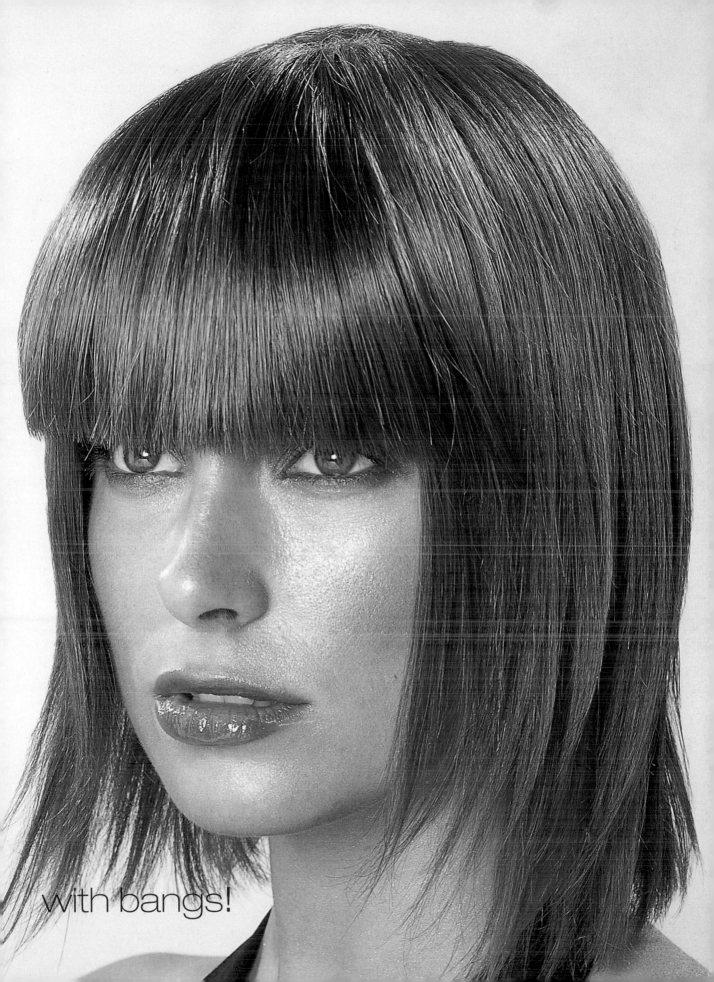

with bangs!

from long…

to short!

disco divas party on

Jaz simply could not believe her luck. Squashed up at the bar of Shaft with Laura, while attempting to order yet another round of Cosmopolitans, she'd struck up a conversation with a girl called Imogen, who turned out to be...wait for it...the fashion editor on *Gloss* magazine.

"Sweetie, I love your two-tone hair," Imogen had declared to Jaz by way of a conversation opener. Jaz, in return, had admired Imogen's fluorescent pink mules, and before she knew it she'd been offered an (unpaid) work placement on *Gloss*. Jaz didn't think twice about accepting. She would quit her job at The Flag on Monday, even if it meant taking a second job to pay the rent.

In another corner of the crowded bar, Chrissie had Steve the record producer well and truly under her spell — or so she thought. She had been flirting with him relentlessly all evening, purring into his ear and batting her eyelids until she was dizzy. "Honey, this is a fabulous party... so glad we were able to come along... there are always so many invitations on Saturday nights." Laura and Jaz listened in to snatches of the conversation, most impressed by Chrissie's small talk, if not by her taste in men.

"OK, Chrissie," Steve was saying. "Here's the deal. I'll arrange the interview with Pout. But there's something I want to ask you in return."
"Yes, honey?" Chrissie flashed him her most winning smile. The audition was in the bag; now he was going to ask her out on a date.
"I was wondering if we could go out to dinner. Sort of a double date — you, me, your roommate and a friend of mine, John. You see, I really like...Laura." Laura! Chrissie practically fell off her skyscraper heels, but thought quickly. Not only was it in the interests of her pop career to go on a double date with Steve, but over three courses and a few bottles of wine she knew she could convince him that it was she, Chrissie, in whom he should be interested. Not boyish Laura.
"Oh, I'm sure I can fix up something," Chrissie purred through gritted teeth.

"No way," whispered Laura to Jaz. "He wears leather pants and he looks like a creep. I'm not going on a date with him." But she hadn't factored in Chrissie's powers of persuasion. By the time the girls left Shaft at 3 am the audition, the double date and a job on *Gloss* were all secured. Result all round — if not exactly what Chrissie had planned.

Across town, poor Kate was swallowing the truly disastrous news that her color palette should be oyster pinks, peach and...biscuit. Yep, apparently she had to dress in the same shade as a stale digestive in order to get herself noticed at Crunch Cookies. Life was so unfair; no doubt Prissie Chrissie would be a strawberry-cream or a chocolate-coated cookie.

Meanwhile, Polly's plane was about to touch down in Miami. She hadn't had a wink of sleep — too many glasses of water and trips to the ghastly toilet. And she'd also been too busy feeling guilty about Harry and wondering if cyber-suitor Simon was as sexy as he sounded in his e-mails. Very soon, she would find out.

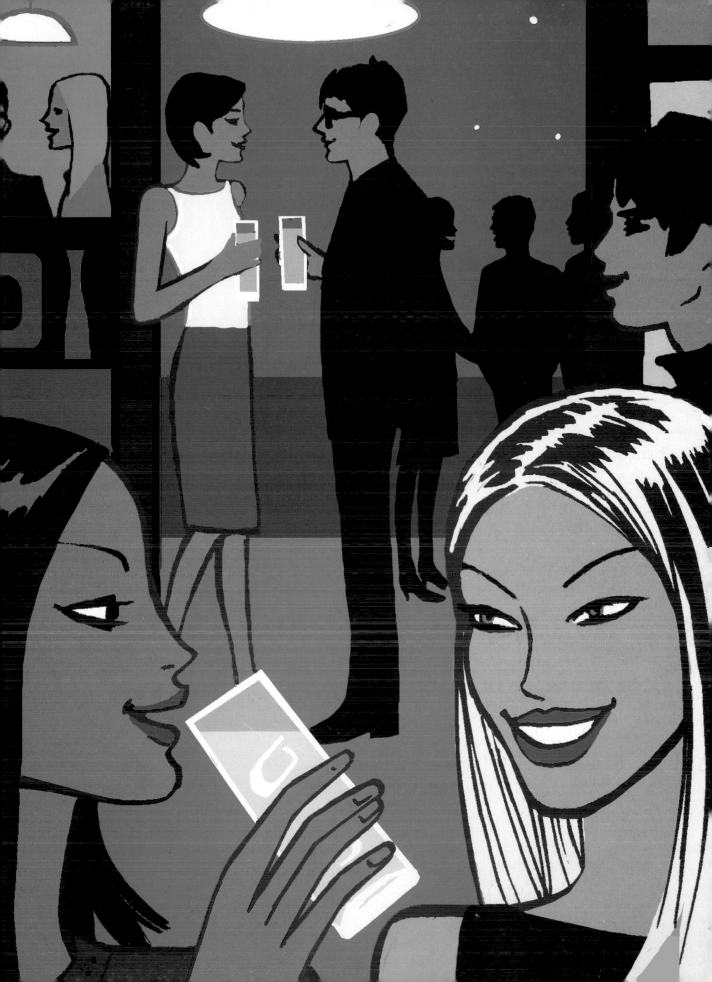

big date hair

Glamourtime hair is fun — there's nothing like
transforming the way you look and feel with a blast
of hairspray, a few pins and a bit of styling know-how,
and Big Date Hair is the ultimate feel-good experience.
It covers your every hair need — whatever the
invitation — whether you want to twist up your
tresses in a ladylike updo to meet his parents for
dinner or gutsy up your mane for a rock chick
look that's got to last for as long as you do.

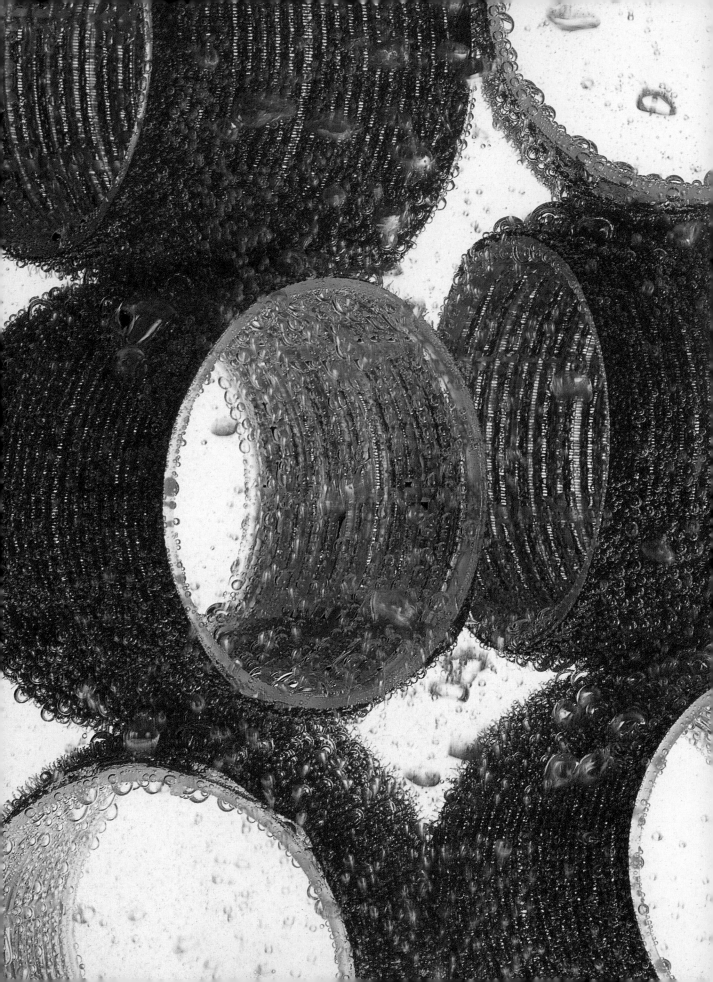

styling basics

the girls catch up

"So it was results all round," said Chrissie with a self-satisfied smile as she retold the tale of the previous week's party at Shaft, the trendy new bar in Soho. The girls were sitting in Café Marron, their local coffee shop and favorite haunt, filling Polly in on all their news. Or rather, Chrissie was filling her in on their news while the other girls sat sipping their lattes, unable to get a word in. "So Jaz got lucky on the job front; Laura was asked out on a date; and I've finally got my audition," Chrissie recapped triumphantly.

Kate groaned to herself. Chrissie hadn't stopped talking about her audition for this stupid new girl band, Pout, all week. Frankly, she was sick of it and it didn't help that she was so bored at work that she was now eating half-pound bags of caramel delights (misshapen and bought at staff discount) daily. It seemed that she, Kate, was destined to spend her days stuck in a dead-end secretarial job, piling on the pounds at Crunch Cookies, while Chrissie led a fast, glamorous life. She tried to change the subject. "So, Polly. How was your work trip?" Polly was stirring her cappuccino a little dreamily.

"What? Oh, um, fine, fine," she said, turning pink and looking a bit flustered. If truth be told, Polly's thoughts were still in South Beach rather than in Café Marron. But she couldn't possibly tell the girls about her little moment of passion with Simon, her sexy colleague. She blushed again as she remembered the long, lingering kiss...

Her roommates eyed her suspiciously. For someone who had stepped off a flight from Miami just a few hours earlier, Polly was looking intriguingly good. Her skin was glowing, her hair looked fashionably disheveled and she was wearing stiletto boots with a pair of new, tight, bootleg jeans. Polly, sensible Polly, was looking rather foxy. "So did you miss Harry dreadfully?" Kate persisted. "Harry?" said Polly.

"You know, your boyfriend," quipped Laura, sarcastically.

Fortunately, Polly was saved from answering by Chrissie's burning dilemma. "I simply can't decide what to wear for my audition," she was saying. "It's a toss-up between my lucky red dress — the strapless one — and my snakeskin-print jeans. Jaz, maybe you could style me?" Jaz had been practically bouncing up and down with excitement for the past half hour (and it wasn't the effect of the caffeine).

"Oh, I'd love to. I start my work placement at *Gloss* on Monday, so maybe I'll be able to borrow a designer outfit for you to wear."

Polly's ears perked up. "Work placement? But Jaz, what about your job at The Flag? You do know that a work placement means you don't get paid, don't you?"

"*Gloss* is going to pay my travel expenses," said Jaz, hugging her fuchsia fishnetted knees with excitement. Laura — who had long thought that Jaz came from a completely different planet — stifled a snigger. "Only travel expenses? How are you going to pay your rent?" asked Polly, dragged back suddenly from her daydream. She was, after all, Jaz's landlady.

"Oh, I'll get an evening job in a bar or something," said Jaz, her eyes shining at the thought of meeting the world's top fashion designers and models, and traveling across the globe on *Gloss* fashion shoots.

Polly sighed. Life in Tribeca was certainly going to be interesting in the next few weeks. Not least, she thought with a pang of guilt, because sexy Simon had promised to call.

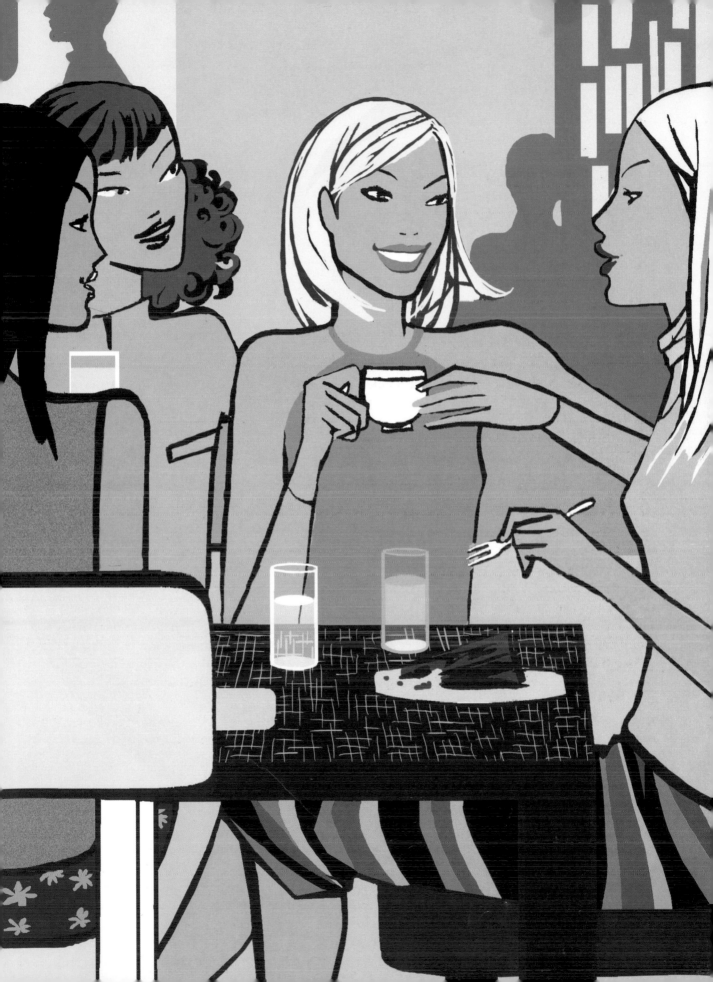

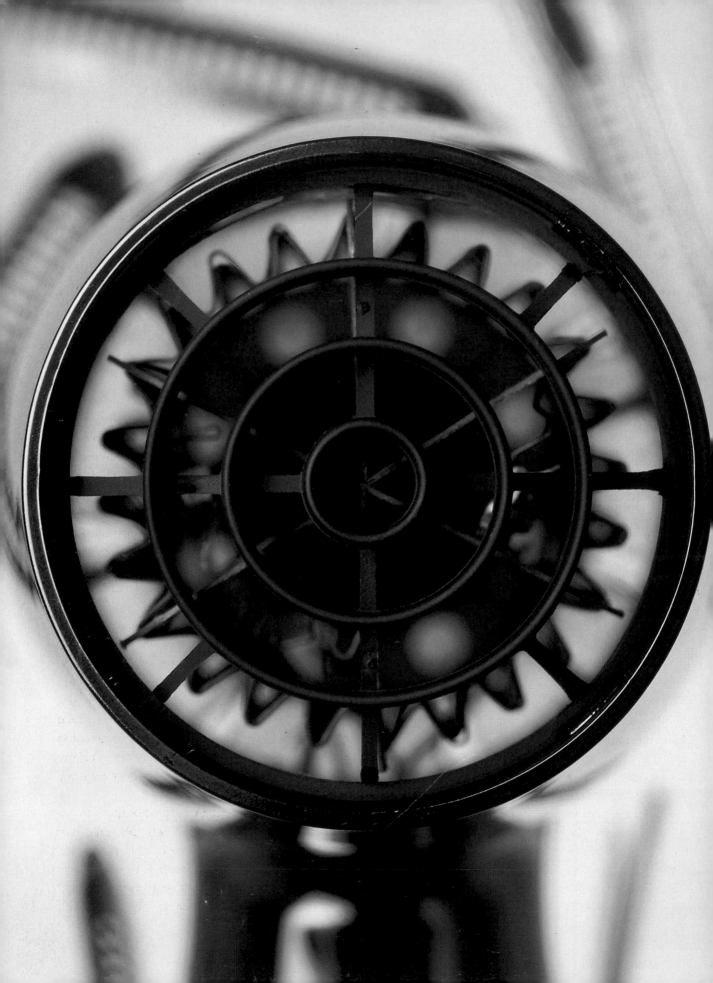

stylist's tool box

You don't need a new haircut or a visit to the salon to achieve wow-factor hair. With a little know-how and the right tools you can perform mini miracles at home. Girls born without curls, for example, can win the battle against nature and give themselves Julia Roberts-style corkscrews. Similarly, those who are blessed (or cursed, depending on your point of view) with a surplus of kinks and curls, can make their hair stick-straight, simply by using the right styling products and drying technique. Hair is the ultimate fashion accessory. The golden rule is that if it looks good, you'll feel good. Here's what the professionals have in their tool box:

the gadgets

hairdryer

Not just for blasting wet hair dry, a hairdryer can make your hair sleek and straight, or give it more lift than a pair of Manolos. Make sure yours is at least 1,500 watts, otherwise you will spend valuable date time drying your hair and possibly even damage it in the process.

diffuser

This big, dish-like attachment is used to dry curly hair. It disperses the flow of air so that curls, natural or otherwise, aren't straightened by its sheer force.

brushes

Styling is about shaping the hair, so don't think you can use the same brush as for everyday grooming. Styling brushes come in many shapes and sizes. Flat brushes, which have bristles on one side only, are good, all-round tools, but are not precise enough to curl or straighten the hair. Round brushes, with bristles all the way around, are for curling, straightening or adding volume. Use small-diameter brushes for short hair and large-diameter ones for straightening kinks out of long hair. Broad, flat paddle brushes are great for blow-drying straight or wavy long hair, as well as for styling hair to a poker-straight finish.

combs

You need a good, all-purpose comb for detangling hair, dividing it into sections and for backcombing.

curling iron

These create curls for girls who don't have them. Use a small-diameter curling iron for short hair or for making tight curls, and large ones for creating looser curls in long hair. You can also get heated curling brushes, which have bristles rather than a clamp to hold the hair in place. Use curling irons on dry hair only.

straightening iron

This is used after blow-drying to give a blunt, sleek, straight look. The two flat, heated plates are clamped over a section of hair and slowly drawn down to the ends. It should not be used too often as they are very dehydrating.

crimping iron

As well as creating the distinctive "corrugated" wave that goes in and out of fashion faster than flared pants, these irons can also be used on the under layers of dry hair to boost volume, or at the roots to lift limp hair.

rollers

Rollers, which can be used to add volume to hair as well as make it curly, have become very hip. And hurrah for the fact that — unlike your grandmother's generation — you don't have to go to bed wearing them. Heated hot rollers (for use on dry hair only) are a speedy way of creating strong curls. For loose curls, take out the rollers while they are still warm. Velcro rollers are non-heated but you can put them into dry or damp hair to add lift at the roots.

hairpins and sectioning clips

Small hairpins are essential for securing updos and small sections of hair — use matte ones, which are less slippery, in a color that matches your hair. Big metal clips are useful when you need to hold larger sections of hair up and out of the way for styling.

Chrissie is leaving nothing to chance. Tomorrow is her big audition with Pout, so she's locked herself in the bathroom for yet another experiment. She knows it's going to annoy Kate, who's already started to make snide comments about Chrissie hogging the bathroom all the time, but it just can't be helped. Chrissie's determined to turn her fine blonde hair into big hair and the way to do it, she's read in one of her many beauty books, is to use extra-large rollers. Standing in front of the bathroom mirror, she finishes rolling the last big Velcro roller snugly

...chrissie tries big hair for size

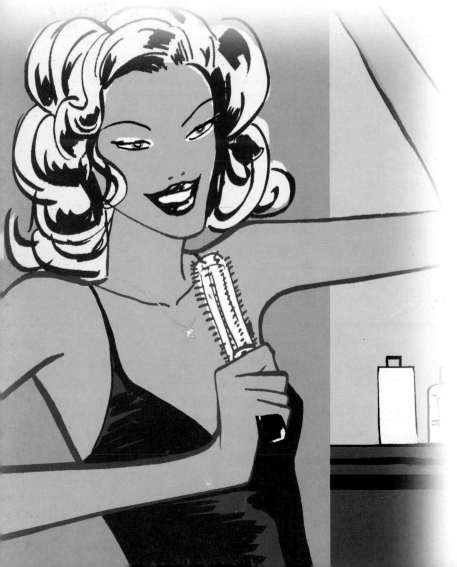

against her scalp (for maximum volume) and spritzes her hair with styling spray. Ten minutes later Chrissie carefully removes the rollers and admires herself with a satisfied (almost smug — Laura would call it narcissistic) smile. Not only does her hair look bigger and bouncier, but the strapless red dress shows off her fake tan to perfection. Jaz has tried to convince her to wear her python-print jeans and a pussy-cat bow blouse, but Chrissie knows better. The other girls from Pout practically live in snakeskin-print jeans, and she wants to look different. In her tight scarlet dress (holding her hairbrush to her mouth in mock singing/karaoke mode) and with her limp blonde locks transformed into big voluminous hair, there is no doubt that Chrissie is going to stand out from the crowd...

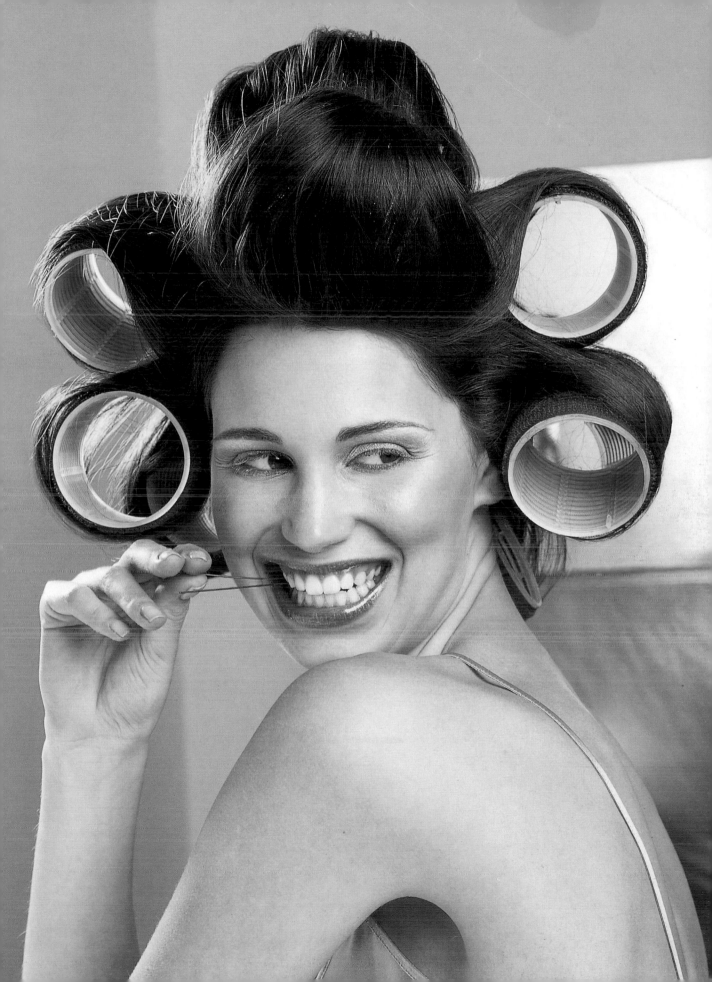

the products

If you don't know a styling lotion from a shine spray, the range of styling lotions and potions out there is enough to make your hair curl. But you don't need a whole battery of products: the contents of your personal tool box will depend on your particular hair type and the style that you want to achieve.

wax and pomade

Wax and pomade are designed to add definition and hold. They come in numerous strengths, holds and consistencies, so it might take a while to find the best one for you — but once you've found it, you won't ever want to be without it.

anti-frizz serum

This is the product for eliminating frizzy, flyaway bits and for making unruly hair behave. It contains silicone, which coats the hair shaft and smooths and seals the cuticle. Use it on wet hair before styling or to smooth down dry hair. Styling lotion can be mixed with other products to give extra-shiny drying and extra protection.

curl revitalizer and activator

These perk up deflated curls by adding moisture — but only if the curl existed in the first place. These products tend to come in gel form, and the more product used, the more defined the curl. Test these products before a big night out, as too much can sometimes overload the hair.

styling cream

Similar to leave-in conditioner, this cream limits damage if you apply it to the ends of the hair before using heated appliances. Volume control or non-chemical relaxers normally come in a cream form and should be used sparingly.

shine enhancer

This usually comes in spray or liquid form and contains silicone to coat the hair shaft, smooth the cuticle and add the magic shine factor. Shine spray is an absolute must-have for perfect, shiny, glamour hair.

mousse

A light and airy foam that is used to add oomph to fine hair (apply it to the roots before blow-drying) or to shape and control dry hair. Mousse comes in varying strengths and can be used for softer setting techniques.

These pump up the volume on pancake-flat or very fine hair by swelling the hair shaft. They work best when applied near the roots before blow-drying. They tend not to overload the hair, since they are designed for fine hair. So, for more volume and hold, use more product.

gel

Gel can be used to slick back unruly hair, giving good hold and a glossy finish. Light-hold gels may also be used in curly hair to define the curls, or in fine hair to add volume.

hairspray

The original styling product, this is still used after styling to hold hair in place. Useful for updos and styles that need to keep their shape. Hairsprays come in different strengths, so choose one for your desired hold. Hairspray also helps to reduce static.

back to basics

Before you start transforming your tresses with rollers, braids and updos, master the fundamental styling techniques for best results. For great curls, see page 60 and for super-sleek straight hair, see page 63.

big hair

you need

Hairdryer • volumizing mousse or blow-drying spray • sectioning clips • brush with a detachable bristle roller • hairspray

1 After shampooing and conditioning, blow-dry the hair roughly until it is 70 percent dry.

2 Apply the mousse or blow-drying spray, working it evenly through the hair with your fingers.

3 Pin up the top layer of the hair with sectioning clips so that you can access the layer underneath. Dry the hair section by section, using the roller brush to hold the roots at right angles to the scalp as you do so to give maximum volume.

4 Unclip the top layer section by section and dry each one in the same way, this time unclipping the handle of the brush and leaving the roller in the hair to set in volume. This creates a soft fullness that lifts the hair away from the head. It also smooths and softens the hair cuticles, maximizing shine.

5 Give the hair a blast of cold air to set, then gently remove the brush head once hair is completely cool.

6 When you have finished drying all the hair, shape it with your fingers and lightly spritz with hairspray.

textured hair

you need

Medium-hold gel • comb • hairdryer

1 A quick, easy way of adding texture to hair of any length is to apply a little medium-hold gel to your roots. You can do this on wet hair or dry hair.

2 Using a hairdryer, direct the heat at the roots and use your fingers to lift the hair as you do so.

3 Once the roots are dry, take the heat through to the ends of your hair, combing it with your fingers. This gives a slightly messy and windblown look.

4 For ultimate "rock chick" texture and great volume, finish by tipping your head upside-down and gently roughing up the hair with your hands.

styling secrets

Always finish blow-drying your hair with a quick blast of cold air. Not only does it "set" the new shape in place, but it closes the hair cuticles which maximizes gloss and shine. (When the cuticles lie flat, they reflect light better.) Now that's a cute tip!

For best blow-drying results, gently dry the hair until it is 70 percent dry before attempting to style it — trying to style and shape wet hair is just a waste of time and effort.

Be careful when you dry your hair upside-down – it can rough up the cuticle which leaves the hair looking dull. Only do it occasionally when you want to build up huge volume.

When using waxes and styling products, the secret is to start off with a tiny amount and add more gradually if it is needed.

Always use a clean hairbrush — not one that is clogged up with hair and product. You should wash your brushes once a week in a little shampoo and warm water.

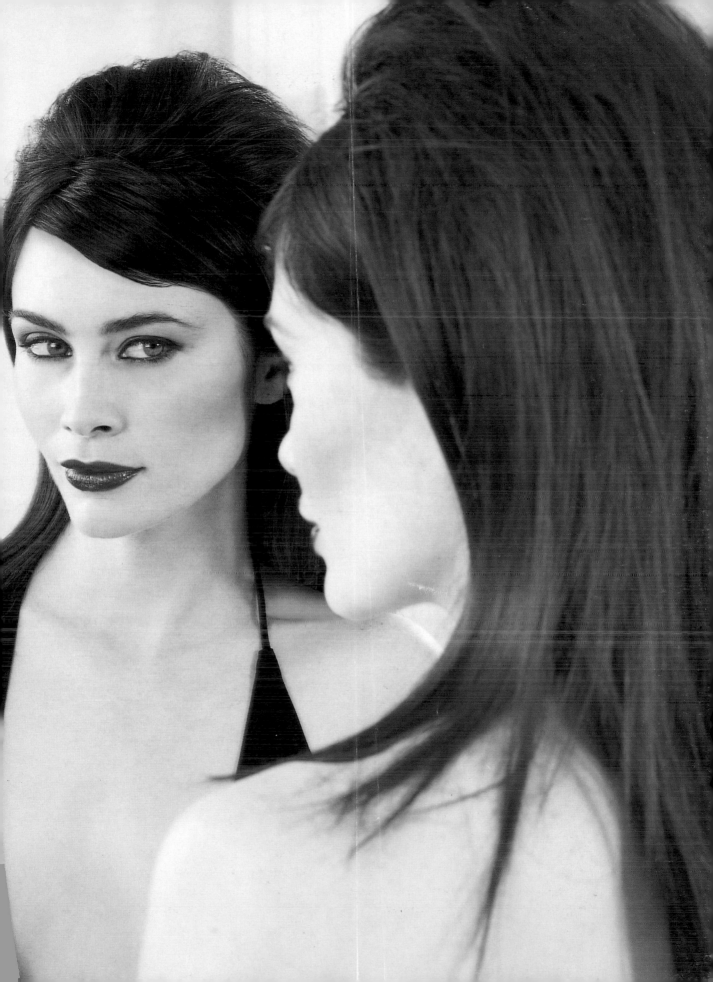

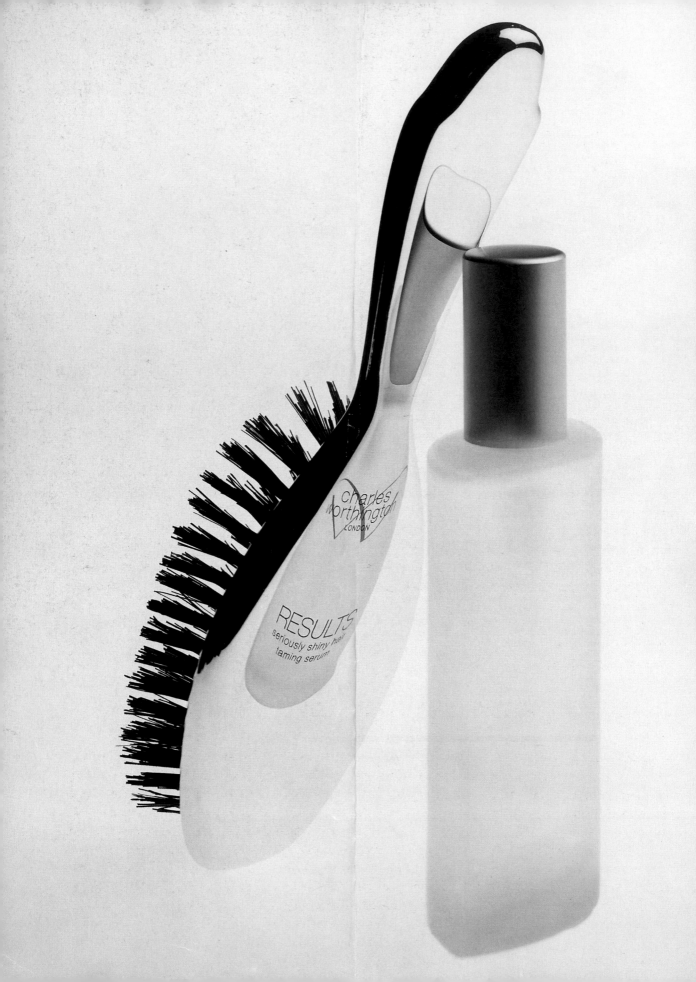

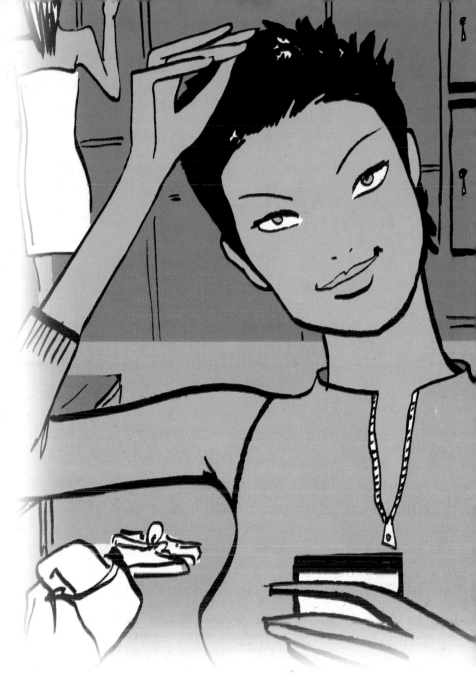

"It must be the effect of living with looks-obsessed Chrissie and Jaz," thinks Laura as she towel-dries her hair at the gym and contemplates making her gamine crop ... well, a little more interesting. Laura normally relishes the fact that she can jump out of the shower, blast her short hair dry and pull on her combat boots — all within ten minutes of finishing her kick-boxing class. Tonight, however, she has half an hour

...laura glams up her gamine crop

to kill before setting off for an important work party. "Well, I might as well give it a go," thinks Laura as she reaches into her gym bag for the little tub of styling wax that Chrissie gave her the night before. "It'll gutsy-up your hair," Chrissie had said — whatever that meant. Laura

usually has little time for Chrissie and her unsolicited beauty tips, but she wants to make an effort tonight. She works the wax into the ends as Chrissie had instructed, then blasts them dry, using her fingertips for lift. By the time she's finished, her hair looks sexy and tousled — as though

she's just climbed out of bed. Laura's impressed (in a rather understated, Laura kind of way). John, the devastatingly attractive assistant producer from Current Affairs, is likely to be at the party — and Laura's more than ready for a spot of networking — if that's what you want to call it.

color me beautiful

Adding a touch of color, whether it is permanent, semi-permanent or temporary, is a great way to perk up hair that is looking dull and lifeless, and a brilliant way to change your look or revolutionize your style. If the words "shrinking" and "violet" could never be used in the same sentence to describe you, then try adding a shock of bright color — this adds punch to any hairstyle. The more faint-hearted can either boost and enhance their natural hair color or get a little adventurous with some creative color. How about a few strands of a contrasting shade around your face, for example? Or, what about getting just the very tips of your hair dipped in a daring bright color? Either way, don't be afraid of color; it can be really fun and opens up plenty of opportunities for transforming yourself — à la Madonna, the mistress of reinvention.

something for the weekend?

The great thing about temporary color is that it's, well... temporary. It provides the perfect opportunity for trying out something new or for making an impact without causing any long-lasting and irreversible consequences. There'll be no crying over spilt milk with temporary color!

It is always a good idea to pick your hairdresser's brains about color before you launch yourself into the rainbow of choices and techniques available. Find out what colors they think will suit your skin tone and what formulations and techniques will have the best effect and results on your hair type.

color wash

This easy wash-in, wash-out color rinse lasts for just one shampoo and is good for subtle shade enhancement. Color washes are also known as vegetable colors and are excellent for refreshing faded color and conditioning the hair.

semi-permanent color rinse

This is a vegetable-based dye that lasts for up to approximately 12 shampoos. You can only go darker or warmer than your natural color.

colored spray

As well as adding oomph to simpler styles, such as braids, this can be used to create an all-over effect. You could, for example, spray hair in a mist of silver to match a silver party dress. Barbarella, eat your heart out!

color mousse

This is good for toning down brassiness or changing your color for the night. It is best to seek professional advice as some leave a colored "cast" on the hair.

wax and pomade

These are applied after the hair has been dried and styled. It's always advisable to do a test strand with stronger colors to make sure it doesn't stain the hair and will wash out — especially if you have blonde or bleached hair. This product is best used on small areas.

hair mascara

The wand makes it really easy to streak color through your hair. Use it around the front section of your hair and on the strands framing your face for best results. Be warned: test hair mascaras at the cosmetic counter first as a color that looks pretty in a tube can look pretty dull (or unnoticeable) on your hair.

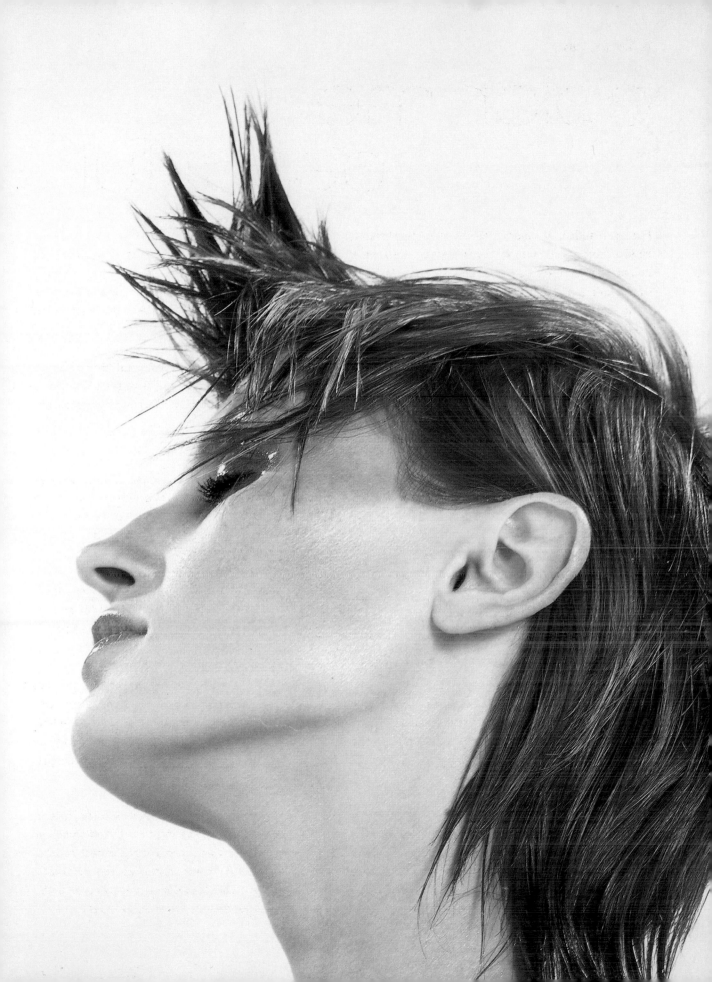

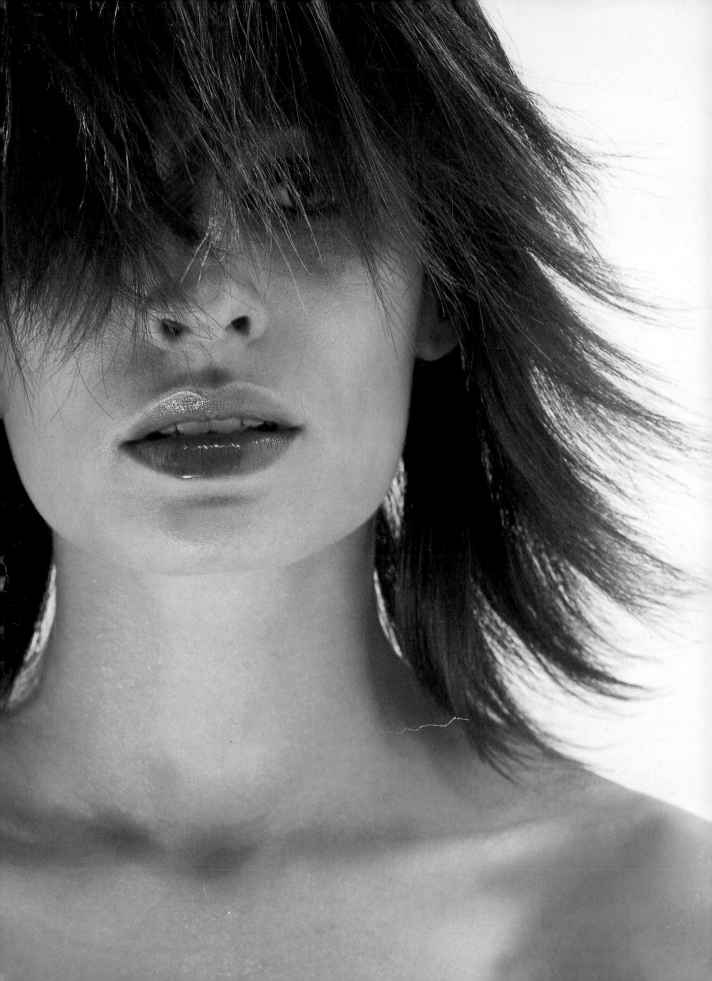

creative color

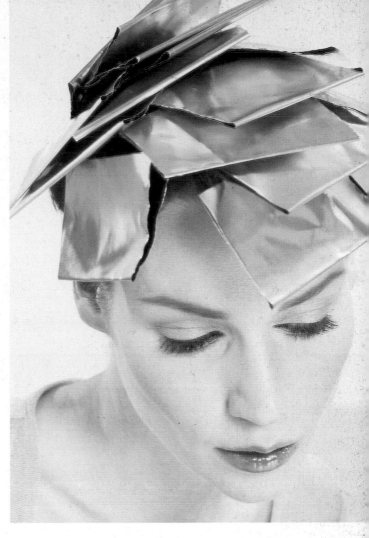

Creative color, as it's known in the salon, tends to be semi-permanent or permanent, so it's a great choice if you're feeling funky and want a look that's going to last longer than a couple of washes. As its name suggests, creative color is where a hairstylist gets creative and even more artistic — your hair is a canvas on which color application and technique converge. Some creative-color techniques can produce radical results, so talk it through with your hairdresser and make sure you know exactly what to expect. Your gorgeous tie-dye locks may not be appreciated if you work in a bank or law firm!

If you're longing to try techniques like dip-dyeing or tie-dyeing but think they sound a bit radical and long-lasting, you can cheat by coloring hairpieces and then weaving them into your hair.

dip-dyeing

This technique (left), inspired by the art of dip-dyeing clothes, is where just the very ends of your hair are colored. It works best on natural, mid-length to long hair and you can use either subtle or vibrant colors. For the most dramatic results, have your ends dip-dyed in a contrasting color to your natural shade. For example, if your hair is dark brown or black, dip-dye the ends bright red.

couture color

Your hair is shaded with color to personalize and complement your haircut, making it unique to you. This type of color enhances movement and emphasizes a dramatic line.

tonal blast

This is a more subtle version of dip-dyeing that works best on short to mid-length textured haircuts. The ends of the hair are colored and then a semi-permanent color wash is applied over the top to give extra brightness and a strong tone of color. A tonal blast can be done on all natural or colored hair, with the exception of hair that has already been dyed black.

3-D lights

Slices of hair are colored with shades of blonde all over the head; darker blonde is applied at the roots and lighter blonde to the ends to give a sun-kissed look. This works best on short to mid-length hair and can be done on all shades of natural or colored blonde hair.

hidden color

Sections of hair are taken from underneath and colored, which makes "work-to-play" hair easy — clip up your hair to reveal the drama below. This works best on all natural hair colors and on mid-length to long hair.

duo color

The hair is either colored lighter on top and darker underneath or darker on top and lighter underneath. This can be done on all natural or colored hair and works best on mid-length to long hair. Trio color involves using three contrasting colors.

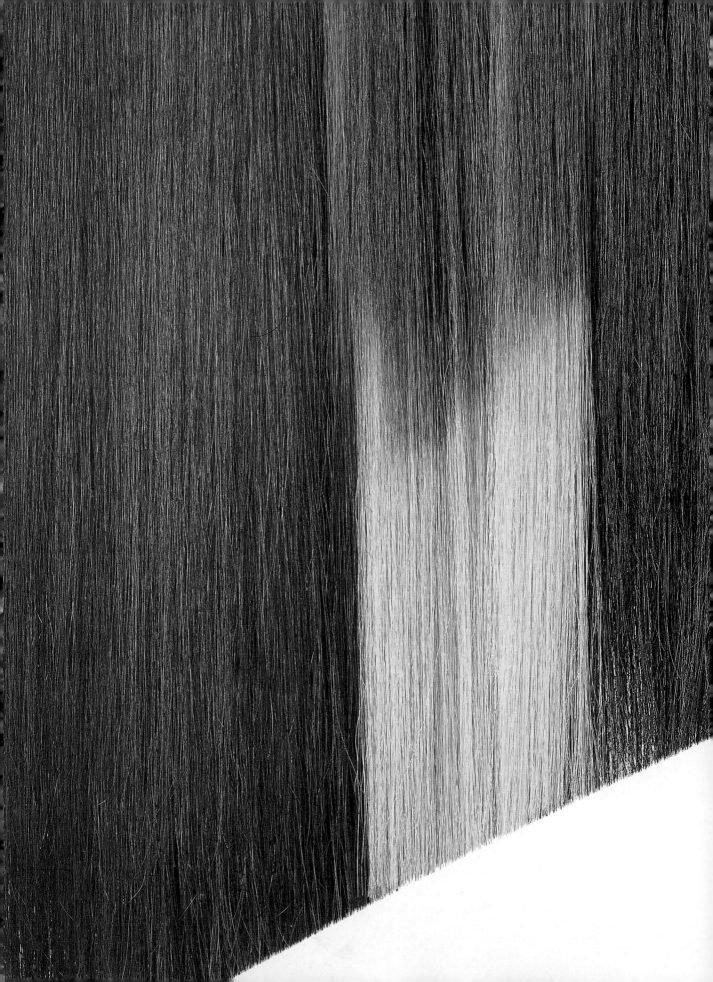

hang loose

spoiling themselves at the spa

Wrapped in fluffy white robes, the girls sat clutching cups of calming herbal tea while having their toes pedicured in the calm cream reception area of their favorite spa. Their faces were as long as Chrissie's newly-painted acrylic nails. It had not been a good week, so they had decided to cheer themselves up with a little bit of pampering. Good old Polly had even offered to pay for Jaz, who could not afford to go otherwise. The soothing tinkle of the feng-shui water wall and the prospect of a massage with hot stones (the latest beauty treatment) had already helped to lift their spirits.

"Poor Jaz," thought Polly. Her dream work placement on *Gloss* magazine had not turned out to be quite as glamorous as she had expected. For the past week she had been incarcerated in the windowless fashion cupboard, sorting out the tights and set free only to fetch organic wheatgrass juice for Imogen, the fashion editor. As for meeting a fashion designer, she was about as likely to meet Elvis.

"Pass me that copy of *The Rainbow*, please Jaz. I need to work on my new image," barked Chrissie. She had become even more obsessed with her looks since Pout had proclaimed her "too womanly" to join their band. She was devastated about it but, in true Chrissie style, only for about two seconds. Instead, she had accepted the job of receptionist at Devastation Records that Steve had offered her by way of compensation. He had hinted that if she took the job, there was a chance that she might be "discovered". "Too right I will," Chrissie had thought, resolving there and then to be the most glamorous (and girliest) receptionist ever. "And to think I wore my lucky red dress," she thought aloud to herself, while admiring her newly-painted, mink-colored toenails (the perfect accompaniment to her long, honey-colored calves, she thought).
"Yes, but look at what you wore with the red dress,"

pointed out Laura, characteristically as blunt as the cut of her boyish crop. "Those turquoise tights that Jaz persuaded you to wear looked ridiculous!"

"Laura, don't be mean to Chrissie," said Polly, looking up from the work file she had brought along with her for light reading — anything to take her mind off the fact that Simon had not called. Worse still, his once-flirtatious e-mails had become very brisk and matter-of-fact. And to top it all, Polly was feeling really guilty about Harry, who seemed to have finally woken up to her existence. He had actually paid her a compliment about her new "messy" hair (as he called it) and had even presented her with a bunch of flowers — even though they were carnations.

"I think I might go for the slimming seaweed wrap," declared Kate, who had been scanning the menu of beauty treatments. Of all the girls, Kate secretly had something to celebrate. She had managed to lose a bit of weight since switching to a new, low-fat brand of cookie that was being trial-tested at Crunch. Matthew was currently racking his brains, trying to think of a name for them. Kate, however, had already thought of one. It was time to convince her gorgeous boss that her talents stretched to more than just typing letters and doing the filing.

Laura was also studying the treatments on offer. Beauty spas were not usually her thing, but she had willingly agreed when Polly suggested it. She had to do something to get John's attention. At the TV party where she had planned to "bump" into him, he had spent the entire time talking to a girl with long, curly hair who was wearing a flowery frock. "Chrissie's worried about looking too womanly, but maybe my problem," thought Laura, as she helped herself to an apple, "is that I'm not womanly enough." Still, it was never too late for a cynical 26-year-old TV researcher to learn a beauty trick or two.

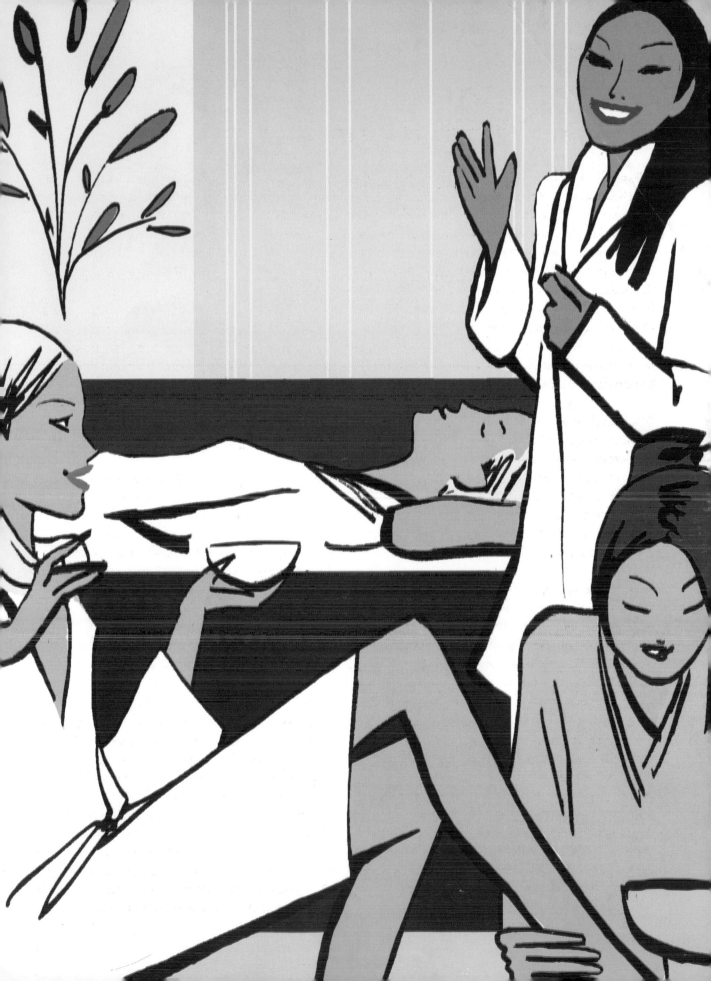

straight talking

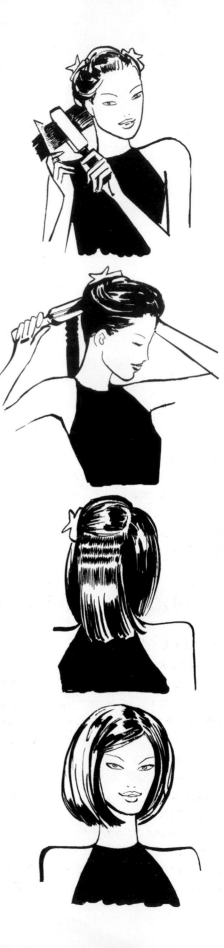

Straight is not as straightforward as you might think. You can take your pick from straight and disheveled, straight and sleek or straight with plenty of volume. There are as many ways to wear your hair loose as there are shades of lipstick. Hair worn down is a great seduction tool: you can indulge in flirtatious ploys, like tossing it back or running your fingers through it (although strictly speaking, this is a no-no as it can make hair look greasy). That said, the secret to great date hair is a style that somebody else wants to run their fingers through...

big straight hair

Big straight hair is all about boosting thickness without weighing down the hair. Here's the lowdown:

you need
Wide flat brush (ideally a paddle brush) • hairdryer • crimping iron • straightening iron • sectioning clips • non-aerosol hairspray

1 Follow the instructions on page 63 for blow-drying and straightening your hair with straightening irons.

2 Pin the top layers of your hair out of the way, using the sectioning clips.

3 Take the underneath layers, section by section, and lightly spritz the root area with hairspray to protect it from the heat of the crimping iron, then crimp the hair close to the roots.

4 When you have crimped the roots of all the underneath layers, gently comb the crimped sections out and then let the hair you have pinned away fall over the top.

Spurred on by her weight loss (it was a good start) and her indulgent day at the spa (she definitely felt more toned after the seaweed wrap), Kate decides that Sunday night is going to be

...kate's power bob goes straight

"an achieve salon-style hair at home" night. She furtively eyes the shopping bag that contains her latest purchase. It's over a month since she walked into her hairdresser's and demanded a power bob. What she had been given — a shoulder-length bob-shaped cut — was as close to a power bob as you can get when you possess flowing, unruly red locks. But Kate longs for bone-straight hair — the mark of the sleek, sophisticated

career babe. She is positive that with the right hair she could get ahead in the Crunch marketing department. Like a woman with a serious mission, she plugs in her new straightening iron to let it heat up while she sections off her hair as instructed by the accompanying booklet. She can hardly believe the transformation that takes place as she carefully runs the iron down each section. In less than half an hour she goes from

pre-Raphaelite maiden to a smart, take-me-seriously hotshot. She knows that she can't do this sort of thing too often (overuse of straightening irons is very damaging to the hair), but once in a while can't possibly hurt. Delighted with her new image (she even looks as sharp and business-like as Polly), she decides that tomorrow is the day to broach the subject of accompanying Matthew on that important conference.

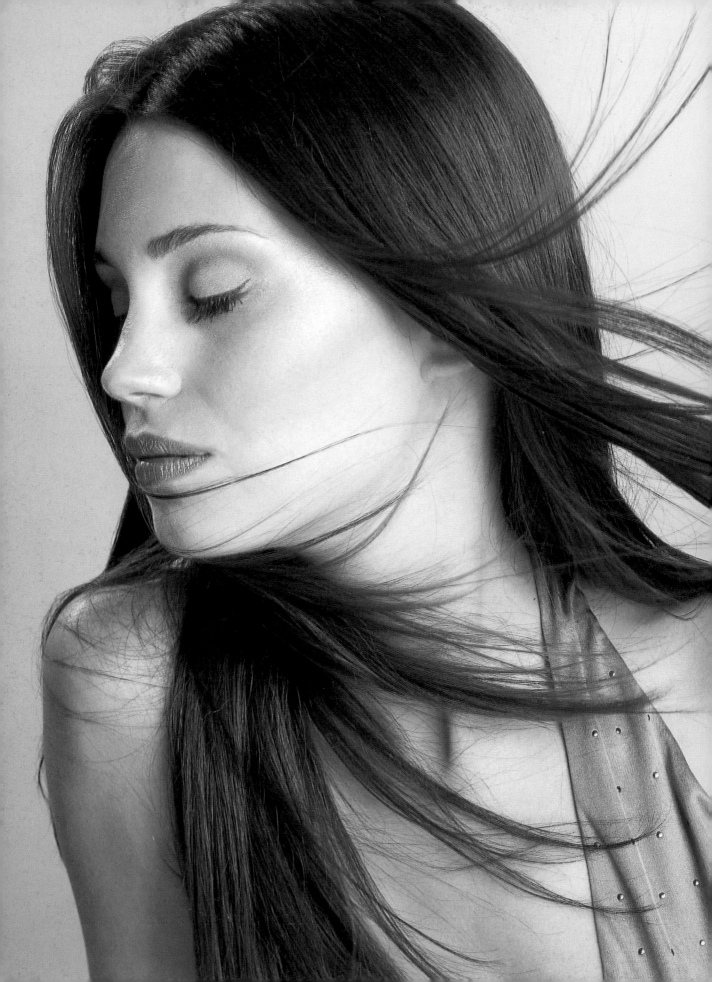

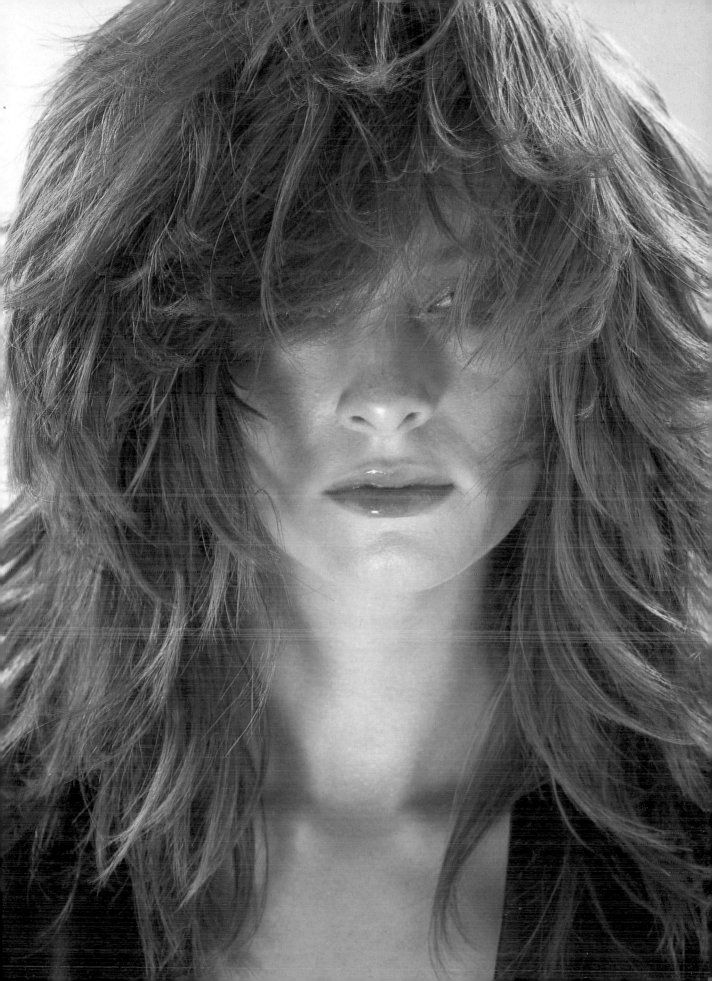

blades

There's straight, there's big straight and then there's "Gucci-style" straight, which leaves your hair looking like blades of grass all over. (Hence the salon-speak for this look is simply "blades".) It's a very sharp look that makes your hair seem almost crispy. But be warned: this technique involves a hot straightening iron and is potentially dehydrating to the hair if used regularly, so it is best saved for big dates only.

you need
hairdryer • straightening brush • pump-action hairspray • straightening iron

1 Follow the instructions on page 63 for blow-drying your hair straight.

2 Using a pump-action rather than an aerosol hairspray, spritz the hair until it is quite damp. (A pump-action hairspray releases a higher volume of product, which makes the hair damper.) Do this evenly down the entire length of your hair.

3 Take a small 1-inch (2.5-cm) wide section of hair and slowly run the straightening iron down it, from the roots to the ends.

4 Repeat this process all over the head, being sure to straighten the underneath layers and not just the top section. This should leave the hair totally separated into small individual "blades".

bed-head hair

There is something very sexy about slightly disheveled or shaggy hair, also known as "bed-head hair" because it looks like you've just climbed out of bed and not bothered to brush it. On long hair, this look is also labeled "Rock Chick" — messy, but sexy, as sported by Chrissie Hynde, Courtney Love and Marianne Faithful.

you need
Light-hold mousse or gel spray • hairdryer • paddle brush • hairspray

1 Apply a little mousse or gel spray to the root area of the hair using your fingers to work it through.

2 Rough-dry the hair. Instead of sectioning off the hair and blow-drying each piece separately, randomly blast the hair with the hairdryer, gently roughing it up with your fingers. This maximizes the volume and give a really shaggy finish.

3 Lightly spritz with hairspray to hold the look.

short and spiky

Don't think that just because you've got short hair, you have limited styling options. There's a lot you can do with short hair — you can make it soft, sexy and tousled; slick it back neatly for understated shiny elegance; decorate it with pretty hair clips; or spike it up for a groovy, street-chick look — all you need is a range of good styling products, some basic tools and a little bit of know-how. This funky textured look (right) is a great way to make short hair more gutsy, and will certainly get you noticed.

you need
Strong-hold gel • hairspray • hairdryer and diffuser

1 Apply a generous amount of strong-hold gel to wet hair, using your fingers to distribute the product evenly to the ends and gently work the hair into spikes.

2 Dry your hair with your head tipped over, using a diffuser to help keep all of the spikes intact.

3 Finally, spray your hair with hairspray for extra hold and shine.

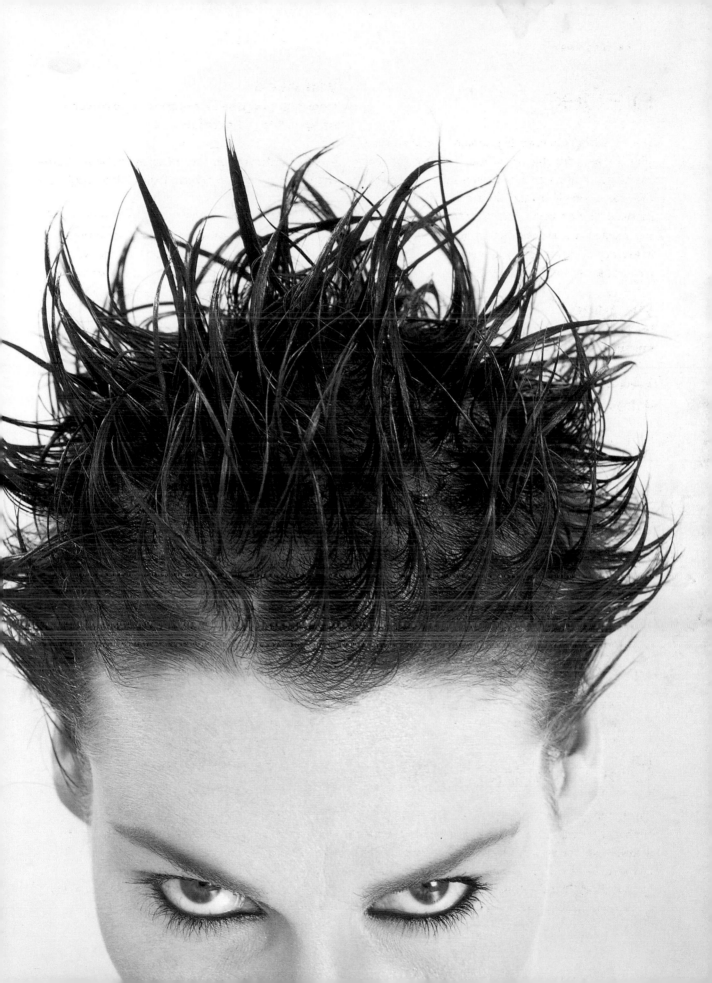

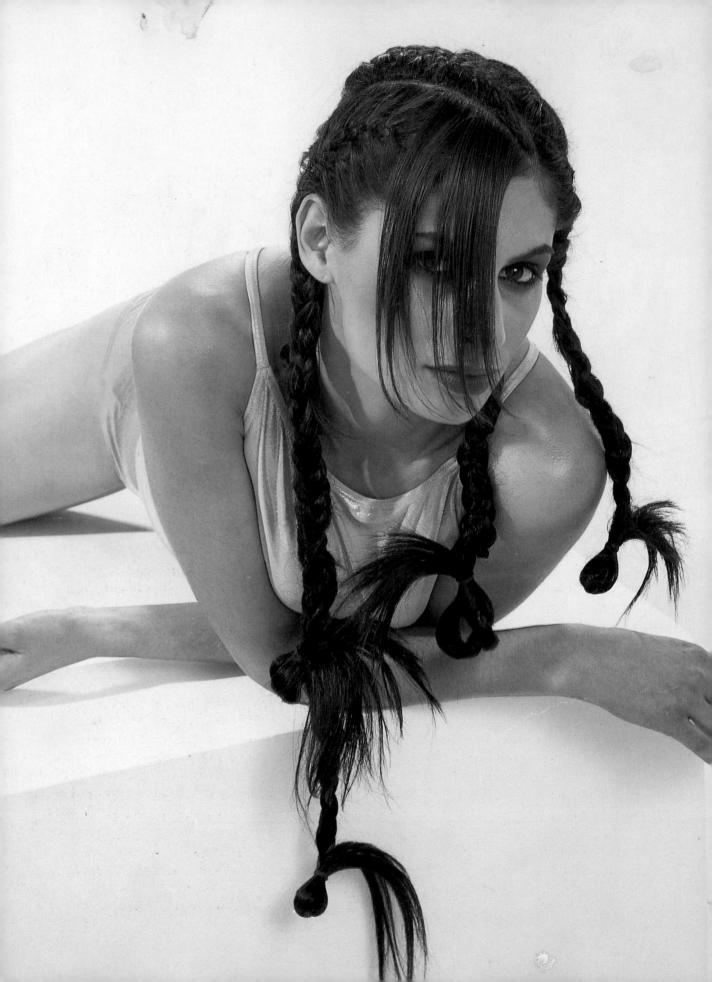

braid it

Braids are not just for schoolgirls — they can look very elegant, very hip or very sexy. There are loads of variations — from a single braid hanging straight down your back to a whole headful of braiding finished with beads. If you don't want all of your hair in a braid, just do a small section of the hair anywhere you like to add extra texture and interest. The most popular way to do this is to braid a small section on either side of the face and then take these around the side of the head and clip them at the back. Very Guinevere!

the multibraid

This is a very beautiful, very simple style of wearing your hair down your back in a neat, elegant, textural braid.

you need
Comb • sectioning clips • three covered elastic bands • hairspray or anti-frizz serum

HAIR SNIP
TO AVOID HAVING A BIG CHUNKY BAND AT THE END OF YOUR BRAID, FINISH IT OFF BY LIGHTLY BACKCOMBING THE TIPS OF THE HAIR. ALTERNATIVELY, USE CLEAR, SNAG-FREE ELASTIC BANDS FOR LARGER BRAIDS OR BEADS FOR SMALLER ONES.

FRENCH BRAIDS WILL LOOK NEATER AND STAY TIGHTER FOR LONGER IF YOU ADD IN VERY SMALL SECTIONS OF HAIR AT EACH TURN. ALWAYS BRAID THEM TIGHTLY AGAINST THE SCALP.

FOR BRAIDS WITH A DIFFERENCE, WEAVE IN COLORFUL RIBBONS OR STRIPS OF LEATHER, YOU CAN ALSO DECORATE THEM WITH FLOWERS AND FEATHERS.

1 Divide your hair into three sections: one on the left, one at the back and one on the right.

2 Divide the left section into three, braid it near the nape and secure it with a hair band.

3 Braid the right section in the same way, leaving the middle section unbraided.

4 Then braid all three sections together for an interesting combination of textures.

5 Finally, use hairspray or an anti-frizz serum to smooth any stray hairs.

sexy braids

These are sexy, bad-girl braids!

you need
Comb • sectioning clips • three snag-free elastic bands • shine spray • straightening iron

1 Divide the hair into three sections from the front of the head to the nape, leaving out a small section at the front to flop seductively over one eye.

2 French-braid the first section tightly onto the scalp, following the shape of the head. This is important as it will ensure that the braid is tight towards the nape.

3 Leave about six inches unbraided at the end. Fold this back and secure it with a snag-free elastic.

4 Repeat with the other two braids, then spritz the hair with shine spray (see opposite).

5 Finish by straightening the loose front section.

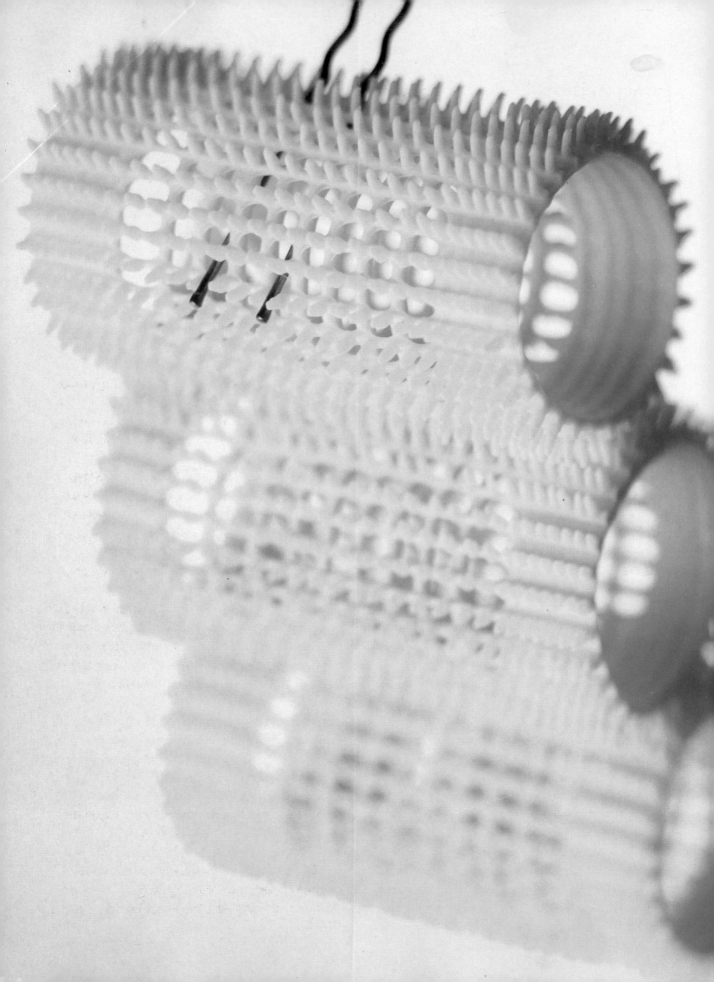

girls with curls

In the same way as girls with the most beautiful curly locks at times lust after flat-ironed hair, those born with naturally straight tresses long for a cascade of tumbling curls. Maybe it's because the grass is always greener... Straightening or curling, you can't defy nature permanently, but you can have a lot of fun.

Curls come in many different guises: from the softest Madonna-style wave to tight corkscrews and romantic Jane Austen ringlets. Even if your hair is naturally as straight as a ruler, it's easy to create the curls of your dreams at home.

wavy hair

The best way to achieve long-lasting, shiny curls is to use a curling iron. It is important to work on freshly washed hair (too much product on the hair will make it look dull when you use the iron).

you need
Comb • hairspray • curling iron • shine spray

1 Starting at the nape of the neck, divide the hair into quite chunky sections (about 9 cm/3½ in wide).

2 Lightly spray the first section with hairspray to ensure a longer-lasting curl.

3 Comb it through to remove any product build-up before clamping the curling iron over the ends of the section, making sure they are completely tucked in.

4 Gently wind the curling iron up, making sure that all the hair is covering the metal barrel. Hold for about 4–10 seconds, depending on the heat of the iron and the curl required, then gently unwind. (Be careful not to run your fingers through the curled section.)

5 Repeat this process until all of your hair has been curled, then lightly spray it with a light glossing spray to finish.

ringlets

If you have naturally curly hair, creating ringlets is easy. This technique is also a good way to avoid frizzy curls.

you need
Styling lotion • styling gel • comb • finishing spray

1 Simply rub styling lotion and gel together in the palm of one hand. Apply to wet hair and comb it through.

2 Leave your hair to dry naturally and the hair will form ringlets. For a bit of extra help, take sections of hair and twist them around your finger before leaving to dry.

3 For a glossy finish, lightly spritz with finishing spray.

If you have straight hair, there are several methods of creating ringlets. The old-fashioned technique of "ragging", using ripped strips of cloth (J-cloth works especially well), has made a 21-century comeback. Once mastered, it is quicker and better than using rollers.

you need
Medium-hold styling spray • strips of cloth • hairdryer and diffuser (optional)

1 Start by spritzing the hair with medium-hold styling spray (use plenty to give a firm, springy curl).

2 Beginning at the nape of the neck, divide the hair into sections depending on the size of ringlet required. (Continued on page 118.)

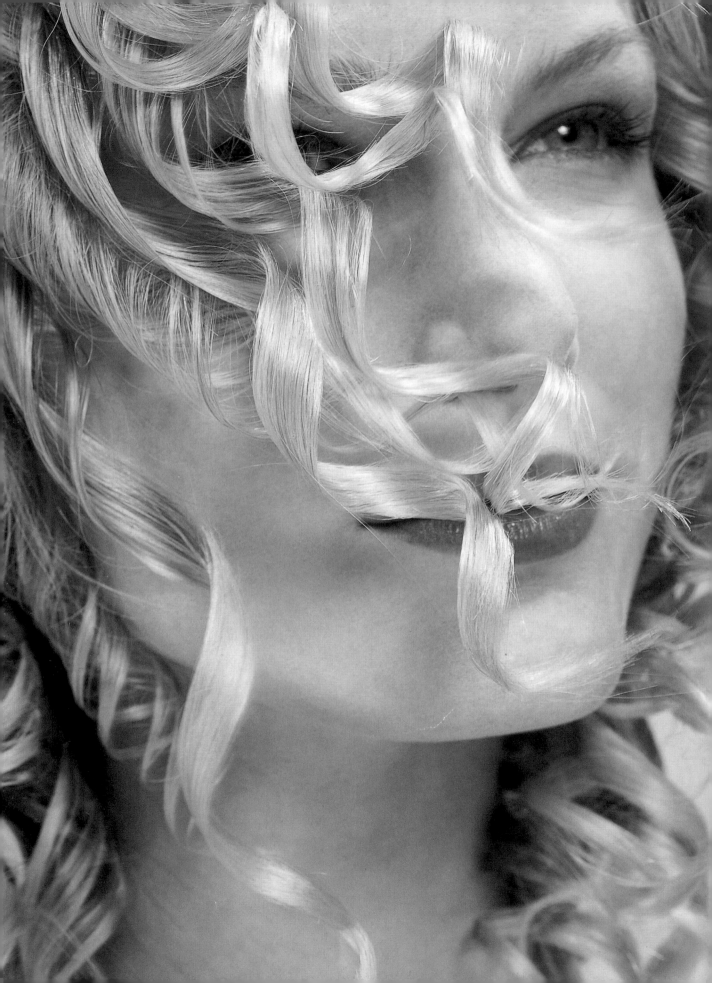

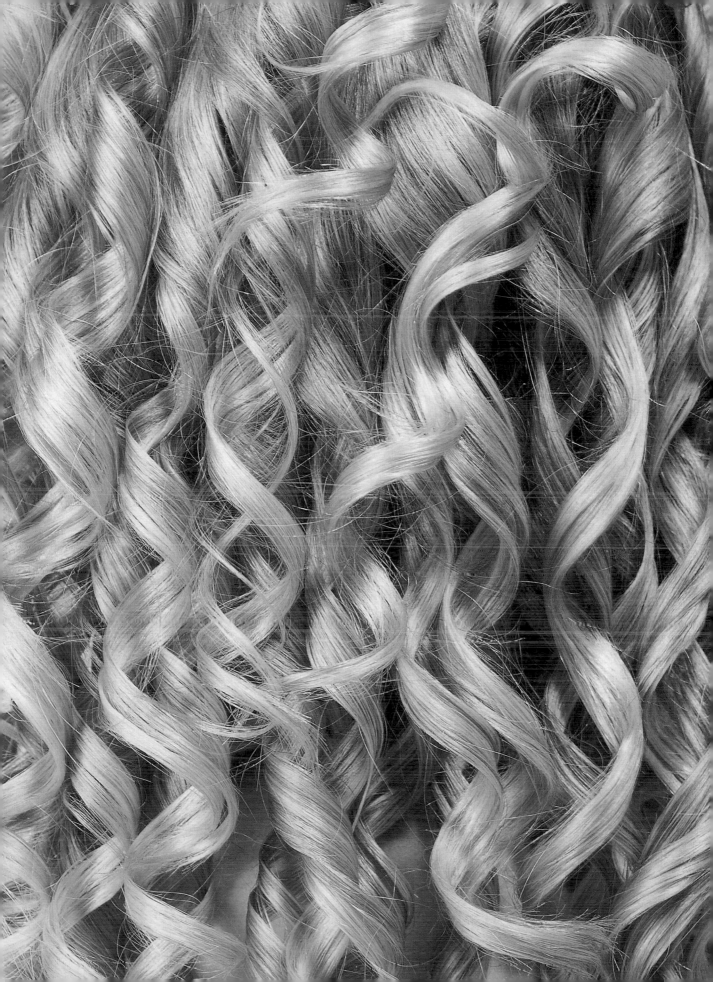

3 Wrap the hair around the cloth, being careful to tuck in the ends neatly. For a more defined ringlet, slightly twist each section as you wind it up.

4 Once the hair is wound tightly around the strip of cloth, snug to the scalp, tie the two ends of the cloth together.

5 When all the hair is tied, either leave it to dry naturally (the rags are comfortable enough to sleep in), or use a hairdryer and diffuser — but this can be time-consuming.

6 When you are sure that the hair is dry, start to remove the rags, beginning at the nape of the neck.

7 When all the rags have been removed, use your fingers to gently break up the curls, depending on how curly or defined you want the final effect.

afro-style

You don't even need to have curly hair to create a cloud of tight Afro curls. Even very-straight tresses can be transformed to get this effect.

you need
Strong setting lotion • strips of aluminum foil • wide-tooth comb

1 Spritz the hair thoroughly with strong setting lotion to give a more defined curl.

2 Follow the instructions for ragging (see above), but take much smaller sections of hair and instead of winding the hair around strips of cloth, use small pieces of foil.

3 When you remove the pieces of foil, instead of running your fingers through the hair, use a wide-tooth comb. This will totally separate the curls, leaving you with a perfect Afro.

big curls

If you're not satisfied with Madonna-style waves or a headful of ringlets, then big curls (with a capital B) are the order of the day. Reach for the hot rollers for a bit of va-va-voom.

you need
Mousse • hairdryer • hairspray • hot rollers

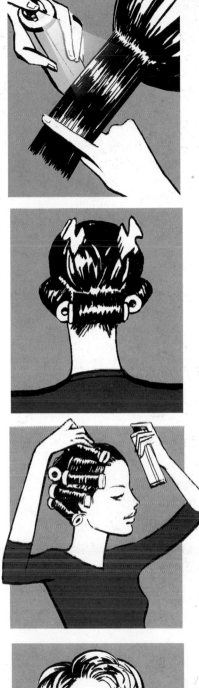

1 To create the perfect foundation for a hot-roller set, apply mousse to the roots of freshly washed hair. Then, using the warm setting on your hairdryer, dry the mousse into the hair.

2 Take a section of hair, making sure it's not wider than the actual roller, and spray it evenly with hairspray.

3 Wind the section around the end of the first roller, tucking in the ends. Make sure that the roller sits firmly against the scalp as this will create root lift and a much bouncier curl.

4 When you've finished putting all of the hair in rollers, apply a coat of hairspray evenly all over. Leave the rollers in for about 10 minutes before gently unrolling them. Don't tug or pull the rollers out.

HAIR SNIP
MAKE SURE THAT THE ENDS OF THE HAIR ARE TUCKED IN WHEN YOU CURL THE HAIR AROUND THE ROLLERS, CURLING IRONS OR RAGS, OTHERWISE YOU WILL END UP WITH A FISH-HOOK EFFECT AT THE END OF THE CURL.

WAIT FOR THE HOT ROLLERS TO GO COLD BEFORE REMOVING THEM AS THIS WILL CLOSE THE CUTICLES OF THE HAIR AND SET THE CURLS.

SPRAY EACH SECTION WITH SHINE SPRAY AS YOU REMOVE THE ROLLER TO GUARANTEE SHINY AND VOLUMINOUS CURLS.

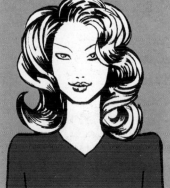

Jaz is dreading the prospect of another boring afternoon in the fashion cupboard, bagging up clothes from the glamorous shoots that she never gets to go on. Imogen announces that she's simply has to go home with another one of her stress headaches (although Jaz can't see exactly what stress her boss is under since all she does is chat on the phone all day to her friends, dahling).

She wonders, would Jaz mind going to the launch of Blast, Jean-Paul's new perfume, after work in her place? Jaz would just about manage…Stifling a squeal, she tries to look nonchalant, but not very effectively. Anyway, the coast is now clear for the rest of the afternoon and she has a party to get ready for. Jaz has been dying to try on that amazing purple dress from Coletta, and perhaps a new hairstyle would be just the thing to cheer her up. Emboldened, she manages to get herself an appointment with *Gloss*'s favorite hairstylist, Adam, and begs him to create something awesome for the launch that night. He patiently crimps every bit of her long, dark shiny hair, backcombing

…jaz goes crazy with the crimping iron

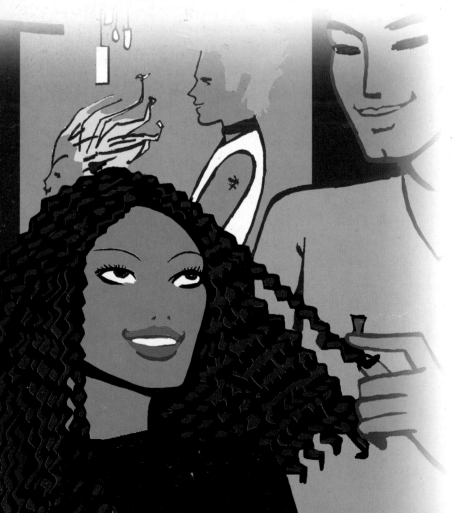

it at the roots for extra volume. "Hmm, not bad," thinks Jaz. Flicking through a back issue of *Gloss*, she spots a great photograph of a catwalk model with braids wrapped around the side of her head. Adam obligingly braids the front sections of her hair into four small braids, tying the ends with colored ribbon. The effect is Kate Bush meets Guinevere–altogether quite pleasing. Jaz is thrilled. Falling off her precarious stiletto heels, she rushes out of the salon towards her oh-so-chic destination, but not before giving Adam a massive hug in gratitude. "I'll do you a favor," she shrieks, almost tripping up as she tries to hail a cab. "I won't hold my breath," thinks Adam, "but she is a real cutie."

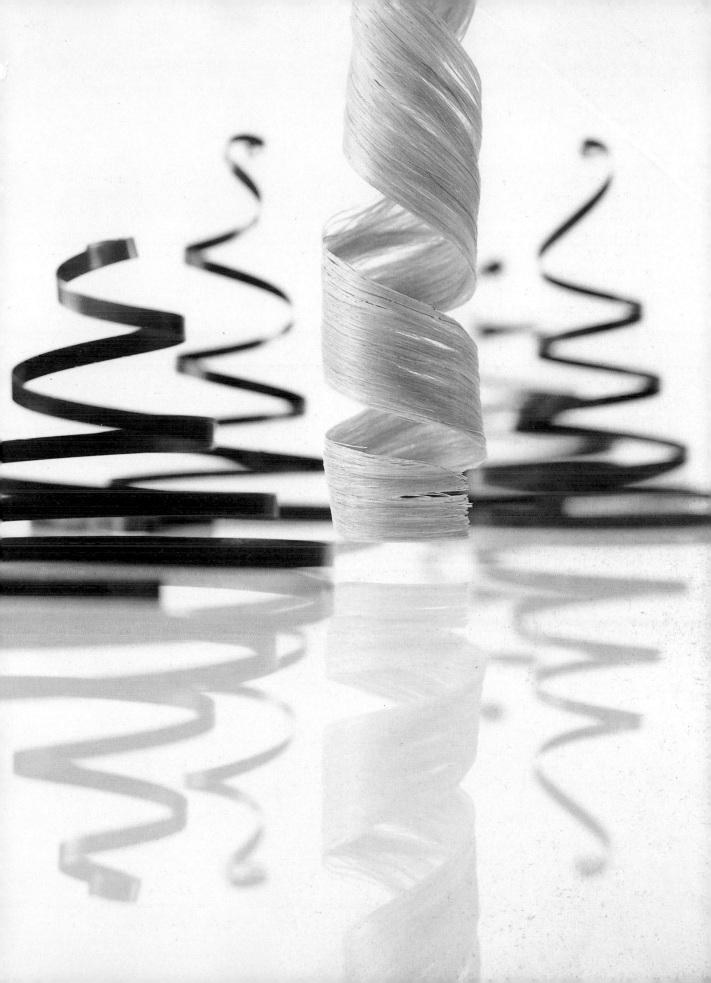

glamourtime tips

1 Accessorize, accessorize, accessorize. There are so many clever, simple accessories on the market that can be used to make an instant change from dawn to night.

2 Glam up any style by using a sparkle gel or spray glitter along your part.

3 If you are going to a hot, sweaty party, backcomb the hair at the root to keep the hair big all night.

4 Outshine any rivals: to polish the hair and make it super-shiny, rub a few drops of shine enhancer into the palm of your hand, then sweep a large make-up brush across your hand and smooth it down the hair shaft. This is especially effective on long hair.

5 Apply colored hair mascara — in gold, copper, blonde or a shade lighter than your own — to strands around your face for instant do-it-yourself highlights.

6 Scent your hair by spraying a cloud of perfume into the air and then walking through it. Hair holds perfume really well, so this seductive little trick should create wafts of gorgeousness every time you flick your hair or turn your head.

7 Hold your hair away from your face with beautiful jeweled clips, or pin it back with a big fake flower.

8 For a super-quick, super-dramatic solution, use a ponytail extension (see page 144).

9 Gently curl the ends of ruler-straight hair using the curling iron to create contrasting texture.

10 Randomly crimp sections of your hair to create volume and a multitextured look.

11 Twist curly sections into full bundles and secure them with glitzy hair grips.

12 Jazz up very-straight hair by randomly braiding sections throughout, even braiding colored ribbon into them.

13 If you're working the party circuit and styling your hair a lot, you may find that your hair becomes heavy and limp due to a build-up of products. Simply use a detoxifying shampoo for a thorough cleansing.

14 Experiment with a wig — why not be someone else for a night?

15 Overuse of heated styling appliances can damage or dry the hair, so always make sure that you follow instructions carefully. If you are concerned that your hair is becoming dry, use a rich, conditioning hair treatment or mask once a week to replenish moisture.

16 To give your naturally straight hair a bit of texture, braid damp hair before you go to bed. When you wake up, apply a little styling lotion to your fingertips and run them through the hair to undo the braids. Or, for a quick fix, apply hairspray to dry hair and braid it. Leave it for half an hour and then undo the braids to get crinkled waves.

17 When choosing your part, look at what you're wearing. Pick out a feature like the shape of your neckline and follow this when styling your part.

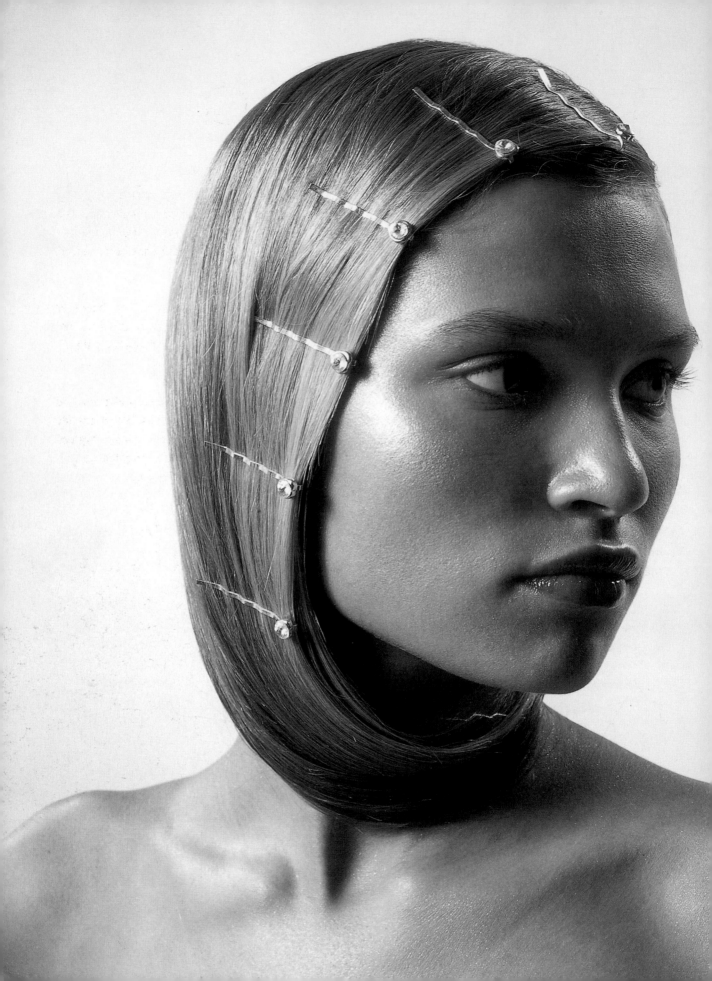

hair dressing

Hair accessories, like bangs, are a very personal thing. Some might love a big fake lily poking out from behind the ear; others may not. Hair clips, feathers, flowers and all sorts of glittery bits and bobs can make a great finishing flourish, but they go in and out of fashion faster quickly, so don't waste money on expensive pieces, and be sure to play around with them first before buying them.

tiaras and headbands

Tiaras can look great with long or short hair, but the trick is to wear them with irony (think Courtney Love rather than royalty). We can thank fashion gurus for the revival of headscarves and bandanas. A brightly patterned scarf worn bandana-style over long, straight hair can look very cool. (It's also a great way to cover up on a bad-hair day!)

Head bands come in a range of widths, materials and finishes, whether you want to opt for a minimal strip of leather or a kitsch band with beaded flowers attached to the side. Make sure they fit properly and comfortably.

do-it-yourself accessories

It's amazing what you can make in the way of hair accessories using old pieces of jewelry. You can wire brooches onto combs; glue beads or sequins onto clips; or thread beads onto wire and attach them to bobby pins. You can even use a rhinestone necklace or bracelet to decorate your hair — simply drape it over your hair and secure it in place with a few bobby pins.

Glue decorative colored feathers onto thin strips of leather — either natural or dyed a bright color — and then attach them to bobby pins.

Wrap fine florist's wire around the stems of fresh flowers, individually or arranged in small bouquets, and attach them to hair clips, pins or combs.

clips

Beautiful glittery, jeweled, beaded or feathered clips are one of the best and easiest forms of hair ornament. They can either be attached randomly throughout the hair or placed at the side to keep hair back from the face.

flowers

A big flower — real or fake — pinned behind the ear or at the back of the head is a great way to "dress up" not only your hair, but also a simple outfit for a big date.

glitter sprays and gels

You only have to look at the big trend for iridescent and glittery face and body make-up to realize that sparkle and shine are definitely "in". Try adding a bit of glitter to strands of hair around the face to brighten up your complexion and put you in the party mood.

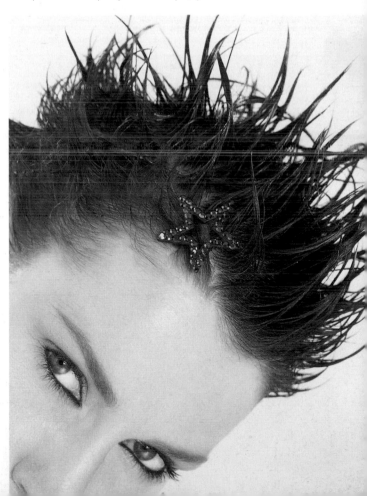

great lengths

If you want to hang loose but your hair doesn't even reach your jaw line, don't despair. You don't have to wait for your hair to grow, you can get a head start by faking it with hairpieces, extensions and wigs. No longer the domain of the follically challenged, these hairpieces are amazingly realistic, and, more to the point, they allow you to experiment with looks you could otherwise never achieve. Sport a sexy, gamine crop by day and a Rapunzel-like mane by night!

faking it

Clip-on extensions and hairpieces are a great way to add volume or length to your hair. But in order to weave some practical magic with a hairpiece, you do need to have a bit of length already, as they look better when they blend with existing hair (see page 144 for instructions on how to attach them).

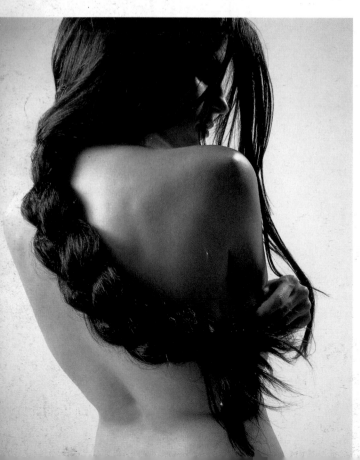

To achieve "extreme long hair", attach five to 10 narrow 23-inch hairpieces from the nape to the crown of the head using toupee clips. These are slightly rounded so they sit nice and flat on the head. If your hair is shorter, you could try fake ponytails or braids, which are attached with clips or combs.

wig tips

1 To make a wig look more natural, have it cut on your head by your hairdresser (razor-cutting techniques tend to work and look best).

2 To give a wig extra body and to make it look less fake, try crimping the roots.

3 If you have a long, straight wig in a color that is a close match to your own hair, a great trick is to cut small sections out of it and pull strands of your own hair through it. Blending the wig with your own hair in this way not only makes the wig look more convincing, but also prevents it from slipping off your head.

4 If you are wearing a wig over long hair and want it to sit closer to the scalp, cover your head with the foot of a nylon sockette and put the wig on over the top.

5 When washing wigs or hairpieces, always seek professional advice; not all wigs are made from human hair and they may need special care and attention.

6 Be very careful when you handle wigs and hairpieces — they are woven onto a weft so they are very delicate.

7 Ask to see the actual wig or hairpiece you wish to buy, as natural hairpieces are different in color and may vary from the color chart.

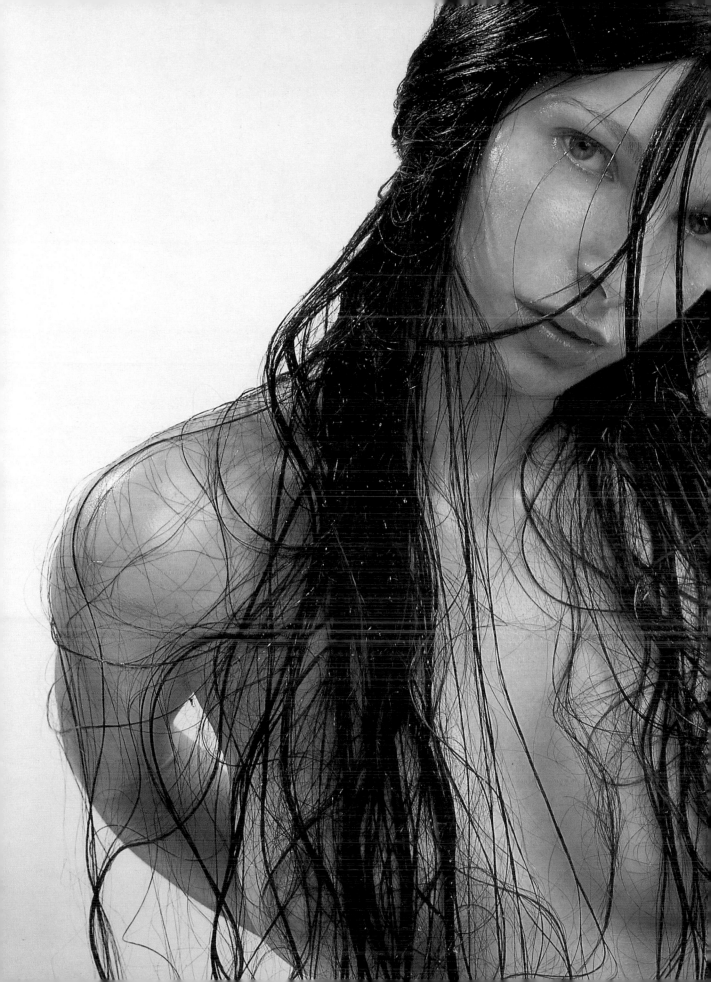

emergency quick fixes

1 To revive or add volume to hair when there is no time to wash it, simply spritz the roots with blow-drying spray and then dry the hair, focusing on the root area.

2 If your hair starts to droop, tip your head upside down and spritz the roots with hairspray. Don't be tempted to put too much product on the ends of the hair as it will just drag it down.

3 A handy trick: if your hair has collapsed from too much energetic dancing at a night club, or if you don't have access to a blow-dryer, spritz the roots with hairspray and use the hand-dryer in the bathroom to dry it.

4 When you are pinning up your hair with hair clips, lightly backcomb the roots to give a longer-lasting hold.

5 If all else fails, tie your hair back in a low ponytail, securing it at the nape. For an extra-tight hold, wrap it with a piece of wet string instead of a hair band — the string contracts as it dries.

SOS tool kit

Make space for the following in your purse and you need never have another bad-hair moment again!

comb or brush

This one goes without saying.

covered elastic band

With one of these, you can always pull your hair back in an emergency.

multifunction styling spray

Use this for holding updos in place or giving an emergency lift to hair that's looking a little limp.

five bobby pins

These will enable you to fix your hair in a sleek chignon or updo and go straight out from work to play. They don't slip out of the hair and don't show as much as shiny ones.

shine enhancer

This silicone-based wonder product will smooth out any frizz and give a sleek, shiny finish.

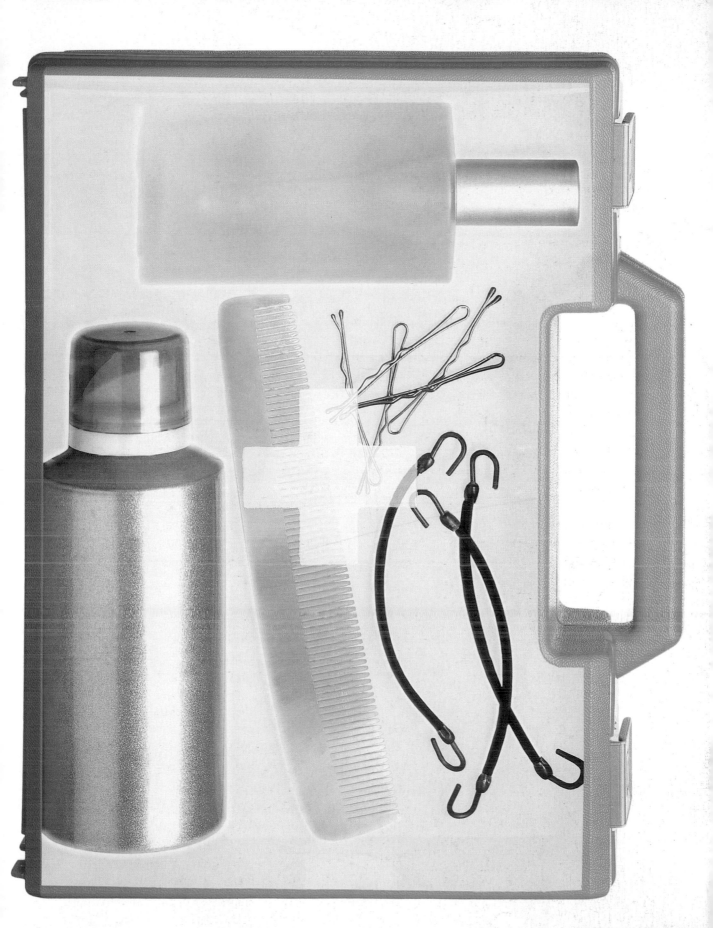

updos

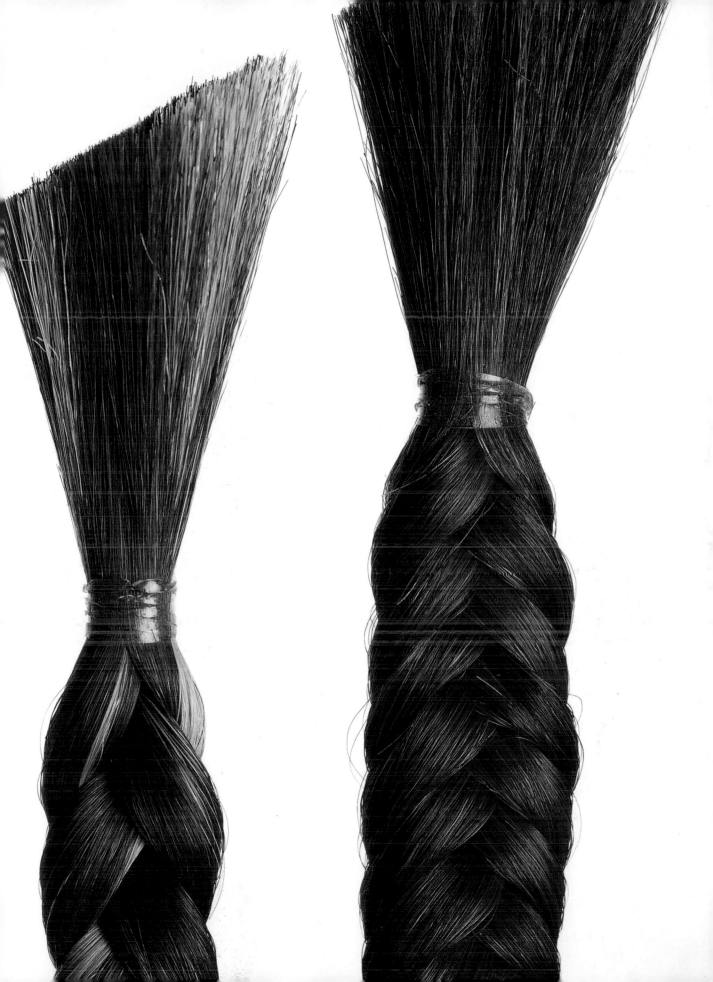

a quiet night in washing hair

"The pizzas have arrived," yelled Polly, entering the kitchen with a stack of boxes. It was Thursday and the girls were having a quiet night in washing their hair. Things were looking up for all of them. Chrissie had finally cajoled Laura into going on that double date — drinks and dinner in the Rush bar tomorrow. Meanwhile, Kate's boss had asked her to attend the cookie conference in Chicago. This — she couldn't believe her luck — was to be followed by a gala dinner. "OK, so it's not exactly a date," she had told the girls, "but I'm certainly not planning to talk to Matthew about cookies all night!"

The girls plonked themselves down on the floor around Polly's chic, Balinese-style coffee table to eat their pizza. "Oh God, I'm almost too tired to eat," said Jaz, slumped on a white beanbag, a vision in a beige-and-lime print shirtdress. She was permanently exhausted these days, ironing tights at *Gloss* magazine by day and mixing cocktails in a trendy Soho bar by night to pay the rent; that was on top of her late night at the Blast launch, which had indeed turned out to be a blast. But she, too, had an important date pending. Adam, the complete sweetie, had put in a good word for her with Astrid, fashion guru at Aristo PR for the assistant's job. Jaz had offered her services faster than you can say "mood-boosting bracelet" and an interview had been set up.

"No pizza for me, thanks," said Kate, who was sporting a seaweed face-pack and a fetching flowery shower cap (having just applied a deep-conditioning treatment to her new power bob). Tomorrow she wanted to shine — and not just on the career front. "It's unlike you to turn down carbohydrate, Kate," said Chrissie, smiling sweetly and flicking back her long, blonde hair. Kate gritted her teeth. "How much longer is Chrissie going to be living under the same roof?", she wondered. Out loud, she said: "I wish you wouldn't make such a mess during your temporary stay here, Chrissie." It was water off a duck's back. Chrissie, to Kate's great annoyance, had taken to performing a nightly one-woman fashion show as she tried to decide what to wear to work the next day. She was loving her new job at Devastation Records. She had to compete with the fish tank in reception for attention, but she was certain she'd be "discovered," even if it did mean getting up an hour earlier than she would have liked to do her hair and make-up in the mornings.

Chrissie had decided to make a special effort for tomorrow's date with Steve. True, it was Laura who Steve was interested in — Chrissie's (blind) date was supposedly Steve's old school friend. But she was planning to win Steve's undivided attention by the end of the first course. After all, Laura, wearing her TV researcher's uniform of jeans and combat boots, was no match.

But Chrissie almost dropped her slice of pizza when Laura picked up a pink slingback from under the table and asked to borrow it. Laura didn't give two hoots about tomorrow's date. As far as she was concerned, Steve was ghastly. Anyway, she only had eyes for John, the elusive assistant producer. She'd agreed to go on this date partly because she was a clever networker who rarely turned down invitations, but also because she was planning to trial-run a whole new look (Chrissie and Jaz must be getting to her).

"So Pol, what are you up to tomorrow?" asked Kate. "Oh, nothing much. Harry's out with the boys so I'll probably watch TV," was the reply. Secretly, Polly was very excited. Simon had phoned that afternoon to say that he would be in New York for the weekend and had invited her to dinner. Needless to say, she had already booked a manicure and leg wax, and a blow-dry with Charles for Saturday morning.

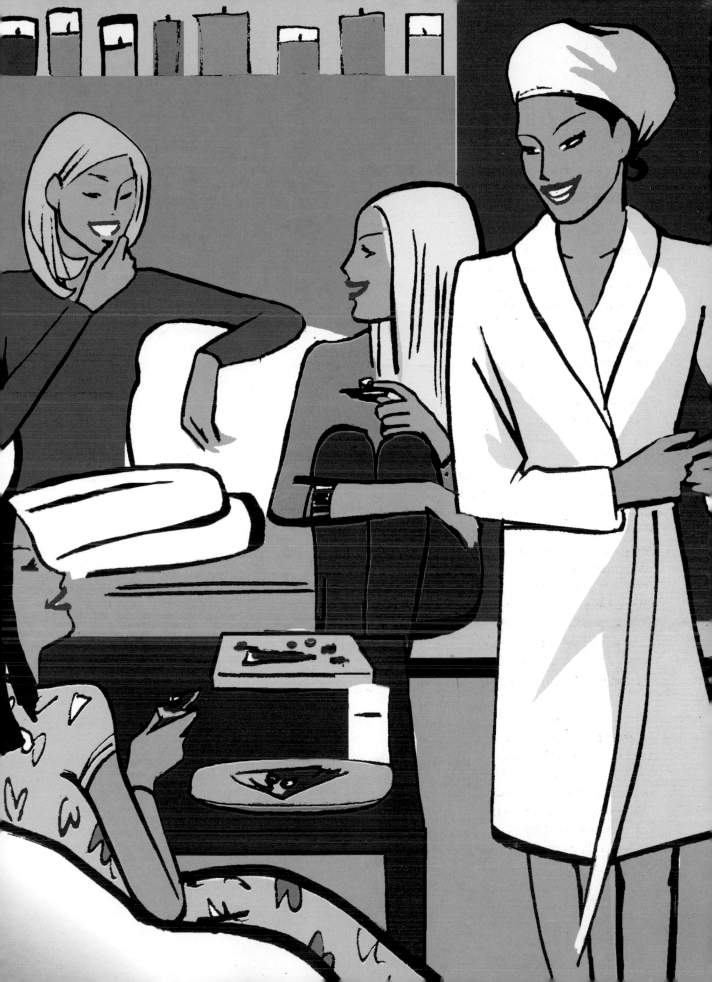

praise the updo

Whether it's a simple top knot or a polished French braid, an updo can make you feel really pulled together and glamorous. Putting your hair up can give you a big confidence boost. Not only is it an instant fix for a bad-hair day, but if you are going out after work, an updo can help you to switch instantly into out-to-play mode. And don't think that putting your hair up is only for formal events. Björk-style twists and scrunched-up top knots are great for clubs and hot, sweaty atmospheres. (It's one way to ensure that your hair stays up as long as you do!) If it's a really big date, nothing beats going to the salon to have your hair put up professionally. But even at home, mastering the art of the updo is a cinch.

the high pony

Ponytails, worn high on the head, Versace-style, can look great for evening. The effect can be super-sexy, rather than sweet and innocent. An added advantage is that a high, tight ponytail is renowned for its instant face-lifting effects. This style works best on unwashed hair because it is easier to work with.

you need
Smoothing brush • covered elastic band or piece of wet string • bobby pins • shine enhancing spray

1 For a sleek look, brush your hair, pull it back and fix it on top of your crown with a covered elastic band. Alternatively, use a wet piece of string, which shrinks as it dries, holding the hair in place securely.

2 Cover the band with a scarf or take a piece of hair from the ponytail, wrap it around the band and secure it underneath with a hair pin.

3 Smooth the hair with shine enhancing spray.

the chignon

Chignons — as worn by Audrey Hepburn, Eva Perón and Grace Kelly — are just *so* chic. They're also a great way to look groomed on a bad hair day.

you need
Gel or hairspray • a covered elastic band or a piece of string • bobby pins • a hairnet if your hair is layered • styling lotion

1 Apply a little gel or hairspray to smooth back the hair and sweep it into a ponytail at the nape.

2 Twist the hair around the elastic band or string as if making a figure-eight shape to create a neat bun.

3 Fasten with clips and cover with a hairnet to keep the ends neat. Or leave off the hairnet and pull a few strands forward to soften the look.

4 Smooth a couple of drops of styling lotion over the surface for extra shine.

french braid

Arguably the the most elegant way to put your hair up — think of Catherine Deneuve's neat French braid in the film *Belle du Jour*.

you need
Medium or firm setting lotion • hairdryer • bobby pins • hairspray

1 Set or blow-dry your hair loosely, using a medium or firm setting lotion. (Continues on page 137.)

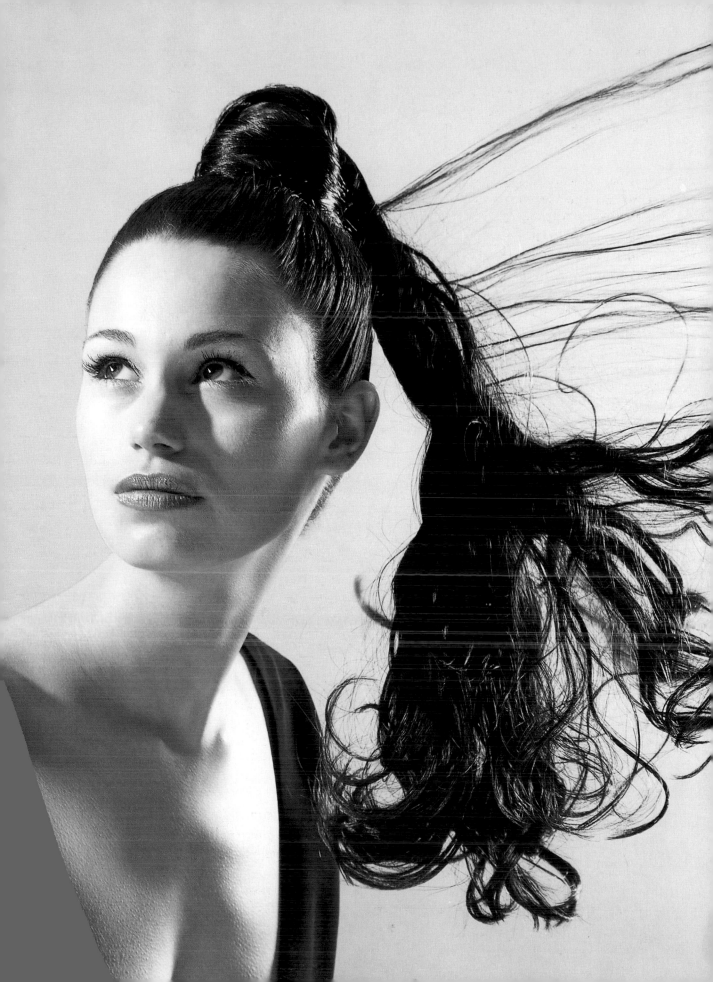

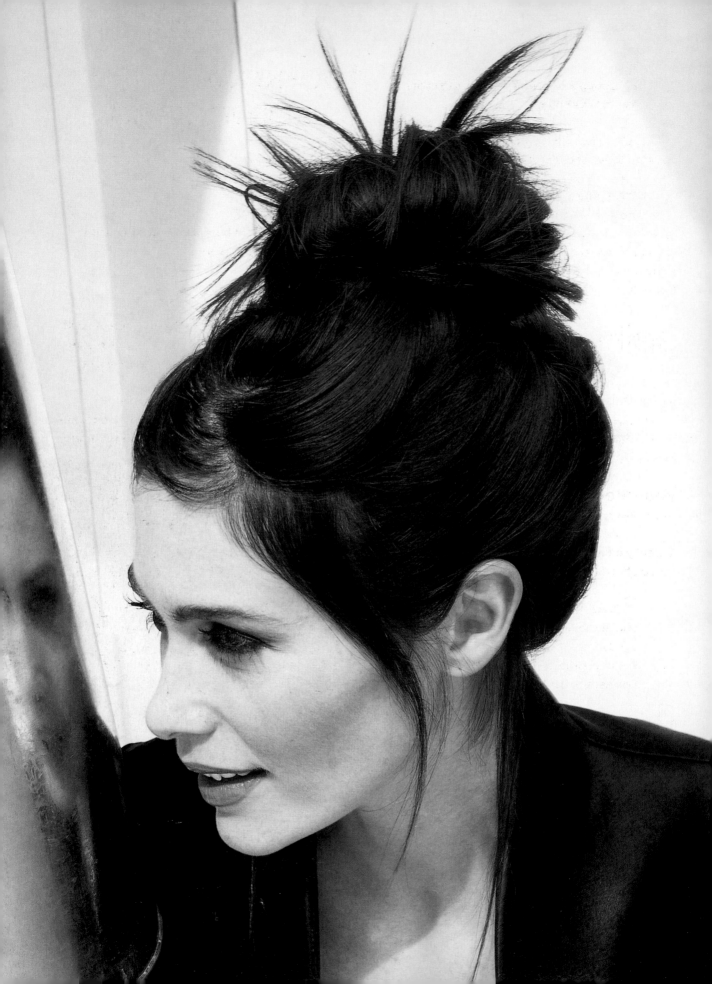

2 Gently run your fingers through your hair to break it up.

3 Twist the hair up the back of the head and, holding it tightly, secure it in place using bobby pins.

4 Spray the hair with hairspray to hold the style in place.

5 For a modern take on the classic French braid, splay out a few ends from the top section to give the style a slightly disheveled finish (left).

spiky twists

This funky hairstyle works best on medium-length hair. It is a great look for clubbing and parties and is actually a lot easier to do than it appears. Make sure, though, that this style complements the shape of your head and face.

you need

Comb • strong-hold hairspray • bobby pins

1 Gently backcomb the hair and spritz it all over with a strong-hold hairspray.

2 Take random sections of hair, about one and a half inches in size, and twist them tightly from the base to the ends. Keep twisting each section until it coils back against the scalp forming a top-knot.

3 Using bobby pins, secure the twists against the head, allowing the ends to work themselves loose to create a spiky effect. It's a good idea to cross the pins as this will give maximum support and hold.

4 Continue in this way until the whole head is covered with top-knots.

5 Gently tease and fan out the ends of the hair to create a spiky effect (see right).

top-knot scrunchies

This is a similar style to the spiky twists (below left) but end result is a head full of neat little top-knots.

you need

Comb • strong-hold hairspray • bobby pins • firm-hold wax or pomade

1 Follow steps 1 and 2 for spiky twists.

2 Secure the top-knots firmly to the scalp using bobby pins as before, but make sure that the ends of the hair are neatly tucked under.

3 To finish, apply a little firm-hold wax or pomade to each scrunchie to smooth down any stray hairs.

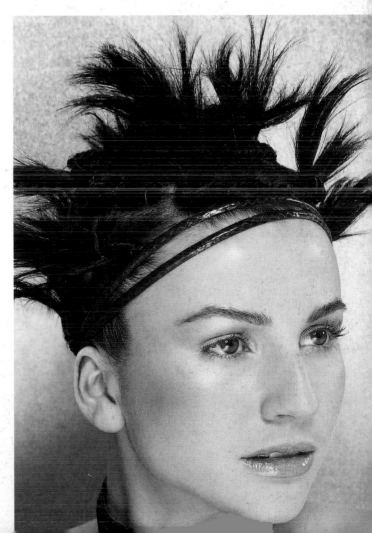

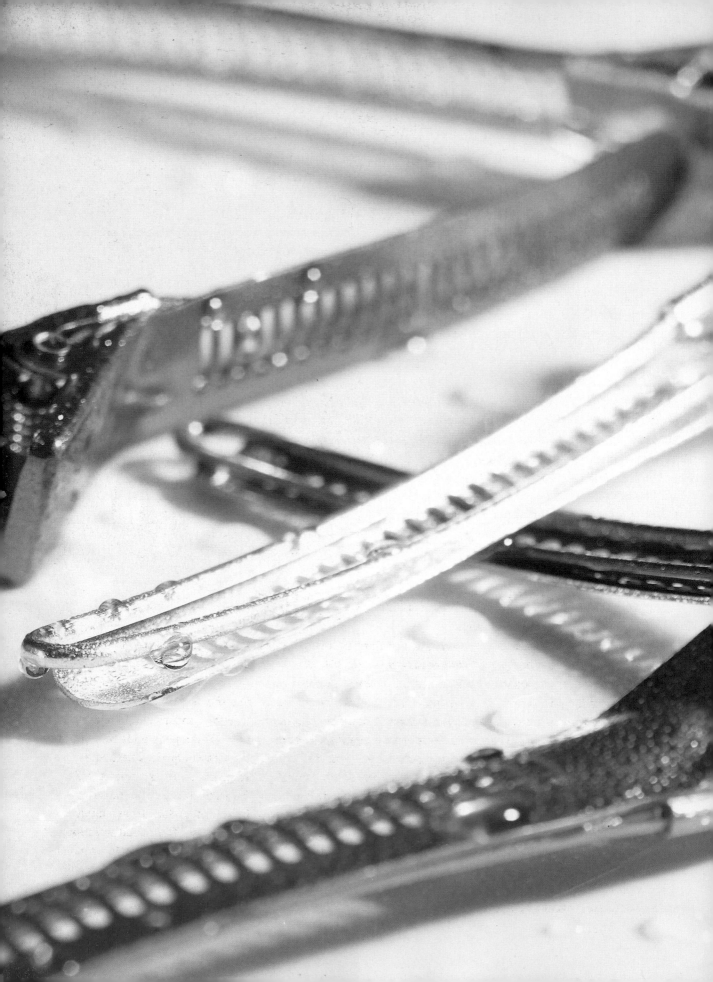

...polly tries a funky updo

Polly leaves the other girls downstairs and retreats to her boudoir for a bit of peace. She sits down in front of her dressing-table and tries out some of Jaz's new glittery eyeshadow in preparation for her date on Saturday. (Jaz, in true form, had left her make-up strewn all over the bathroom.) She's dying to tell the other girls about sexy cyber-suitor Simon and their little fling in South Beach, but she knows it isn't a good idea. She feels so guilty about Harry and anyway,

both Jaz and Chrissie are terrible at keeping secrets. Still, she tells herself, there's no harm in having dinner with Simon as he passes through town on his way to Geneva. The eyeshadow looks a little out of place with her layered, shoulder-length blonde hair. Polly feels like throwing caution to the wind. After all, on Saturday she'll be off-duty and for once not wearing a neat little suit. Absentmindedly, she twists a section of hair around her finger and pins it to the crown

of her head (as seen in one of Jaz's copies of *Gloss*). The effect is very funky and very un-Polly, but she likes it. She carries on twisting random sections of hair, allowing the ends to work themselves loose, creating a spiky effect. By the time she's finished, the effect is more funky urban chick than frumpy city banker. The added advantage is that if she bumps into anyone she knows on her illicit date, they almost certainly won't recognize her.

updo dos and don'ts

DON'T try and put up freshly washed hair since it is too slippery and floppy to handle.

DO soften a chignon or bun by loosening some wisps of hair around the face, otherwise the overall effect can appear a bit harsh.

DON'T try anything to create a style that is too complicated or too structured so that it looks as though you've tried too hard. (Ivana Trump's beehive is not the look to aim for!)

DON'T use hairpieces for the first time on a big date. It's best to experiment with them beforehand. Your hairdo slipping into your soup is not going to make a good impression.

DO remember to backcomb the roots of your hair. This will set a firm foundation for the perfect updo.

DO use accessories. They are perfect as a quick cover-up for a not-so-perfect updo.

DO use colored hair mascaras to brighten up selected pieces of hair.

DO carry a handbag-size can of hairspray and some bobby pins with you at all times to rescue your updo in an emergency.

DO use an invisible hairnet around a bun to keep the hair in place, especially if your hair is layered or has straggly ends.

DON'T try too hard. Sometimes the quickest and messiest updos look the best.

DON'T use accessories that are too heavy as they pull down an updo and ruin the look.

DO make the most of long hair if you have it. There are times when bigger is definitely better.

HAIR SNIP

FOR SALON-STYLE HAIR AT HOME IN AN INSTANT: TO MAKE LONG HAIR LOOK FABULOUS IN NO TIME AT ALL, HERE IS A QUICK, SIMPLE HAIR-UP TRICK. SECURE THE HAIR IN A PONYTAIL HIGH ON THE CROWN USING A COVERED ELASTIC BAND. AS YOU PULL THE PONYTAIL THROUGH, CATCH THE ENDS IN THE BAND TO FORM A LOOP. ARRANGE THE ENDS INTO A FAN SHAPE AND SEPARATE THEM WITH GEL. IT DOESN'T MATTER IF THE STRANDS WORK THEMSELVES LOOSE, THIS ONLY ENHANCES THE LOOK.

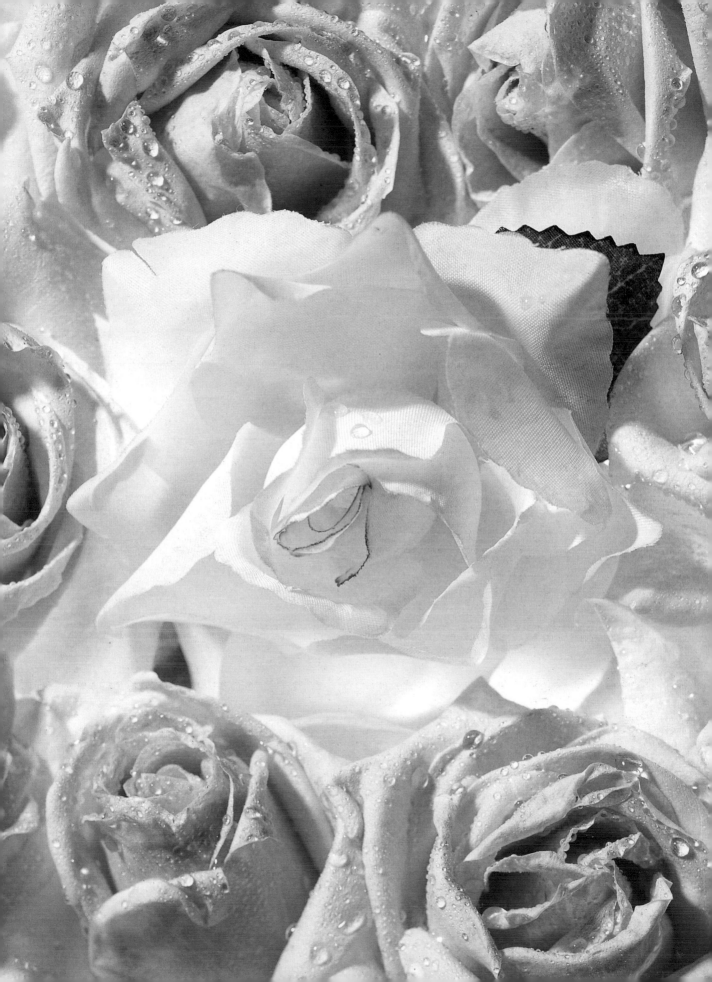

corn-rows

This is a very groovy look, but be warned: you need to have an elegantly shaped head as this can be quite a severe hairstyle. If you want to try this style for the first time, it's a good idea to go to a salon and have it done professionally, but if you are good at braiding, try doing it using the following instructions.

you need

Comb • sectioning clips • snag-free mini elastics (colored bands or hair beads, optional) • bobby pins

1 Section the hair into many small "rows" from the forehead to the nape, holding them out of the way with sectioning clips.

2 Starting at the forehead, braid each section into a mini French braid, keeping them tight against the scalp.

3 Secure each braid with a mini elastic band. Different colored bands or beads can be used for a quirky effect.

4 If you find it too difficult to braid, just twist each section tightly instead and secure it using bobby pins.

bun rings

A speedy, easy way to put long hair up is to use a bun ring (you'll find them in most large drug stores).

you need

Smoothing brush • snag-free elastic band • hairspray • hairdryer (optional) • bun ring • bobby pins • tail comb • light glossing spray

1 Using a smoothing brush, pull your hair back into a low ponytail, securing it at the nape with a snag-free band. Spray hairspray onto a large make-up brush and smooth it over the surface of the hair to control any loose ends.

2 Place a bun ring around the ponytail and secure it with bobby pins.

3 Start to wrap the hair around the bun ring section by section, and secure it with bobby pins.

4 Continue until you have completely covered the bun ring and all the sections are neatly secured in place.

5 When the hair is secure, gently pull a few wispy strands out of the bun using the end of the tail comb and finish by spraying with a light shine enhancing spray (right).

6 Stick a feather or decorative hairpin through the bun if you want to add drama (left).

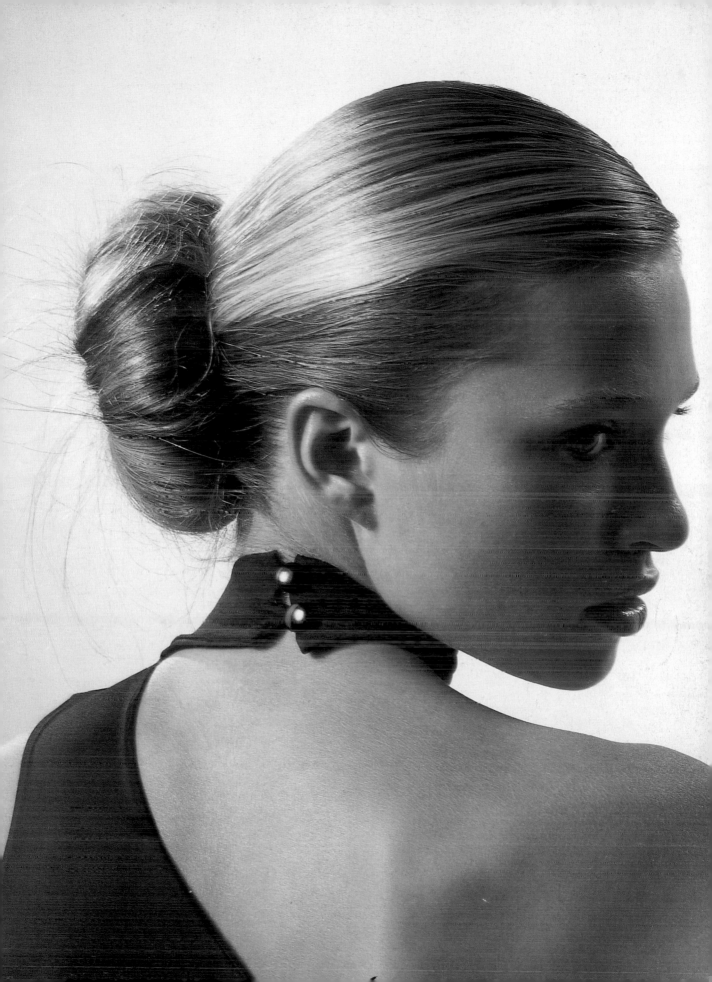

fake an updo

Even if your hair is only medium-length or shorter, it is still possible to create an impressive up-sweep by weaving a little practical magic with a hairpiece.

mane piece

The foolproof way to secure a hairpiece is to take a three-quarter inch section of your own hair at the crown or below. Twist it into a knot and pin it. Then place the comb of the hairpiece into the knot and pin it on either side. For a really slick finish, try the following.

you need

Snag-free elastic • bobby pins • weft of hair approximately 3 ft (1 m) long • fine hairpin

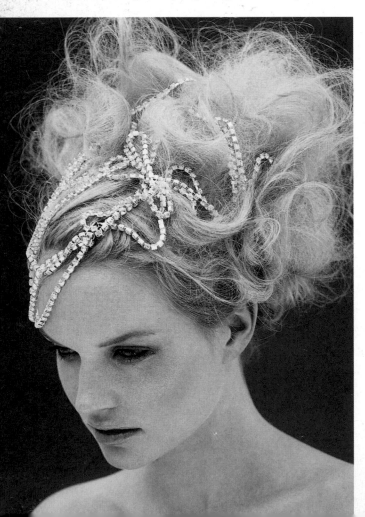

1 Sweep your hair back into a tight ponytail at the nape and secure it with a snag-free elastic.

2 Attach the weft of hair, wrapping it once around the base of your ponytail and securing it with bobby pins.

3 Take a small section of the weft and wrap it around the ponytail a few times to disguise the join and secure it underneath with a fine hairpin.

uptown girl

This is a look that is guaranteed to turn a few heads.

you need

Hot rollers • hairspray • bun ring • bobby pins • hairbrush • long rhinestone necklace (optional) • hairpins

1 Set your hair on large hot rollers and lightly spritz it with hairspray.

2 When the rollers are cool, take them out and let the curls droop slightly.

3 Pile the hair through a bun ring and use bobby pins to hold it in place.

4 Backbrush the hair loosely, until it resembles "candy floss".

5 Sweep the hair randomly around the head, letting tendrils fall across the face. Make sure you retain some height on the crown and hide the bun ring (right).

6 If you want to accessorize, push the hair back and drape a rhinestone necklace over the front of the hair, securing it with hairpins (left).

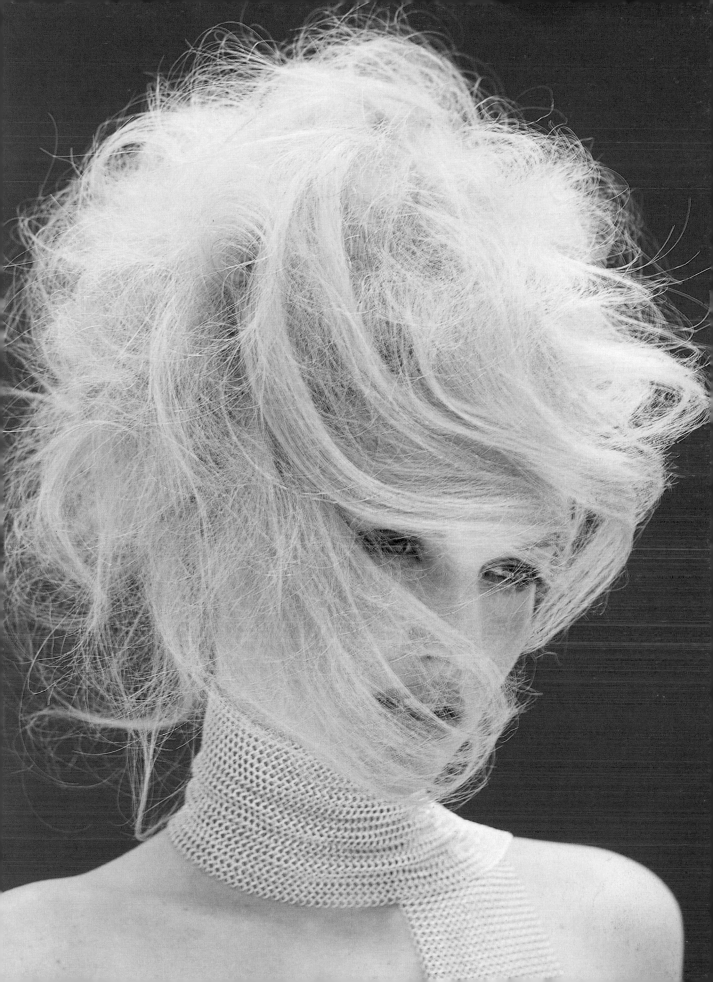

dressing updos

Accessories and hair make-up are just as effective for adorning an updo as they are for dressing up loose hair. Everything from glitter clips and beaded hair pins to feathered combs and a rhinestone tiara can add drama and glamour to even the most understated chignon, pleat or twist. An updo, however, does open up new accessorizing opportunities: beaded hairpins, decorative chopsticks and feathers are all winners.

stenciling

To add even more oomph to an updo for a big night out, try the following stenciling technique.

you need
Stencil • washable body paint • narrow paintbrush • glitter powder • hairspray

HAIR SNIP
ALWAYS CHOOSE YOUR ACCESSORIES TO MATCH YOUR OUTFIT AND YOUR MOOD. IF IT'S A BIG NIGHT OUT, GO BIG, USING FLOWERS — EITHER REAL OR FAKE — FEATHERS AND COLORFUL BEADS. IF YOU JUST WANT TO BRIGHTEN UP A DULL OUTFIT, GO SMALLER AND MORE UNDERSTATED.

CHOOSE STURDY ACCESSORIES THAT ARE TOTALLY SEALED AT THE ENDS. THERE IS NOTHING WORSE THAN A GLITZY ACCESSORY BREAKING HALFWAY THROUGH THE NIGHT, OR NOT BEING ABLE TO REMOVE ONE AT THE END OF IT.

1 Choose your stencil design to work with your overall look. You can either buy a pre-cut stencil from a home-decorating store or make your own by drawing or tracing your design onto a piece of stiff paper and cut it out with a craft knife.

2 Position the stencil on the hair and gently dab on the paint with the brush until you have filled in the design. Then dab a little glitter powder onto the wet paint. Make sure you hold the stencil very still to avoid any smudging or a blurred outline.

3 Carefully remove the stencil and blast with hairspray to set the design (see page 149).

it's a wrap

Ribbons and cords look stunning wrapped around an updo, but you need a lot of height.

you need
Hairdryer • blow-drying spray • comb • hairspray • bobby pins • cord

1 Roughly dry the hair using a blow-drying spray, which is ideal since it's not too heavy.

2 Tip your head upside-down, letting all the hair fall forwards. Lightly backcomb the hair to give it volume and spray it with hairspray.

3 Use a bobby pin to attach the end of the cord to the hair at the nape, then start wrapping it around the backcombed section. You will get a better hold if you do this randomly.

4 Tie the cord around the top section of the hair and secure it with a pin (see page 150).

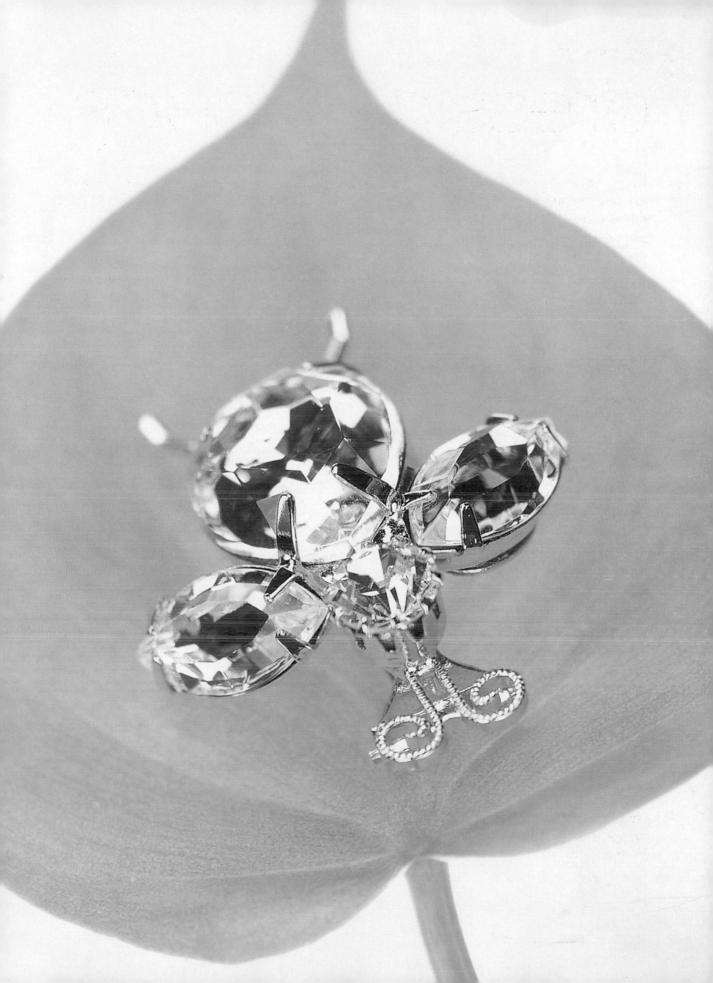

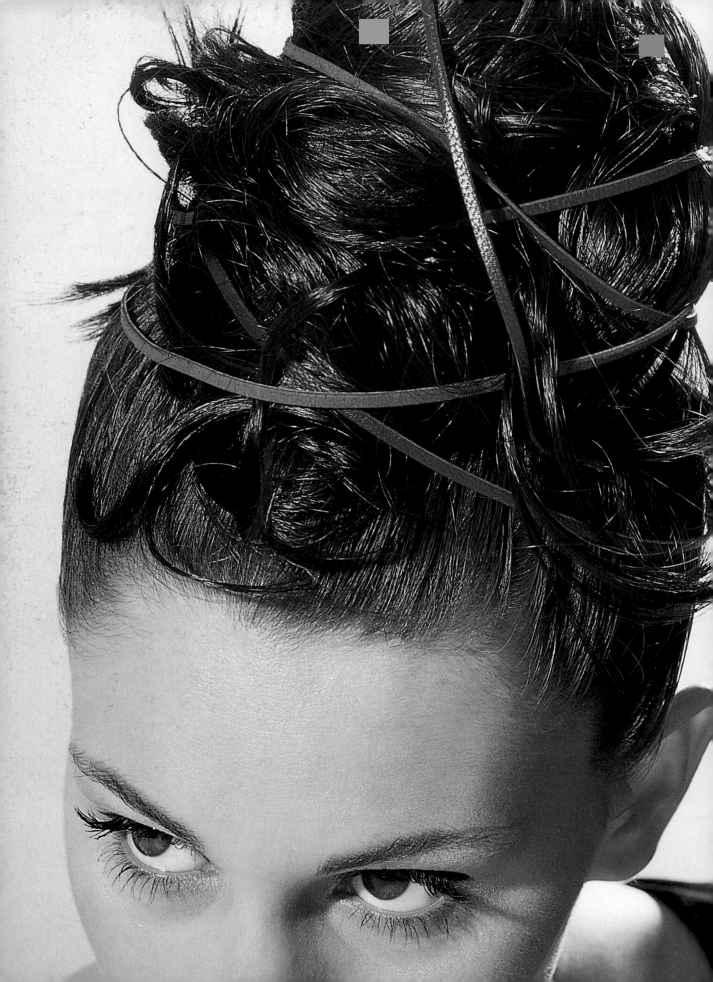

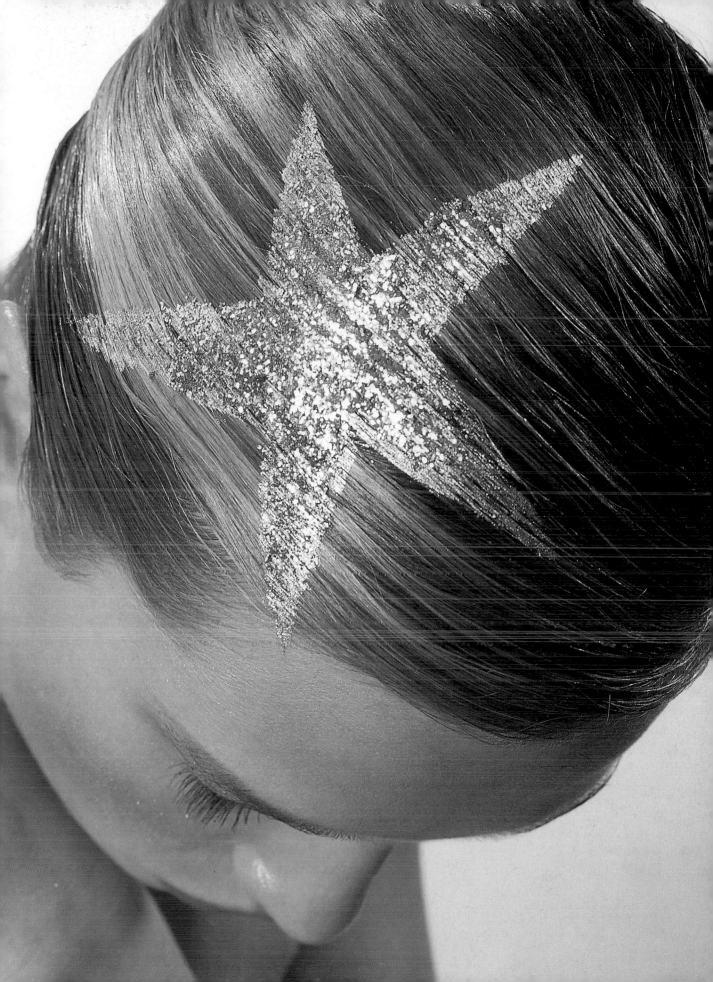

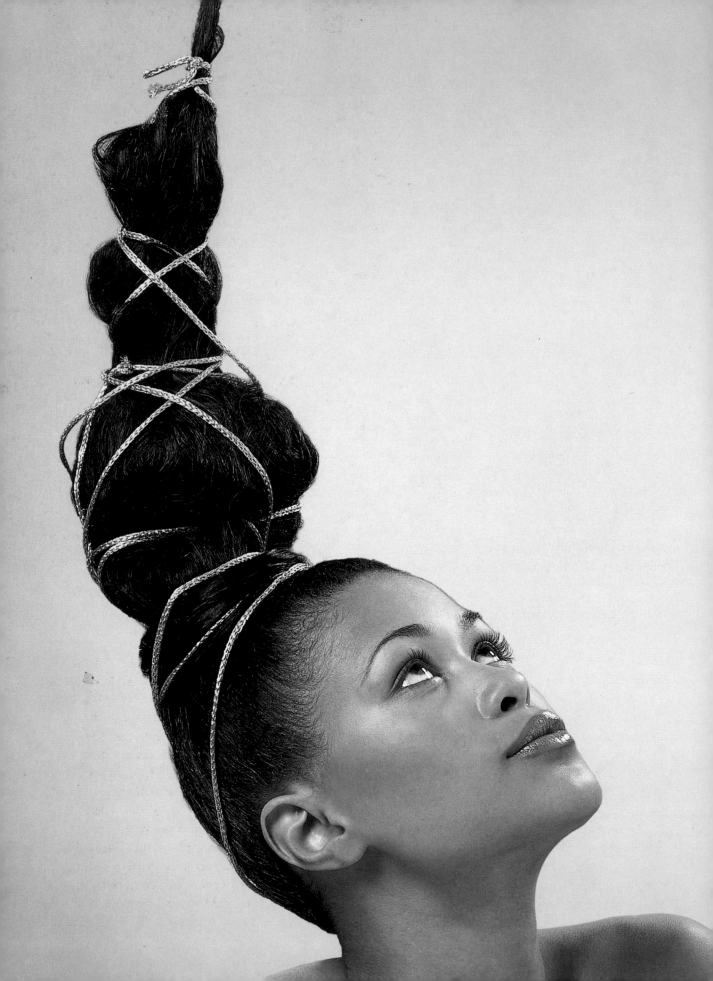

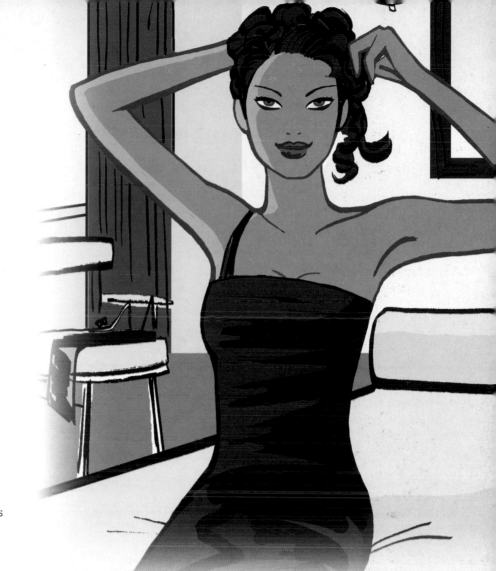

Kate kicks off her power heels with relief and collapses onto the hideously patterned hotel bedspread. God, playing the

...kate does day-into-night hair

part of Miss-Get-Ahead-At-Work is so exhausting. It's 7 pm and the conference has only just finished. Several times during the day's coffee breaks, she had tried to get Matthew to listen to her idea for marketing the new low-fat cookie brand, but to no avail. All he was interested in was whether she had managed to take down all the minutes. Oh well, there's always this evening to further her career... Damn, is that really the time?

She's got less than half an hour to get ready! Preparing to jump in the shower, Kate pulls her hair back swiftly into a ponytail, catching the ends in a covered elastic band to form a casual updo. Glancing in the mirror, she realizes that her emergency shower-do actually looks quite good. It's just as well, as she doesn't have enough time to wash her hair and wear it down — it would take hours to preen all those unruly curls into some

sort of shape. Feeling refreshed and revived from the shower, she climbs into her slinky black evening dress (her favorite floral dresses were just too country bumpkin to cut it on the career front, she's decided). Spiking out the ends of her impromptu updo, she pulls a few strands of hair around her face free to soften the final effect and dabs on some glitter gel. Kate is ready to be the belle of the ball.

...big date night

"Come on, Laura...it's 8 o'clock and we're late," yelled Chrissie, pacing up and down the hallway. She looked fabulously lean and willowy in her silvery sequinned jeans and black halterneck top, her hair pulled into a high, Versace-style ponytail. The girls had arranged to meet at home and then take a cab into Manhattan for their double date. But what was Laura up to? She never took longer than ten minutes to get ready, while Chrissie usually took two hours. "She's probably doing sit-ups or something," thought Chrissie, knowing Laura's passion for working out.

"I'm coming," replied Laura, as she negotiated her way down the stairs in Chrissie's elegant pink slingbacks. Chrissie swayed on her stiletto spikes. In place of the usual combat boots, Laura was wearing a scarlet skirt embroidered with flowers and a stretchy pink top. Her hair looked softer and more flirty than usual and she had little rosebuds clipped into it. "Wow," said Chrissie, somewhat taken aback (and, if truth be known, rather annoyed) by the unexpected competition. She had never seen Laura looking this good. "Oh, by the way, Steve phoned earlier to change the venue to Cirque instead of Rush." Laura shrugged her shoulders as she wondered if Steve's friend could possibly be as dreadful as Steve.

Meanwhile, over at the offices of Bartrum Inc. Bank, Polly was in a panic. Simon had arrived from Miami a day early and had called that morning to ask if she could make dinner this evening. She should have said no. Instead, she'd rushed out at lunchtime to buy a new slinky black dress (well, what were bonuses for?). Now she was in the bathroom getting ready. She hadn't had time to wash her hair this morning, thanks to Chrissie hogging the bathroom. So she resorted to her favorite bad-hair-day fix and pulled her blonde hair back into a sleek chignon. Five minutes later she was hailing a cab in the street outside, "Can you take me to Cirque, please?"

Chrissie walked into the bar at Cirque, followed closely by Laura who, for someone more used to wearing running shoes, had gained command of her high heels remarkably quickly. Steve was waiting at the bar alone, wearing leather jeans, a fake tan and a smug expression. "Well, hello girls," he practically drooled over Laura.
"Where's your friend?" asked Chrissie, sharply. She wasn't going to be able to divert his attention away from Laura if there were only three of them.
"Right behind you." Laura looked over her shoulder and practically fell over.

Standing behind them was...John — the object of Laura's desire. Yep, Steve's single friend and Chrissie's blind date was none other than gorgeous, sexy, elusive assistant TV producer, John.

Upstairs, Polly walked through the door of Cirque, her heart pounding — she wasn't sure whether it was passion or guilt, but she certainly hoped she wouldn't bump into any of Harry's friends. She could already see Simon, waiting patiently at a corner table. He looked heart-stoppingly gorgeous. Aaggh! What would they talk about? He hadn't mentioned their little fling in his e-mails, maybe he wasn't interested in her anymore? Polly still wasn't sure if the tone of this dinner was to be work or pleasure.

Chrissie, meanwhile, was losing patience. Steve wasn't paying enough attention to her. Still, Cirque seemed to be packed with good-looking men. "Time to go for a walk", she thought. "Perhaps to the ladies room upstairs to fix my lipstick." Swinging her slim hips through the restaurant doors, she suddenly saw a very familiar face. It couldn't be — yes, it was. Polly was sitting opposite a gorgeous man who looked devastatingly attentive as he kissed her hand. "Polly," said Chrissie eyeing up Simon suspiciously, "what are you doing here?"

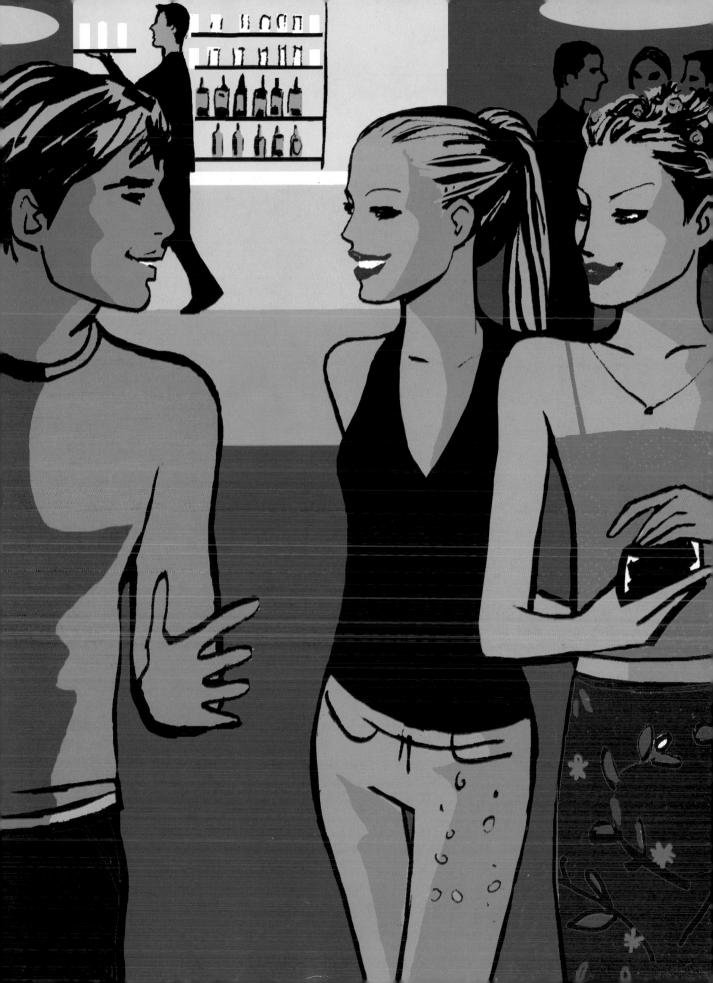

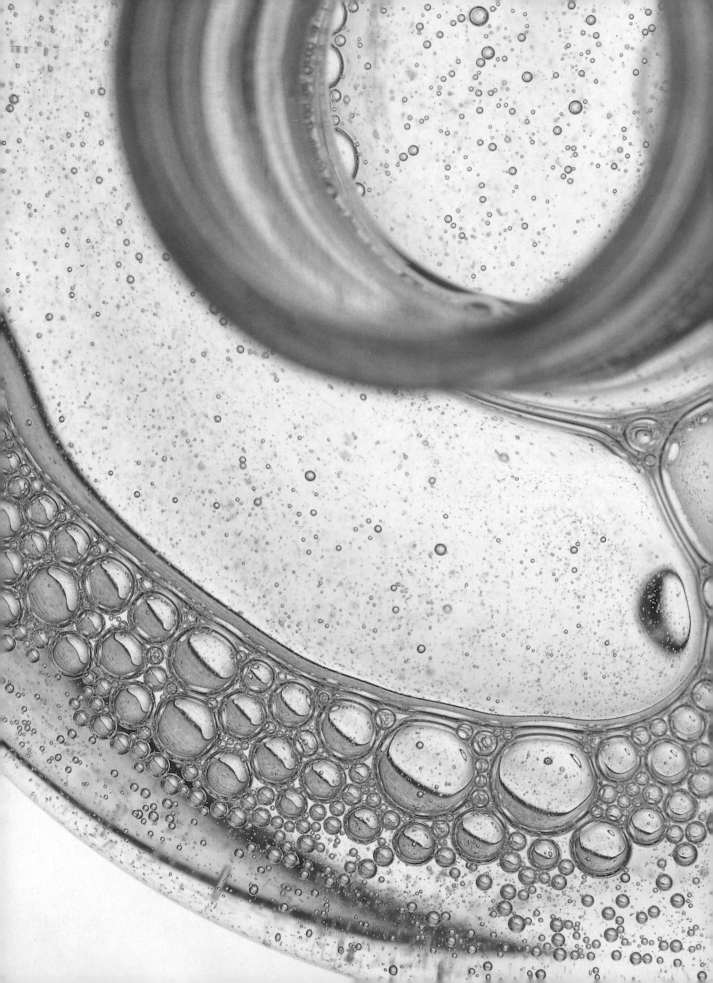

vacation hair

Vacations are a great time to experiment with new styling ideas and products, but they can be damaging to your hair if you don't look after it properly. A change of climate — whether hot and dry, humid or cold — can cause hair disasters, from fading color to split ends. Vacation Hair shows you how to get your hair in peak condition before and after your trip, and provides fantastic styling ideas, whether you're heading for the ski slopes, the beach, a spa retreat or a city.

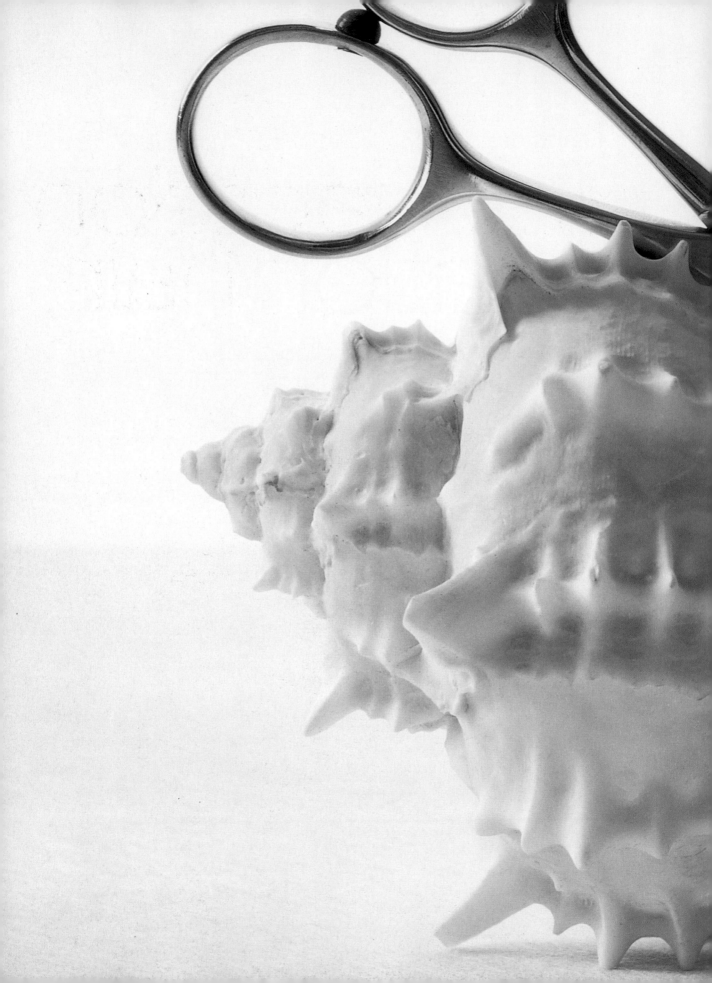

pre-vacation hair

morning after the big date night

"So how long have you been seeing him?" asked Chrissie. She'd been dying to know all the details since spotting "perfect" Polly with a gorgeous man in Cirque the night before. The girls were draped across the couch in their sitting room, feeling worse for wear after their big night out. "Since Miami," Polly admitted. She'd been bursting to tell the girls about her cyber-suitor, Simon, since their affair had started. And now the secret was out. "Are you planning to tell Harry?" demanded Chrissie. How ridiculous of Chrissie to take the moral viewpoint, thought Polly. If she'd met someone as perfect as Simon she wouldn't be letting him go in a hurry. "I'm going to tell him at dinner," answered Polly. "Though I have to say, Chrissie, I thought you'd support me on this. Simon's everything I've been looking for in a boyfriend, everything Harry isn't. I'm sure he's the one." "How about finishing one relationship before you start another?" Chrissie snapped.

Chrissie was jealous. Despite her careful preening and fabulous outfit, Steve had barely noticed her. It was obvious that his attention was fixed on Laura. To make matters worse, Steve's friend John, who was supposed to be Chrissie's blind date, turned out to be Laura's work colleague. It was clear from John's enthusiasm and Laura's flirting that they were keen on each other. Chrissie could hardly believe it — two gorgeous men competing over Laura! Chrissie was used to being the center of attention and yet last night no one had seemed interested in talking to her. Now she could tell that Polly was bursting to talk about Simon and how they had got together, but Chrissie's hurt ego had got the better of her. The details of Polly's affair would have to wait; the two girls fell into a tense silence. Upstairs, Laura was just waking up. She lay in bed for a while thinking over every detail of last night. She'd nearly fallen off her high heels when she'd discovered that Steve's single friend was John, the sexy assistant TV producer at work. The rest of the evening had been fantastic. Her flirty hairstyle and feminine clothes had done the trick — not only had Steve been drooling over her all evening, but John had made it clear that he was interested in more than work chat. In fact, he'd asked for her number before she left the club and she'd watched him write it on a card and carefully tuck it into his wallet. Laura was delighted with herself. She'd played her part perfectly all night: flirty and interesting but just that little bit unavailable at the same time. She smiled to herself. "He'll call me," she thought, "he won't be able to resist."

In her executive hotel room, Kate was suffering with a hangover and crushed confidence. She'd felt so sure of herself when she was getting dressed for the Crunch Ball the night before. Entering the ballroom, she'd caught the eye of her boss, Matthew, and his double take had given her a rush. "You look really… great," he'd managed to say. But just as she'd begun her carefully planned, bright and engaging conversation, Rachel, a leggy brunette from the sales division, had slipped her arm through Matthew's and pulled him towards her. Cutting into Kate's conversation mid-sentence, Rachel had looked her up and down patronizingly and said, "You don't mind do you Kate? Matthew and I have got some important figures to discuss." Without a backward glance, Matthew had walked off with Rachel giggling on his arm. The rest of the evening had been a complete nightmare. Kate had decided to drown her sorrows with complimentary champagne, and she'd looked hot and disheveled by the time she reached her room later that night.

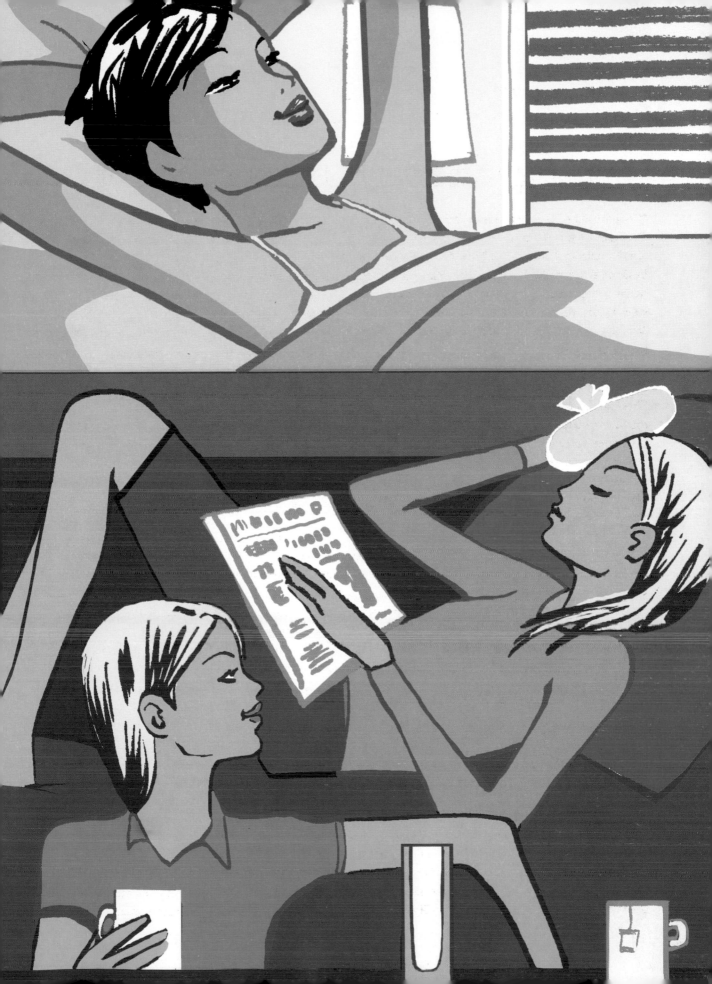

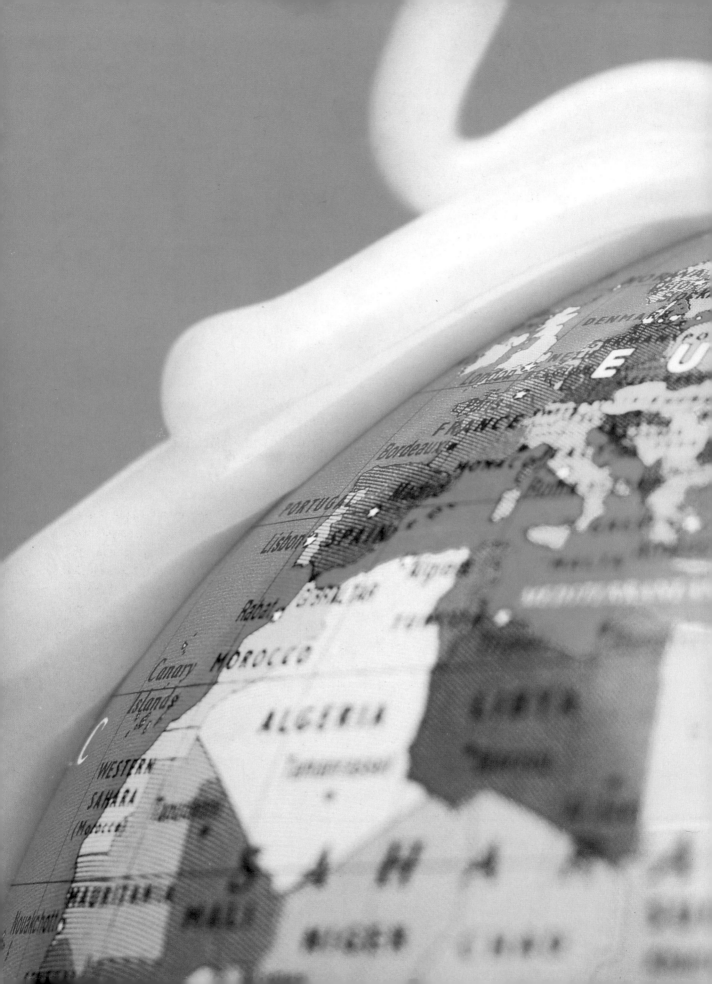

going away

Each year we look forward to our vacations and dream of sun-drenched days, relaxation and the chance to indulge ourselves, pushing our vacation budgets to the limit. We buy new clothes, cosmetics and perfume to look our best while we are away and often leave our haircare to the last minute. Foreign travel — whether it's to a hot destination for some sun, sandy beaches and clear blue sea or to the mountains to enjoy fresh air and crisp snow — will always be good for recharging your batteries, but rarely good for your hair. On vacation you are going to be miles away from your usual hair salon and the creature comforts of your own bathroom. However laid-back you might want to be on vacation, it's likely that there will be moments when you want your hair to look its best. And whatever the climate of your destination, you will probably be outside your usual environment and, as a result, your hair will be under attack from weather that it's not used to.

Your hair, unlike your skin, has no natural defense system. The ultraviolet (UV) rays of the sun, even on a relatively cloudy day, beat down on your head and dry out your hair. UV rays create free radicals, which attack the hair within the hair shaft as well as on its surface. The pigments within the hair (which give hair its color) are damaged by the sun, and daily exposure breaks down the hair's strength, causing a loss in color intensity, shine and vitality. So, when you are away, you should try to think of your haircare routine in the same way as you do your skincare routine. When you go on vacation, you pack a cleanser, moisturizer and sunscreen and after-sun lotions for your face; your hair needs similar treatment. Shampoo, conditioner, sunscreen for hair and a styling product should all make it into your make-up bag. You should condition color-treated hair after every wash — at home or on vacation. Uncolored hair should be conditioned when you are away to prevent damage from the new environment. Remember, you cannot over-condition your hair. Just choose a conditioner to suit your hair type, be it fine and flyaway or thick and curly.

cold climate

Cold weather makes hair very brittle and can cause dryness. The effect on the hair is just as if you were to climb into a refrigerator and cool your hair down extremely quickly — it leaves it weakened and vulnerable to damage. Low temperatures can also cause static or flyaway hair and this is a problem especially for fine hair types, especially those with very straight hair. Many people tend to towel-dry their hair, leaving it slightly damp, and simply tie it back before going outside — a definite no-no for hair in the cold. Keep your hair well conditioned if you are spending time in low temperatures and, whenever possible, wear a hat to keep your hair from exposure to the cold.

fine hair

Use a gentle, everyday shampoo and a light, leave-in conditioner to keep the ends of your hair protected. In extremely low temperatures, always use a heat-protection spray before styling, and work some styling lotion sparingly through the ends of the hair after blow-drying to seal the hair shaft and lock the moisture in. If you find your hair becomes static, spray a little hairspray onto your brush and smooth down the flyaway hair.

curly hair

A good conditioning treatment after shampooing your hair helps to keep your tresses shiny and well conditioned. Again, a heat-protection spray is a must, plus a shine enhancer after blow-drying to keep the hair hydrated.

frizzy hair

This tends to be much drier than other hair types. Use a leave-in conditioner after shampooing and take a deep-moisturizing mask with you on vacation to give the hair an intensive treatment at least twice a week. A heat-protection spray keeps the moisture locked into your tresses and keep the elements out.

humid climate

Whatever your hair type, your hair swells and expands when it's wet and behaves in the same way in a humid climate, where the air is full of moisture. Humidity makes hair fluffy and, if it's prone to curling, it will cause frizziness. All hair types benefit from a pre-vacation conditioning treatment in the salon to nourish the hair and seal the cuticles. Preventing excess moisture from entering the hair shaft in a humid climate is key.

fine hair

This tends to get weighed down by the moisture in the air and looks flat and limp. Just as with other hair types, you need to block out the humidity if you can. A pre-vacation salon treatment will help to reduce split ends and close the cuticles that allow water to enter the hair shaft. Use a light leave-in conditioner on your hair while you are away (apply it from mid-way down the length of your hair to the ends) and seal the ends of the hair after blow-drying with a styling lotion. Be careful not to use too much on fine hair — a blob the size of your thumbnail is more than enough. Hairsprays are a great SOS option for a bad-hair day in humidity — they instantly hold down the cuticle of the hair and prevent moisture from entering the hair shaft.

curly and frizzy hair

Sealing the outside of your hair — the cuticle — is the only way you will minimize the candyfloss look while you are away. A pre-vacation deep-conditioning treatment is a must. Make sure you pack a creamy leave-in conditioner for your trip and use it religiously every morning. Using an anti-frizz serum will help unruly curls behave. It coats the hair shaft with silicone, not only sealing the cuticle but also weighing the hair down a little. If your hair is really frizzy, try working some serum through it while it is still wet before blow-drying. This should add some weight to the curls and seal the cuticles so that your hair does not absorb water, swell and frizz again as it dries. If you decide to go with the flow and make the most of your curls while you're away, mix gel and serum together in the palm of your hand and apply it throughout the hair to give the curls extra definition and shape.

hot, dry heat

The sun can strip the hair of its natural oils and a dry heat will only intensify the problem. Just two weeks in the sun without protecting your hair can weaken hair cuticles, with peeling, breaking and split ends becoming a problem. The sun's UV rays attack the melanin pigment that gives hair its color, as well as the keratin, the protein fibers, within the hair shaft that provide strength and elasticity. A weakened cuticle leaves hair vulnerable to dehydration and the color bleaches and fades. Sun exposure also encourages free radical activity in the hair shaft. The cells of the hair are damaged, as the free radicals cause premature ageing. Deep-conditioning treatments are vital before traveling to a hot climate, especially for chemically treated hair. However, the only way to protect your hair 100 percent from sun damage is to keep it out of the sun — a hat is the best option.

fine hair

Pack a gentle daily shampoo and a light leave-in conditioner with UV protection. A sun-protection spray that contains a UV filter will help shelter the hair from the sun and sea salt if you are sunbathing on a beach. Reapply the spray through the hair after each dip.

curly hair

Pack a gentle moisturizing shampoo to cleanse your hair daily, plus a creamy leave-in conditioner to help guard against excess dryness. If you are sunbathing, apply a sun-protection spray or oil that contains a UV filter to reduce sun damage to the hair, and reapply it regularly, just as you would suntan lotion to your face and body. Take a nourishing hair mask with you to deep-condition your hair.

frizzy hair

Your hair tends to be dry anyway and needs extra care in dry heat. As before, use a sun-protection spray or oil on your hair during the day and make sure you apply a rich leave-in conditioner with UV protection to your hair each morning before going out in the sun. Apply a hair mask at least every other day during your vacation — you can leave it on overnight for an intensive treatment if your hair becomes very dry in the heat.

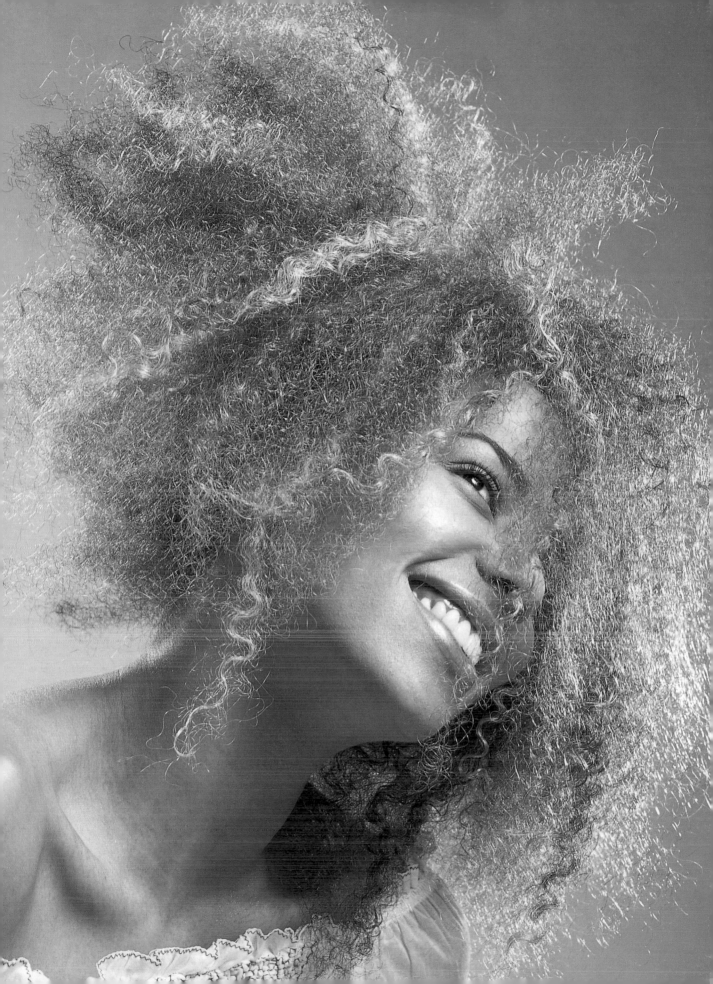

vacation hair enemies

All weather and climate changes bring environmental aggressors that are damaging to your hair. The perfect vacation setting — sun, sea and sand — provides the key elements that damage your hair. For hair to be sleek and easy to style, it must be well moisturized — a difficult task when you are exposed to extreme heat (and conversely extreme cold). A trip abroad is the perfect time to spend some money on good-quality hair products to protect, condition and bring out the best in your hairstyle.

rain

A sudden shower may catch you unaware, so, unless you have an umbrella or hood to cover your hair and prevent it from getting soaked, dive into the nearest café and sit out the storm in comfort. The haircare rules for rain are similar to those for a humid climate: block out the excess moisture or pay the price. If you become drenched in a sudden downpour, only to watch the sun come out afterwards, be careful about letting your hair dry too quickly. The sun's rays heat up the hair shaft, drying out the hair and causing it to lighten. You wouldn't try to blow-dry your hair when it is dripping wet — you would towel-dry it first and then rough-dry it before styling it properly — and the same care should be taken after a rainstorm. Carry a travel-sized bottle of conditioner in your beachbag or knapsack and if you get caught in a storm, smooth a little conditioner through your wet hair to help protect it while it dries naturally. Comb it through to leave it looking styled or tie it back loosely to look instantly groomed. If you have frizzy hair, smooth some anti-frizz serum through it, pull it back into a ponytail and let it dry naturally. When it's nearly dry, brush it straight, secure with hair clips and leave it until it is bone dry. You should be left with soft waves rather than corkscrew curls.

sea

Salt is your enemy here as it roughens up the surface of the hair, leaving it dull, damaged and porous. If your hair is color-treated, the combination of salt water and sun damage will make your color fade rapidly. A leave-in conditioner (which contains UV protection) is effective for protecting hair, as it coats the hair shaft and acts as a physical barrier to the salt. If you are happy to slick your hair back while you lie on the beach, use a sun-protection oil or wax on the hair to hold the cuticle down and prevent the hair shaft from being damaged. Always wash the salt out of your hair thoroughly at the end of each day.

chlorine

Chlorine is extremely bad for the hair, especially when combined with the sun's rays. When your hair is wet it acts like a sponge and is highly absorbent. So when you are in a swimming pool and wet your hair, chlorine enters the hair shaft, leaving it looking dull, dry and brittle. The best way to protect your hair is to wet it in the shower before heading for the pool and cover it liberally with a leave-in conditioner, preferably one containing a UV filter to give extra protection from the sun's rays. Alternatively, try applying a non-water-soluble hair wax, which will act as an effective barrier (this is more suitable for shorter hair). Wash your hair thoroughly every day after swimming.

sand

Tie your hair back while you are on the beach since sand roughens the surface of the hair. Give it a good, long rinse at the end of each day to get rid of any sand, then condition your hair, squeeze out excess moisture with a towel and gently comb it through.

air travel

Ever gone on a long-haul flight and left the airplane with your hair glued to your scalp or crackling with static electricity? The air pressure in the cabin, coupled with the dry air, high altitude, nylon seat covers and magnetic field in the plane causes even thick hair to become static. It's possibly the worst atmosphere for hair. Tie your hair back and place a silk headscarf over your headrest to minimize the static effect on your hair. Always travel with your hair free of styling products so that it can breathe. Take a small can of hairspray or a mineral-water atomizer in your carry-on luggage, plus a small comb or brush. Spritzing water over your head rehydrates and revitalizes your hair during a long-haul flight. Control static hair at the end of the flight by spraying a little hairspray onto your brush and brushing it through the hair to minimize flyaway strands (this works just as well in cold weather when hair can also become static). Drink plenty of mineral water during the flight — it's important for your skin as well as your hair.

wind

A cold, strong wind will cause some dryness. Keep your hair well conditioned and tie it back to keep it groomed and in place.

sun

Sun dehydrates the hair. The overlapping cuticles, which protect the center of the hair shaft (its cortex), peel and break as they dry out in the heat. The cortex is made of keratin, a fibrous protein, which gives the hair its strength and elasticity. The sun's UV rays damage the hair by breaking down its protein structure. When the outer hair cuticle becomes damaged, or porous in the case of chemically treated hair, it's all the more easy for the sun's rays to enter the cortex causing dehydration and fading hair color. Sun exposure also increases free radical damage, causing premature ageing in your hair, just as in your skin. Look for products with built-in UV protection — everything from your conditioner to sun-protection spray for the hair. Or simply use regular sunscreen on your scalp to prevent burns.

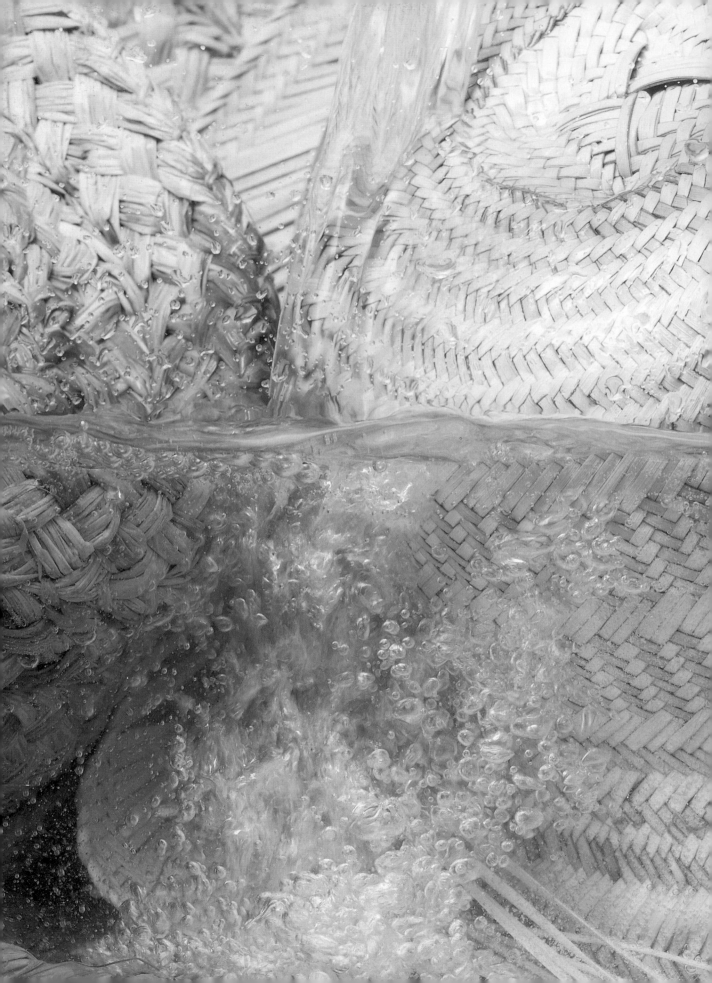

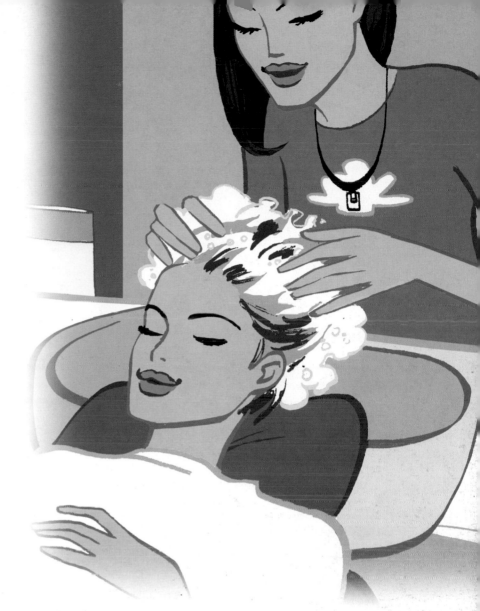

Dinner with Harry goes badly. Despite his recent lack of enthusiasm for their relationship, he's furious that Polly is calling it off. His male ego is taking a beating and he isn't going down silently. With his voice getting steadily louder, he argues through the main course and storms out before coffee arrives. Polly pays the bill quietly and goes home.

Waiting for her on her laptop is a message from Simon: "Come away with me. Flights and hotel booked — leaving Saturday. Surprise destination. Pack for the sun." Romance is exactly what Polly's been dreaming of, but sense tells her that this could be moving too fast. How can she take time off work? Deadlines are non-negotiable. More importantly, her highlights are in desperate need of attention — her natural color's showing through and Polly, ever practical, has no intention of flying

...polly's last-minute hair prep

off for a romantic week with a bad case of root regrowth. Her answer, she decides, will be governed by whether she can get a last-minute appointment with her colorist, Carolyn, before they're due to fly.

Next morning, Polly arrived at work early, determined to keep her mind off Harry (she does feel guilty for hurting him), and off Simon's exciting plans. The salon receptionist gives her an

appointment for a touch-up of highlights and a hair mask. (It pays to be a regular customer.) Her decision has been made for her and, since she's taken so little of her annual vacation, her boss is in no position to refuse her vacation request. Polly e-mails her reply to Simon: "Great idea. See you at the airport. Can't wait."

At the salon, Carolyn puts a few foils along Polly's part and around

her hairline to even out the root regrowth. "The sun will lighten your hair, Polly," she says, "so I'm not going to put too many highlights in now. Let's book you in for a cut and color for your return and we can take a look at your hair color then," she advises. She also applies an extra-rich, creamy conditioning treatment to Polly's hair to give it a remoisturizing boost. Polly is now ready for her trip.

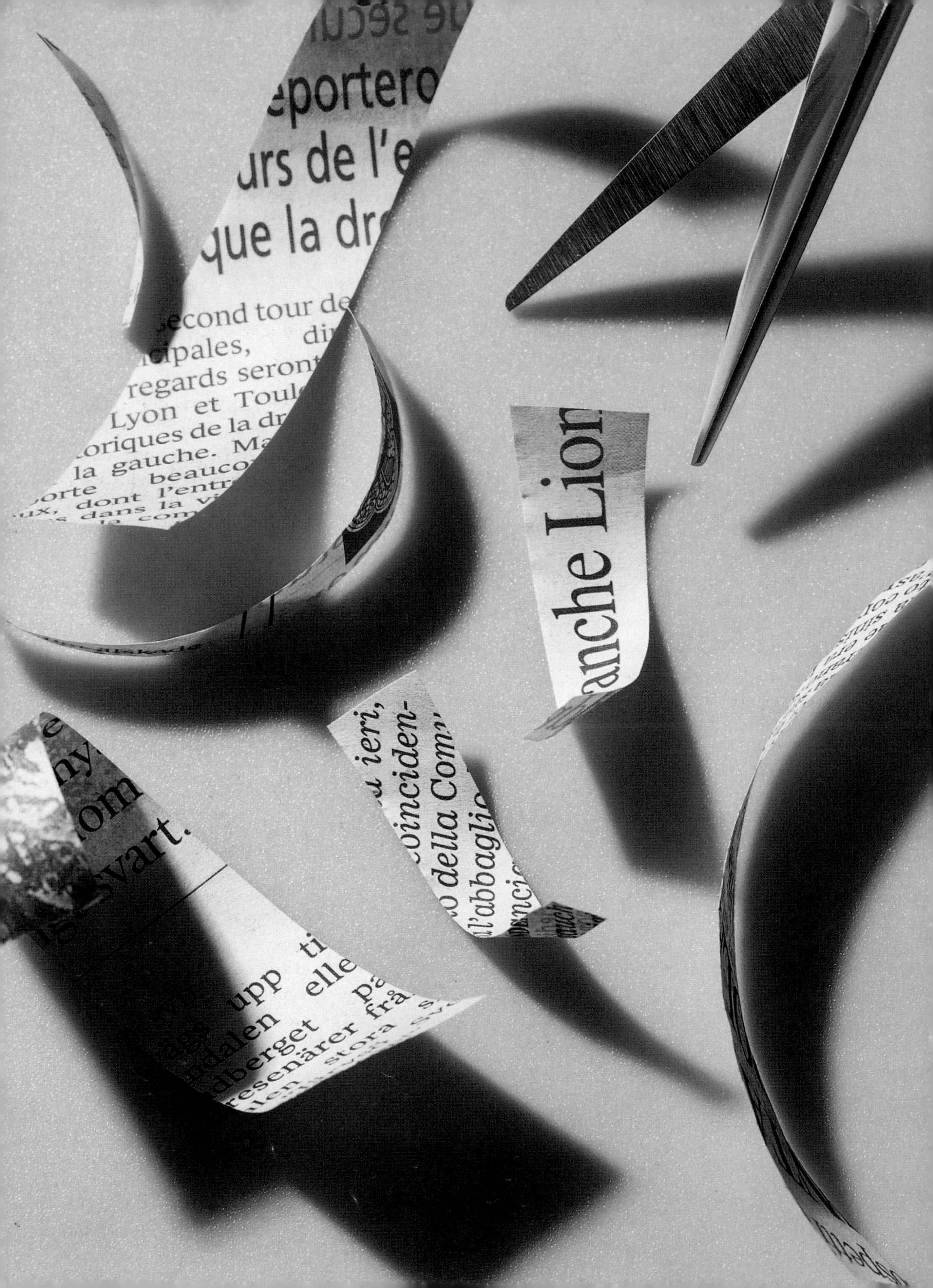

eporterο
urs de l'e
que la dr
second tour de
cipales, di
regards seront
Lyon et Toul
toriques de la dr
la gauche. Ma
porte beaucou
dont l'entr
ux, dans la v
anche Lion
u ieri,
coinciden-
to della Com
all'abbaglio
om
svart.
upp ti
dalen elle
dberget på
resenärer frå
dalen stora s

hair prep

In the days leading up to your vacation, make time to book a consultation with your hairstylist and colorist to discuss your particular hair needs. Your salon can provide professional conditioning treatments that keep your locks in top condition throughout your vacation and minimize the damage caused by various environmental aggressors while you are away. Ask your hairstylist to recommend an at-home intensive conditioning product and make a conditioning treatment part of your weekly haircare routine in the month before your vacation. This gives your hair a head start when it is faced with a change in climate.

Choose your haircare products carefully. Look for shampoos, conditioners and styling products that offer UV protection if you are going to be outdoors and in the sun on your trip. Make the most of the latest travel-sized versions of your favorite products — not only will they save valuable space in your luggage, they will also be convenient to carry around with you for on-the-go styling during the day. A great alternative is to decant your favorite products into small plastic travel bottles (available at drug stores) so you can travel light.

cut

A good haircut compensates for a more casual vacation styling routine, so that you still look well groomed. Your hairstyle should be able to hold its shape even if you opt for minimal styling while you are away and dispense with the daily blow-drying, leaving your hair to dry naturally. Get your hair in shape by having a simple cut that requires only minimal effort to look good. A gently layered style, for example, will literally fall naturally into place and needs very little maintenance. Warn your hairstylist that you are going on vacation so that he or she can work your cut into an easy-to-manage shape and leave enough length to trim away any split ends when you return.

cutting considerations

Type of vacation If you are traveling in a hot climate or will be particularly active on vacation, you may want the option of wearing your hair up. Plan ahead — if your hair is short to medium length decide whether to let it grow longer so that it can be tied back.

Consult your hairstylist He or she might recommend having a few layers cut into your hair (to add shape) so that it looks good and is easy to style while you are on vacation.

Be realistic You may want to inject some freshness into your look, so, as well as buying a few new vacation outfits, get advice from your stylist on different ways to style your haircut. Vacations are a great time for experimentation and trying out different products.

color

Book a consultation with your colorist before your vacation. You may want to have your roots retouched or your color revitalized so that it looks perfect for your trip. To look fabulous while you are away, have your hair color done two to three weeks before you go, so that it is fresh and your hair has time to settle. However, depending on your destination and the climate there, your colorist may suggest waiting for a full-color treatment until your return. Blonde highlights go even lighter in the sun, so warn your colorist if you are heading to the heat. It may be better to put a few highlights around your part and hairline, rather than using bleach on your hair before your trip. Similarly, lowlights and tints will fade in the sun, so your colorist might suggest a revitalizing color treatment on your return, rather than before you go. Remember, chemically treated hair is porous and more vulnerable to the elements. If your hair is color-treated or permed it will lose moisture faster than untreated hair and will need extra care while you are away.

blonde hair

Ask for a quarter-head of highlights rather than a full one before a trip to a sunny climate. This will color the area around your face, on top of the crown and at the sides to refresh your color. The sun will lighten your color further while you are away. If you have many very light highlights through your hair, have a few natural blonde lights put through before your vacation as they will go lighter in the sun, so you will not damage the condition of the hair as much.

red hair

Have your color done two to three weeks before your vacation and ask your colorist to mix a corresponding vegetable dye to take with you to refresh the red during your stay. Alternatively, use a colored mousse (in the same shade as your hair) to refresh any light or brassy highlights. Test the color on a white tissue before putting it on your hair, as some colors can be misleading.

brown and dark hair

Ask your colorist to lighten a few tips of the hair around your face before a vacation to the sun. It looks naturally sunkissed and will lighten a little while you are away, leaving flattering highlights close to your skin.

color considerations

1 Use a shampoo and conditioner formulated for color-treated hair. You need moisturizing products that gently cleanse and condition the hair shaft. Deep-cleansing shampoos will lift color out of the hair faster, so stick to gentle, daily formulas. Many shampoos and conditioners for color-treated hair now contain UV protectants that reduce sun damage.

2 You will always need a hair-color treatment after your vacation, so if in doubt, wait until your return.

3 The ultimate protection for your hair color is a hat or headscarf. Don't forget to tuck the ends of your hair into the hat as they are vulnerable to the sun if left exposed. The only way to avoid color fading is to keep your hair out of the sun altogether.

hats for different face shapes

To properly protect your hair, you need to keep it covered from the elements or out of the sun entirely. So wearing a hat is the most realistic option for shielding your hair while you are out and about. A baseball cap or headscarf will be better than nothing since both cover your scalp and, to some extent, your hair. The best solution, though, is a hat with a good-size brim that will shade your face and neck along with your hair. If you are sitting in the sun, always tuck the ends of your hair up into your hat — they are the driest part of your hair and the most vulnerable to damage from the environment.

oval faces

Virtually any hat shape suits an oval face, as the proportions of the face are even. Choose one that you feel confident wearing, otherwise it will sit unused in your hotel room during your trip.

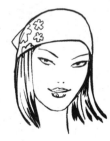

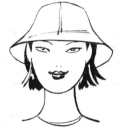

round faces

Balance a round face with a hat that has a good, high crown and a decent size brim. A short crown and small brim makes your face look more round.

long faces

A hat that has a wide brim offsets the length of a long face. Choose one with a low crown — a high crown makes the face look even longer.

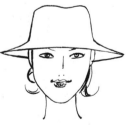

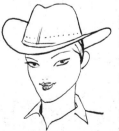

heart-shaped faces

Most hats suits a heart-shaped face, although a medium-sized brim (rather than a wide brim) helps to prevent the jaw line from looking too narrow.

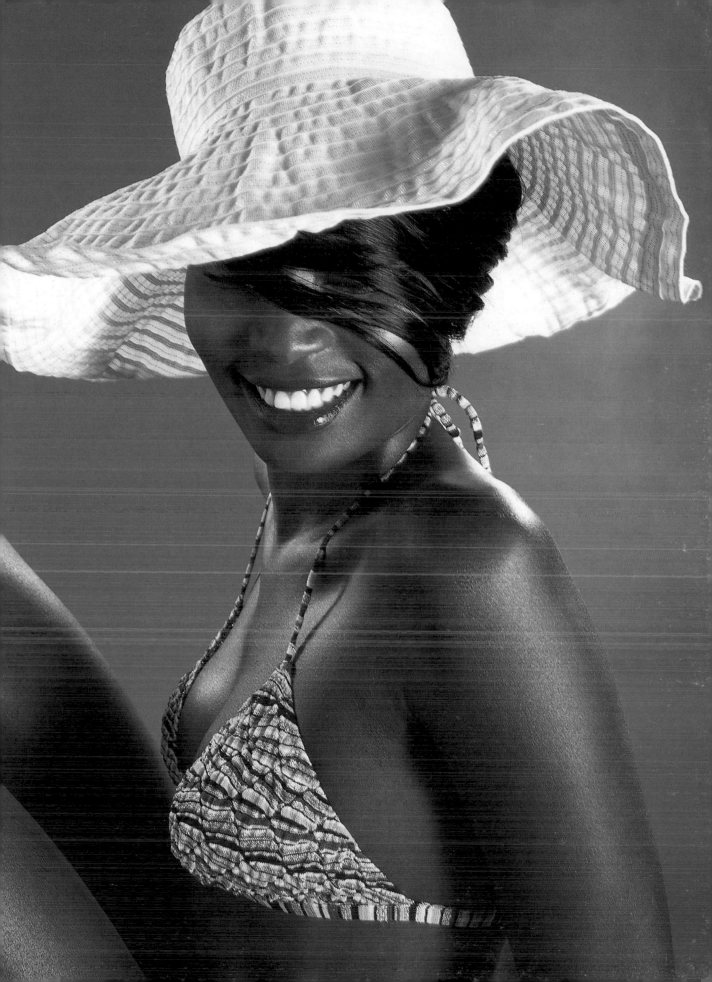

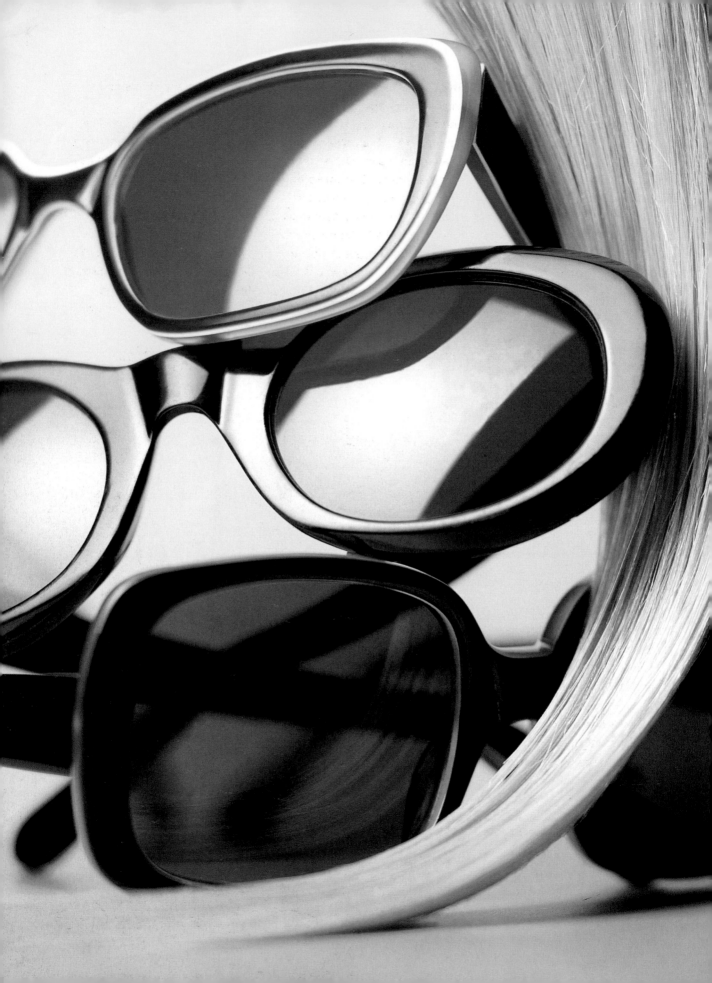

Back at the condo after her interview at Aristo PR, Jaz is packing her overnight bag. Fashion PR guru, Astrid, has offered Jaz a job provided that she makes a good impression on a key client in Paris. They are catching a flight that evening and having dinner with one of Paris's top young designers. Tomorrow they have a meeting with a buyer at Galleries Marais department store to help the designer introduce

Jaz sprays some shine enhancer through her hair and brushes her thick, dark locks into a neat high ponytail. Then she smooths down loose hairs with a natural-hold hairspray. She looks chic and ready for business. Jaz packs Kate's straightening iron. She knows she looks much more stylish with long, sleek hair and it usually has a natural kink when she wakes in the morning. Kate had reminded her that she'll find

complimentary shampoo in her hotel bathroom, so she just packs her own quick-rinse conditioner, as she hates using heavy conditioners on her hair. She finds a travel-sized bottle of mousse, which she pops into her make-up bag. It will help her to style her hair quickly in the morning. She also packs her multipurpose smoothing brush, which she can use when she blow-dries her hair.

...Jaz's trip to the fashion capital

his collection. Having spent months packing up clothes in the fashion department at *Gloss* magazine, Jaz is finally entering the fashion circuit for real. She has to perform well — and look trendy and stylish for the next 24 hours.

Clothes are not a problem — she has Chrissie's wardrobe to choose from as well as her own. She decides to travel in black, low-slung pants and take Chrissie's camel leather skirt and pointed, high-heeled boots, which look great with skirts and trousers. A couple of tops and her new knee-length military coat will cover all the options. What to pack for her hairstyling needs proves more of a problem. She's fairly certain the hotel will provide a hairdryer, but should she take hers in case? Jaz calls Kate to ask her advice. "Why don't you borrow my straightening iron? Don't forget to pack an adapter, so it will work in Paris," she says.

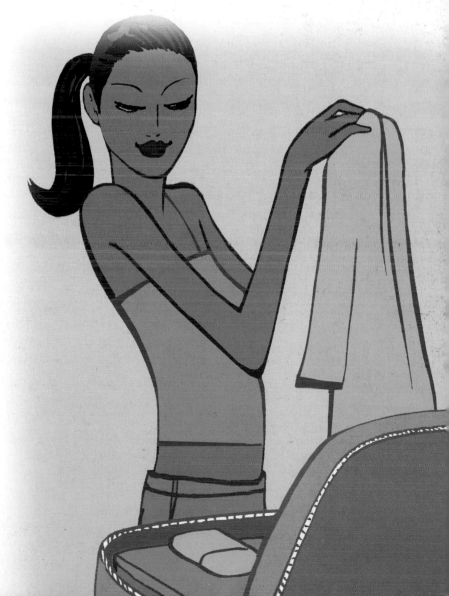

vacation hair tips

maintain the condition

Look after your hair on the plane — you don't want to damage it before you even get to your destination. Use an anti-frizz serum to protect it and spritz it with mineral water to rehydrate. Remember, salt water will dry and dehydrate the hair, so use a detoxifying shampoo to cleanse away the salt and then condition with a moisture mask. If your hair does start to dry out, brush it every night with a natural-bristle brush. This encourages natural oils, which moisturize dry hair. While you are on vacation, remember to eat healthily and drink lots of water. Both your body and your hair will benefit.

protect, protect, protect

Ideally, wear a hat or headscarf to protect your hair from the sun's rays, but remember that heat can also damage the hair, so condition it well to prevent it from drying out. When you are not wearing a hat, make sure that you protect your scalp. It is part of your skin, so use sunscreen to prevent it from burning.

special treatment for colored hair

If you have colored hair, seek advice from your stylist before you travel. You may need to have your color done before or after your vacations, but either way it is very important that you get the right advice to achieve best results and maintain good condition. Delicate blonde hair will suffer if you spend lots of time in smoky clubs while you are away — styling lotion will coat the hair shaft and act as a barrier, while detoxifying shampoo will cleanse away any stains. If you have naturally brown hair that shows signs of fading in the sun, rinse beer through it to add depth and gloss, and then rinse well with water.

accessorize

Take a collection of colored ribbons with you for dressing up your hair for going out. Ribbons make great accessories, are easy to pack and are available in many colors and materials that can be matched to any outfit. Hair fragrance is also very useful for freshening up the hair when you don't have time to wash it.

travel kit

brush and comb

A wide-tooth comb can be used on wet hair and is essential to banish tangles. You should also pack a small all-purpose brush to cope with all your styling requirements.

hair accessories, clips and bands

Pack at least one stunning hair accessory for your vacation. If you're going to a sun spot, a tropical-flower clip would be ideal, whereas a rhinestone comb or sparkly clips might be appropriate for a city jaunt. Bobby pins are useful for pinning your hair up (in a twist or chignon), and covered elastic bands are the perfect quick-fix solution to most haircare problems — just tie your hair back. If you like to leave your hair loose, a wide fabric or zigzag hairband is great for keeping it off your face.

products

If you're going on a beach vacation, take a gentle, everyday shampoo to wash the sun, sea and sand right out of your hair, while a detoxifying shampoo is extra-cleansing for hair that is exposed to city grime or smoky clubs. A good conditioner with a UV filter is the key product for vacation hair. Don't expect to return with your hair in decent shape without it. In addition, pack an intensive hair mask for the ultimate moisture boost. Also essential if you are going to sunny climates is a sunscreen spray. As with suntan lotion, you should reapply this regularly throughout the day, especially after swimming.

travel plug

This is essential if you are heading abroad, since no hairdryer, straightener or electric curling iron will fit a foreign socket without it.

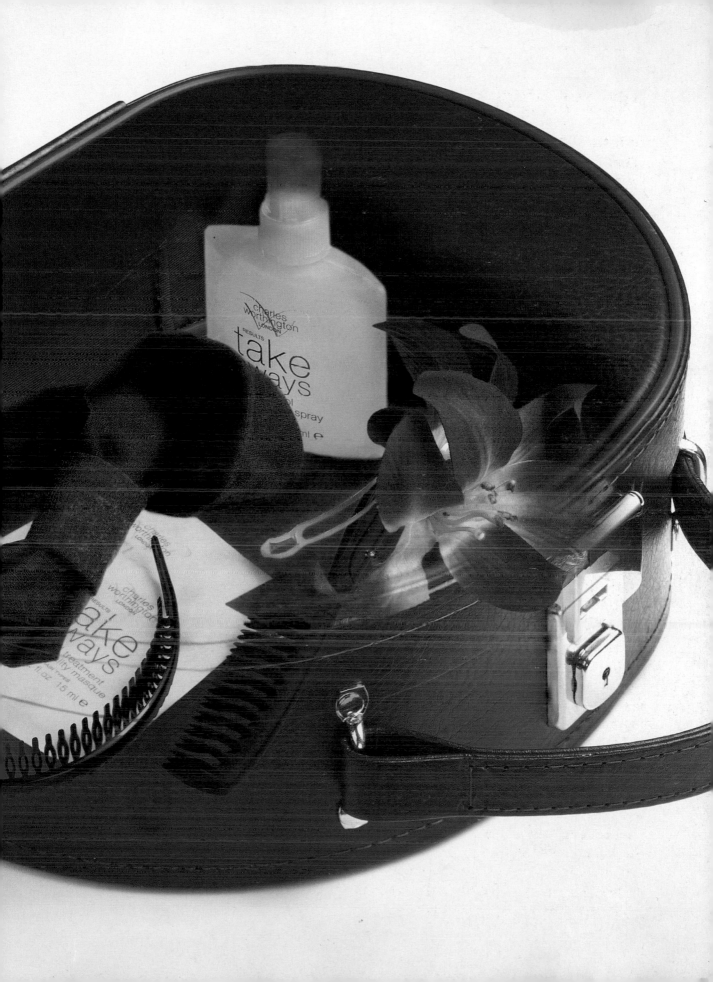

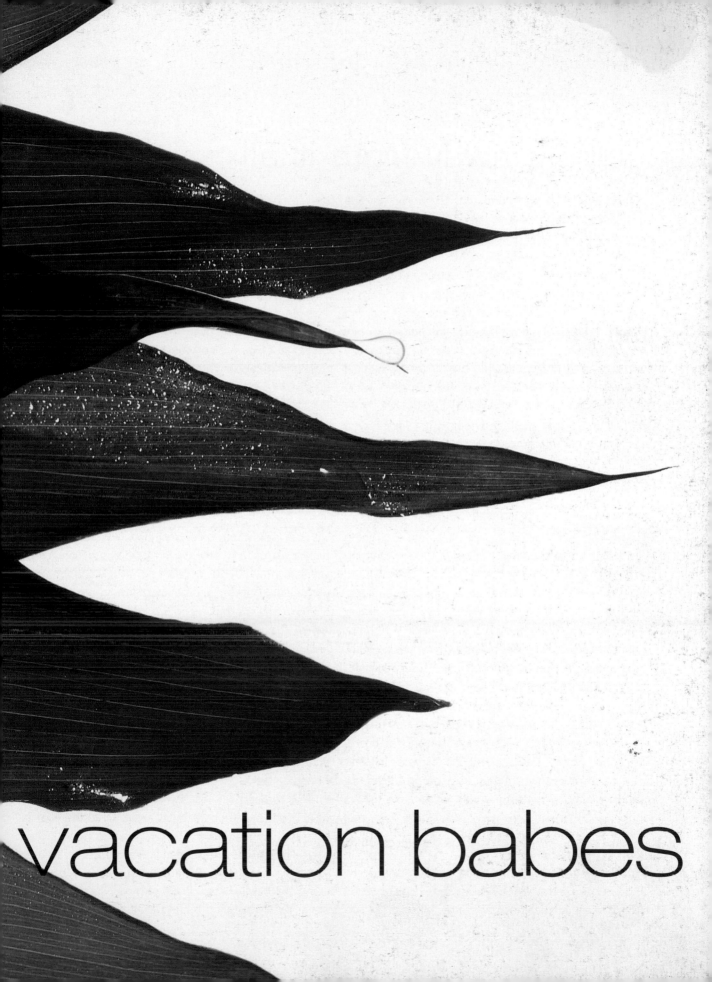

vacation babes

getting away from it all

Things were going from bad to worse in the marketing department at Crunch Cookies. Matthew was too preoccupied with the latest Crunch Creams campaign to listen to Kate's idea for marketing the new low-fat cookie. Kate found herself buried by a seemingly endless stream of marketing figures that she had to input into the system. Feeling demoralized, she opened her second pack of chocolate-chip cookies of the day and tucked in. Gazing around the office she saw all of her colleagues concentrating hard on their work. "They're all so driven," she thought to herself. "And I'm stuck in this dead-end job with a boss who barely acknowledges me." Picking up her bag, she quietly left the office and headed towards the nearest travel agent.

Five minutes later she was clutching an airline ticket. "I'm suffocating in my life, and I'm going nowhere," Kate thought. "Polly's got her high-flying job in the City, Jaz's new job means she'll be surrounded by glamorous designers and fabulous-looking models, and Laura's working on a fascinating new real-life documentary." The daily grind at Crunch Cookies seemed mundane in comparison. "I'm going to take charge of my life," Kate resolved. "A two-week yoga retreat in India is just what I need. I am going to relax and find my inner strength." She walked slowly back to the office, sat down at her desk and vacation request form. Matthew barely read it as he signed it, and mumbled something about organizing adequate secretarial cover while she was away. Kate let his indifference wash over her — at last she had something to look forward to.

That evening at the condo Jaz and Chrissie were in a restless mood. Polly's living room was covered with discarded fashion magazines, open CDs and the remnants of their supper. Laura was in her bedroom with the door closed yet again. She had been mooning around ever since the night in Cirque, was hardly talking to the girls and would rush to answer the telephone every time it rang. Jaz's trip to Paris had given her a taste for the high-life — she was in a total party mood. Chrissie was still smarting over her lack of success with Steve at Cirque. She was also a little concerned that her receptionist's job at Devastation Records was doing more to enhance her telephone skills than her career. She was still no closer to being "discovered." "We need to get away, we need to get some sun," Chrissie whined to Jaz.

"And how are we going to do that?" Jaz replied. "We haven't got any money to spend on a night out, let alone a vacation."

Chrissie knew it was true. Her uncontrollable shopping habit took care of any spare cash; she never could resist a new pair of shoes or the latest handbag. Jaz's unpaid work placement at *Gloss* magazine had cleared her savings account and her new job at Aristo PR put a considerable strain on her bank balance. She had been shopping every lunchtime since she'd started work, trying to put together a fashionable wardrobe for the office. "Well, we do have our Visa cards," said Chrissie, who had whipped hers out of her wallet and was waving it in the air. Jaz looked nervous. "Do you think we should?" she said. "You're only young once," laughed Chrissie. "Let's go and party in Jamaica. We can book it tomorrow." "You can book it on the Internet now," said Laura, who had just walked into the room. "I've just booked mine." "Your vacation?" shrieked Chrissie and Jaz together. "Would you like to tell us where you're going?" demanded Jaz. "And who with?" added Chrissie. "The jungle in Sumatra, and John, as a matter of fact," Laura replied coolly.

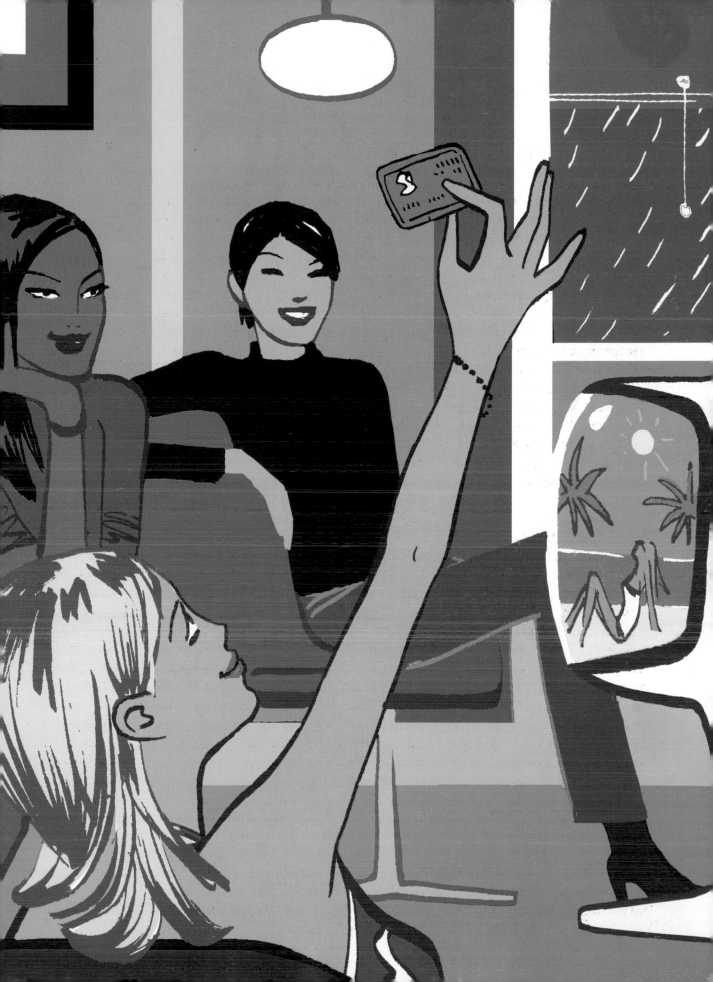

beach babe

There isn't anything you would rather be doing than lying on the beach and soaking up the rays. If you're not curled up on a lounge chair engrossed in the latest best-selling romantic novel, you're strolling along the beach, taking a dip in the sea or enjoying some waterskiing or windsurfing when you have a burst of energy. You're a high-maintenance girl on the hair front: all that sun, sea and sand are going to make your hair drier than the Sahara Desert. That ice-filled cocktail from the beach bar won't help matters either.

hair solutions

Work water-resistant sunscreen or a sun-protection hair product into the roots of your hair and spread it evenly across your scalp and around your hairline. Your head can easily be burnt through your hair by the sun and your hairline is a particularly sensitive area. If your scalp does get burnt, the hairline tends to peel first — not a great vacation look.

The best way to style your hair is to keep it simple during the day. Tie it back into a slick ponytail if your hair is long enough, or just comb it back once you've applied your sun protection through the roots if your hairstyle is shorter. Remember, wearing a hat is the best protection for your hair.

Make sure that you wash your hair thoroughly at the end of each day to rinse out all of the salt, sand and sun-protection product, then give your hair a good conditioning treatment. If you have the time, apply your conditioner or hair mask and spend 20 minutes relaxing before rinsing to give hair a real boost. Let your hair dry naturally if you're having a relaxed evening, or twist it up into a chignon if your hair is long enough for instant chic. Blasting your hair with a hairdryer or styling it with straighteners and a curling iron while you are in a hot climate is going to make dry ends worse. Limit your use of them to evenings when you want to look really special.

vacation tool kit

- Daily-wash shampoo
- Heavy-duty conditioner
- Nourishing hair mask
- Hair-protection spray with UV filter, or sunscreen to use on your scalp
- Snag-free elastic hair bands
- Wide-tooth comb
- Headscarf or hat
- Styling products to suit your hair type

braid it

This is a fun, sexy look for beach parties and barbecues, but it is time-consuming to achieve and you need to set aside plenty of time to do it properly.

you need

Approximately 30 pieces of ¼ inch (5 mm) ribbon • sectioning comb • scissors for trimming ribbon

1 Starting at the front of the hairline, use a sectioning comb to neatly section off a piece of hair about 1 inch (2.5 cm) square.

2 Tie a length of ribbon securely around the section of hair at the roots.

3 Twist the section of hair all along its length, from the roots to the ends.

4 Tightly holding the ends of the twisted section of hair with one hand, wrap the ribbon neatly around the hair, crisscrossing as you go. Tie the ribbon securely around the ends of the hair and trim any excess.

5 Continue sectioning, twisting and braiding all over the head in the same way.

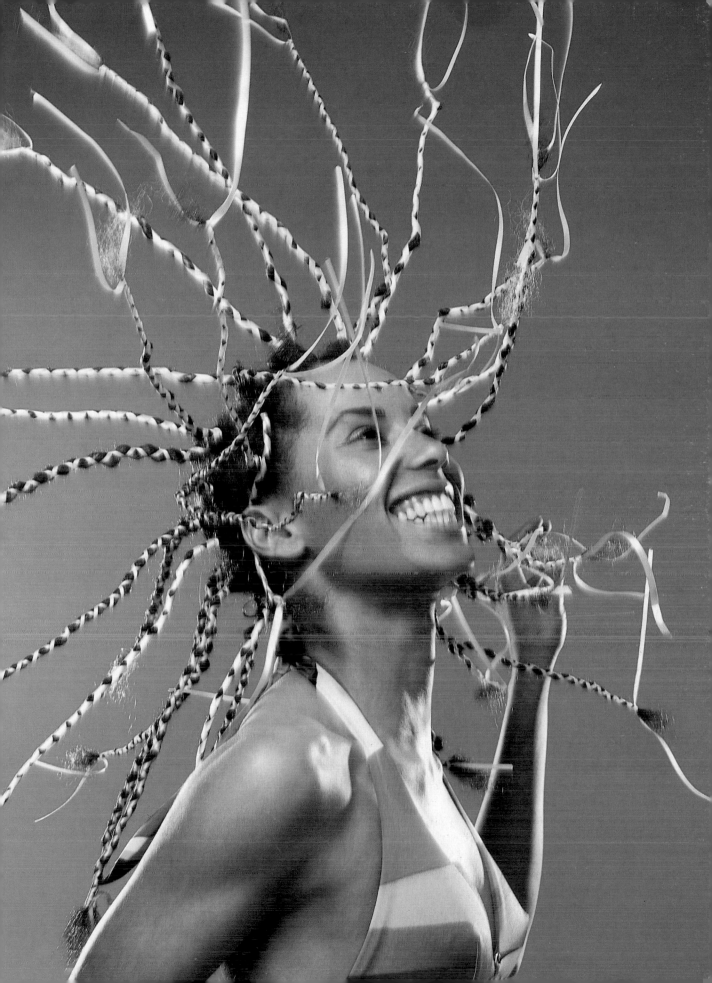

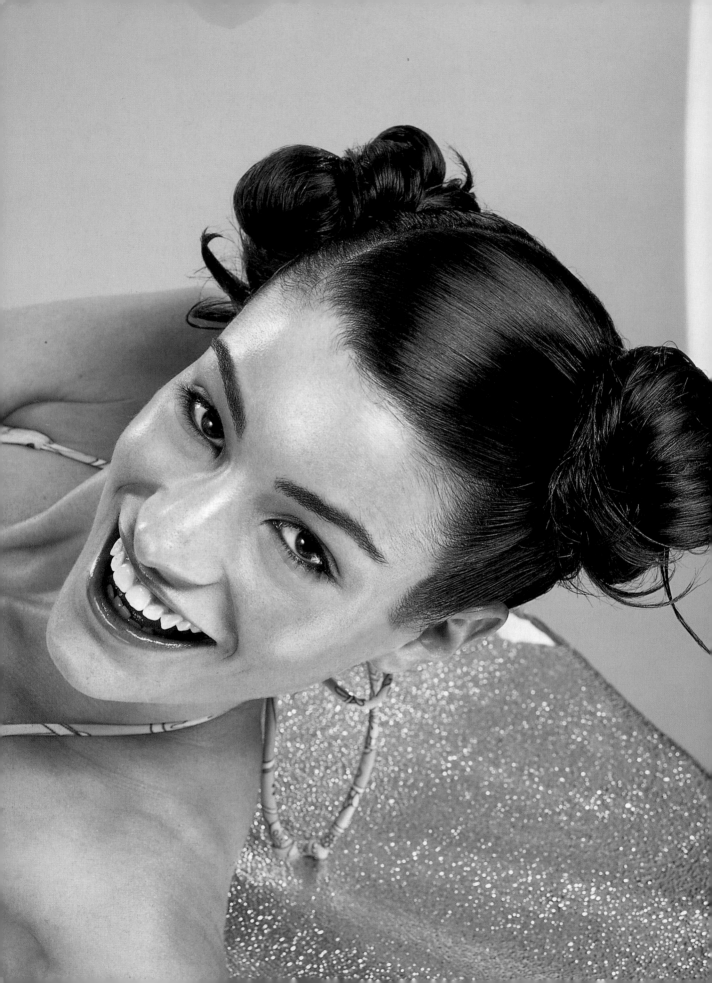

beach bunches

This is an easy style which you can do in no time at all before hitting the local nightspots. It's fun, cute and trendy — and perfect for clubbing, too.

you need
Sectioning comb • two snag-free bands • bobby pins • shine enhancing spray or light-hold hairspray

1 Use the comb to part the front section of the hair to one side. Then take the parting diagonally back to the opposite corner in the nape of the neck.

2 Comb the hair neatly into two ponytails and secure them with snag-free bands, making sure they are tight at the roots. Position the ponytails wherever you like, but for a quirky finish place them at different angles to each other.

3 Taking each ponytail in turn, twist the hair loosely and wind it around the base of the ponytail. Secure the ends of the hair into the ponytail base using pins.

4 Finish by lightly spraying the hair with a shine enhancing spray or light-hold hairspray to smooth any stray ends.

mohican pony

Vacations are all about relaxing and having fun, so if you're feeling daring, let out the punk rocker in you and try this unusual style, which is guaranteed to turn heads wherever you go. You can either use colored bands and cord or, as here, stick to neutral tones.

you need
Sectioning comb • snag-free elastic bands • light wax • lengths of cord

1 Starting at the front of the head, take a section of hair from ear to ear, comb it up smoothly and tie it securely with a snag-free band.

2 Take the next section of hair, from above the ear on each side, comb it neatly to the top of the head and gather in the remainder of the last ponytail. Start to secure with the band as before, but this time leave the hair in a loop.

3 Repeat this process, working your way down the head to the nape of the neck. Leave the last section as a ponytail and smooth it with a light wax.

4 To finish, wind lengths of natural cord around the bands to disguise them.

HAIR SNIP
WHILE YOU ARE ON VACATION, DON'T BE SCARED TO TRY OUT SOMETHING DIFFERENT WITH YOUR HAIR — REMEMBER, YOU PROBABLY WON'T EVER SEE THESE PEOPLE AGAIN. YOU CAN GET PLENTY OF GREAT IDEAS FROM MAGAZINES

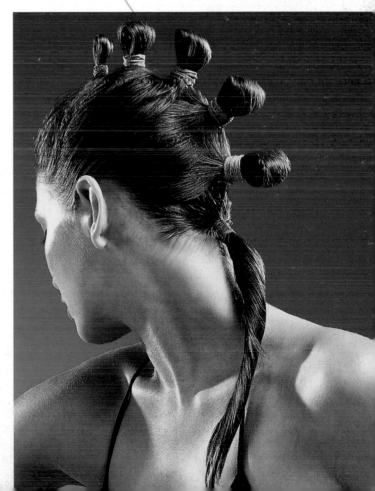

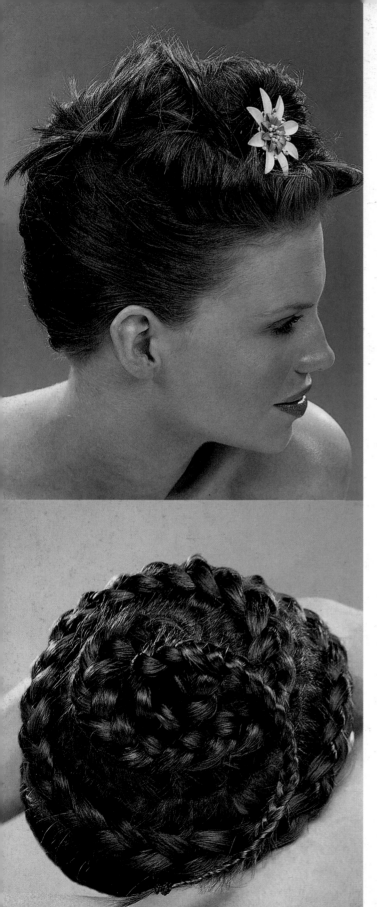

flower girl

Before you start, make sure the hair is free of any knots — you do not have to have clean hair for this style, but it will be more comfortable if you comb out any tangles.

you need

Sectioning comb • clip • bobby pins • flower

1 Section off the top part of the hair and clip it temporarily out of the way, leaving the back hanging loose. Gently pull the sides and back section into a loose ponytail and twist it up to the crown, holding it in place with the hair pins.

2 Unclip the top section and loosely twist it back randomly, securing it with bobby pins.

3 Finally, add a fresh or fake flower and secure it in place.

french braid

You will probably need the help of a friend to do this and get the shape perfect, but once you have got it, it will probably last for a couple of days, and can be accessorized for the evening.

you need

Tail comb • snag-free elastic band • hair clip • light-hold hairspray

1 Start by sectioning a one-inch square piece of hair, parallel with one eye. Using a tail comb, start creating a spiral shape, running behind the ear towards the nape. While you are sectioning the hair, get your friend to start braiding tightly against the scalp.

2 Carry on working towards the crown area, keeping an even spiral as you go.

3 When all the hair is braided, secure the ends using a band and secure the tail of the braid to the top section with a hair pin. Finally, use a little hairspray and the pointed end of the tail comb to push any flyaway hair into the braid.

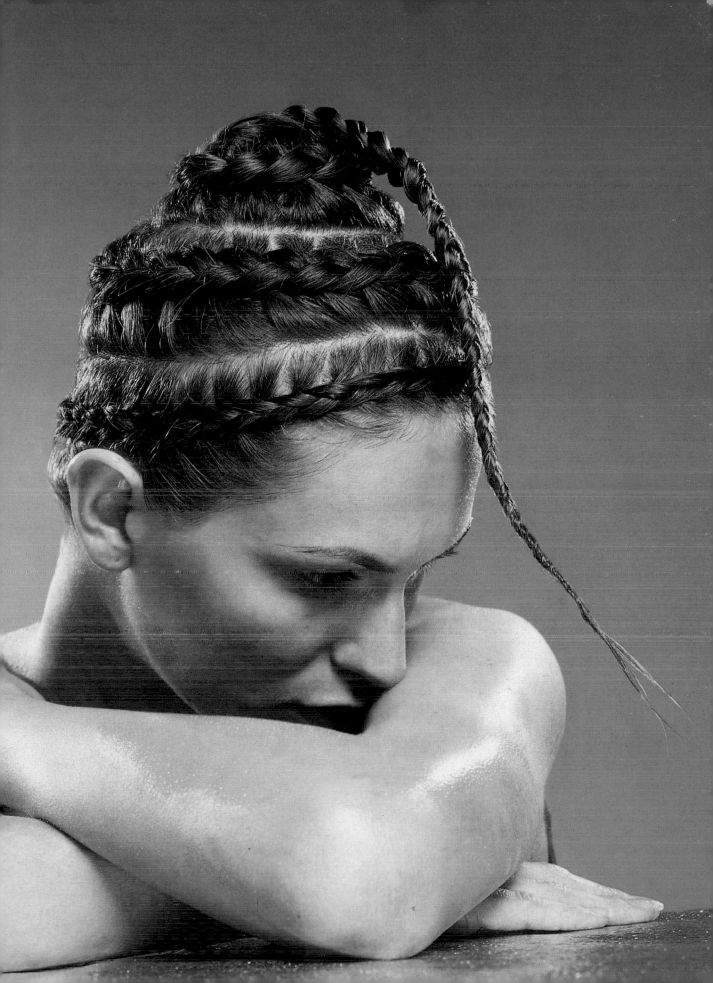

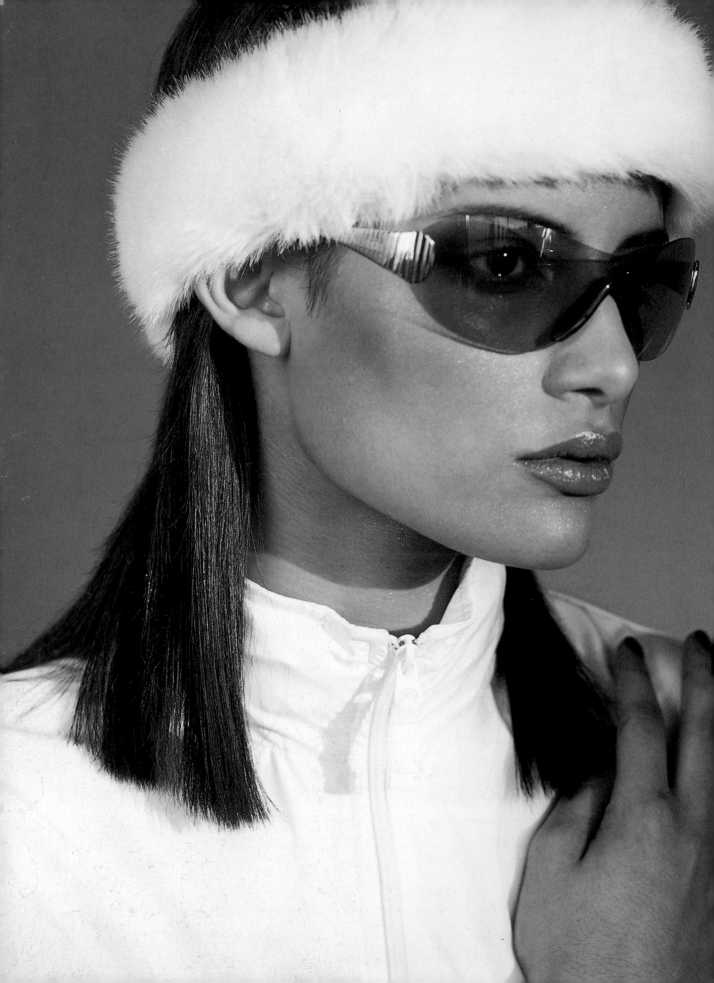

snow white

You can hardly wait to get to the mountains. During the day you keep your hair off your face with a warm hat or headband that covers your ears as you zoom down those mountain slopes. By night, you can be found enjoying the après-ski in a dark, smoky bar.

hair solutions

The snow reflects the sun's rays, making them even more powerful, so protect your hair by using a good, leave-in conditioner with a UV filter. Keep your hairstyle simple, sporty and chic — glamour girls look out of place on the slopes. The cold makes your hair brittle and static, so keep a band or clip in your pocket to pin back flyaway hair.

vacation tool kit

- Daily-wash shampoo
- Leave-in conditioner (with UV filter)
- Snag-free elastic hair bands or hair clips
- Anti-frizz serum and hairspray (to help combat static)

ski chic

Sleek-straight hair is the ultimate in sophisticated cool.

you need
Blow-drying spray • paddle brush • hairdryer • straightening iron • light water-based wax

1 Spritz the hair with blow-drying spray and use the brush to blow-dry it straight, section by section. Glide the hot straightening iron down the length of the hair.

2 Finish with a light wax for extra gloss.

ice queen

This style is a modern take on movie-star glamour. It's quirky yet sophisticated, and easier to achieve than it looks.

you need
Comb • large hot rollers • snag-free band • two hairnets (to match your hair) • hairpins • hairspray

1 Section your hair on large hot rollers to create volume and a good foundation to hold the style.

2 Section off the top rectangle of hair, from the crown to the temples, and sweep the remaining hair into a ponytail above the nape.

3 Backcomb the ponytail and cover it with a fine hairnet to form a bun. Secure with pins and hairspray.

4 Lightly backcomb the top section and twist it round, loosely. Secure the shape with pins and hairspray.

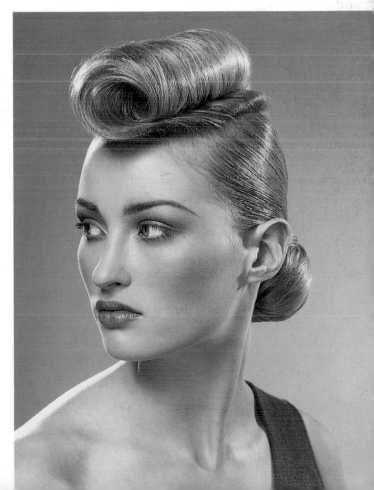

euro chick

Weekend city breaks are your thing. You like the stylish, cosmopolitan look with hair that will take you from chic boutique and café to museums and elegant restaurants.

hair solutions

Pollution and weather are threats, so wash daily with cleansing shampoo and condition hair to put the moisture back in. Carry leave-in conditioner or styling lotion with you in case you are caught in a rainstorm, and use sunglasses to hold hair off your face for a quick fix.

vacation tool kit

- Gentle cleansing shampoo
- Leave-in conditioner (with UV filter)
- Small can of hairspray
- Bobby pins (to control stray hairs or pin hair up)
- Natural-bristle brush (to help keep hair free of dirt)
- Sunglasses (the stylish hair solution)

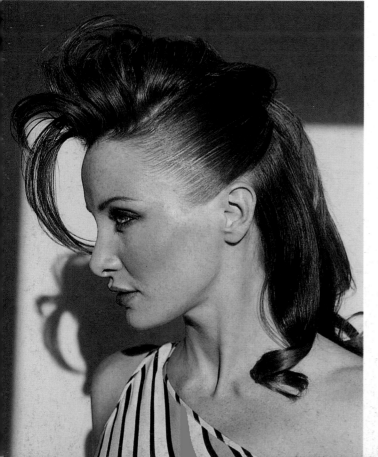

daytime sleek

This is the perfect style for city chic and can be easily adapted for a high-glamour evening look (see below).

you need

Comb • large hot rollers • flexible hold hairspray • natural-bristle brush

1 Section the hair and wind it onto large rollers. The top section should go across to one side, the sides should go forwards and the back should go downwards.

2 Spritz with flexible hold hairspray to give maximum hold and leave to cool.

3 Gently take the rollers out and smooth the hair using a bristle brush. If the hair is static, spray the brush with hairspray. Finish by spritzing with flexible hold hairspray.

evening chic

Simply sweep back the sides and backcomb the top.

you need

Comb • large hot rollers • flexible hold hairspray • natural-bristle brush • sectioning clip • firm-hold gel • bobby pins

1 Prepare as for daytime sleek, above.

2 Clip the top section of hair out of the way and, using a firm-hold gel, comb the sides away from the face and secure with pins.

3 Backcomb the top section at the roots to give maximum lift and clip in place, letting the hair fall loosely over the face. Spritz with hairspray to finish.

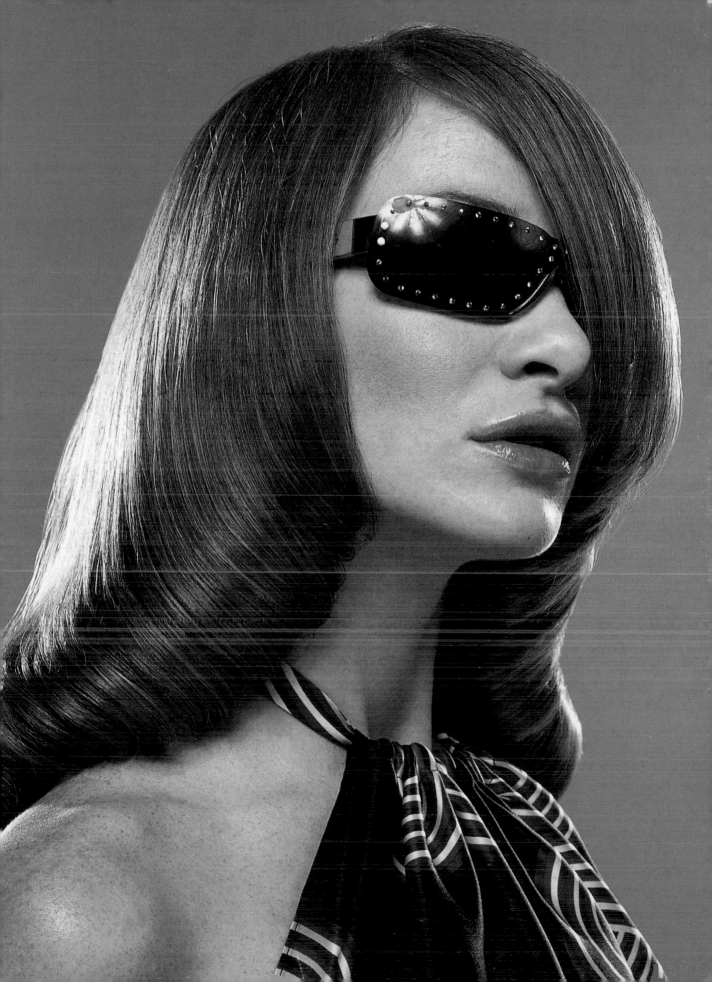

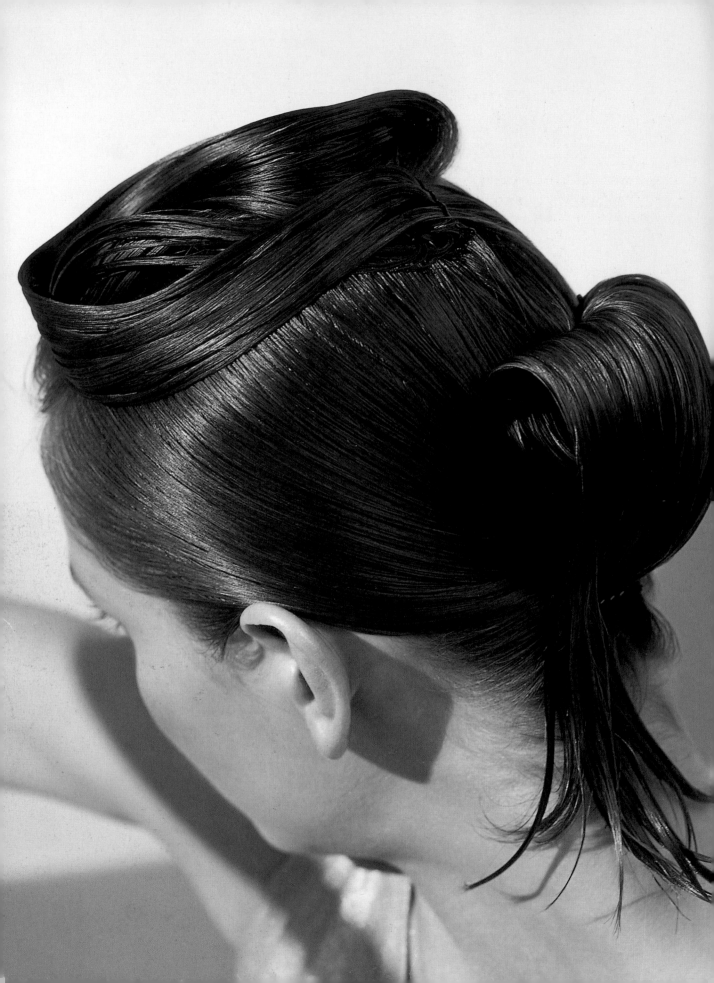

yoga fiend

Whether you're stretching your limbs in a yoga class or lying back for a massage, your hair is the last thing you should be worried about. Go for a natural look — creating big, glamorous hair is not a part of your vacation agenda.

hair solutions

Keep hair low maintenance by tying it back casually or letting it hang free. Pamper your hair as well as your body — apply a deep-conditioning mask, lie back and relax.

vacation tool kit

- Shampoo and conditioner
- Deep-conditioning hair mask
- Wide-tooth comb
- Snag-free elastic hair bands and hair slides

mask it

This is ideal if you need to give your hair a treatment that will boost its moisture levels and combat dehydration.

you need

Comb • deep-conditioning treatment • snag-free elastic band • fine hairpins • clips

1 Comb a moisturizing treatment through the hair, working through the entire length, from the roots to the ends.

2 Twist the top section of hair loosely onto the top of the head, then pin it in place.

3 Secure the rest of the hair in a ponytail at the nape of the neck , and place a clip above and below the band.

hair treat

Even if your hair is in good condition, this treatment is ideal for keeping it out of the way while you pamper yourself.

you need

Comb • deep-conditioning treatment • snag-free bands • fine hairpins

1 Comb a moisturizing treatment through the hair as described previously.

2 Make a ponytail in the center of the head and braid it, securing the ends with a band.

3 Wrap the braid around the head and secure it in place with fine hairpins.

HAIR SNIP

TAKE ADVANTAGE OF THE HEAT, WHETHER IT'S THE SUN OR A SAUNA. HEAT ALLOWS THE TREATMENT TO PENETRATE DEEPER INTO THE HAIR SHAFT.

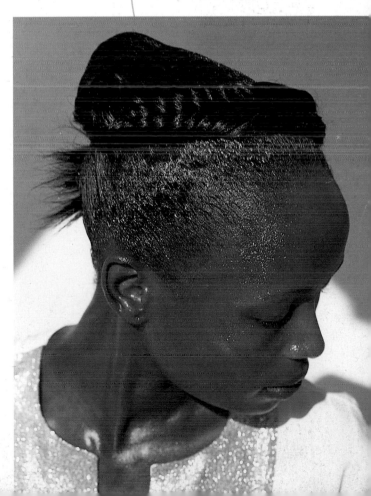

st tropez babe

When you are surrounded by celebrities, rock stars and royalty on vacation, you need a hairstyle that grabs some of the attention for you. Don't be afraid to make an impact with your hair. High-octane glamour is the only way to go — your hair has to be big, bold and full of body to make sure you really stand out from the crowd.

hair solutions

By day, you need to look sleek and chic for lounging on the beach and hanging out in cafés drinking cappuccinos and watching the world go by. Stick to simple styles for low-maintenance elegance and remember, less is more for daytime. Smooth ponytails, neat bobs and understated twists will give you effortless style. But by night, you need to rev up the pace with all-out glitz and glamour — go for big hair every time. The best way to achieve this look is by backcombing or backbrushing your hair, but remember only to backcomb the roots, otherwise you will be left with an uncontrollable bird's nest, instead of St Tropez glam! Remember, too, that sun and nightly hairstyling will take its toll on your hair. Whenever you get the chance on vacation, treat your locks to a nutritious hair mask to keep the shine in your hair.

vacation tool kit

- Medium-hold setting spray and hairspray
- Medium-hold hair mousse
- Deep-conditioning hair mask
- Covered elastic hair bands
- Brush or comb for backbrushing

glamour curls

This hairstyle is truly "big hair" like never before. The curls give great volume and texture, and the finger-styling creates a tousled, backcombed feel. This style works best if you have long hair, as the weight of your locks pulls curls downwards.

you need

Medium-hold setting spray • hairdryer • hot rollers • medium-hold hairspray

1 Spritz medium-hold setting spray evenly through damp hair — the weather will determine how long this style will last, so be generous with the spray and make sure you cover the hair evenly. Then blow-dry your hair thoroughly.

2 Make sure your rollers are as hot as they can get. Then, starting at the top of your head, take medium-sized sections and wind them onto your hot rollers.

3 Spray the hair with medium-hold hairspray to help keep the humidity out. Leave the rollers to cool for as long as possible — use this time to put your make-up on and get dressed.

4 When the rollers are completely cool, gently take them out and apply some more medium-hold hairspray. Then, using your fingers like a comb, pull through the hair to break up the curls. (To make the style bigger, use your fingers to backcomb the hair.)

HAIR SNIP
ADD EXTRA BODY TO YOUR STYLE BY MASSAGING STRONG-HOLD HAIR MOUSSE TO THE ROOTS OF THE HAIR WHILE IT IS WET. FIRST, ROUGHLY BLOW-DRY THE HAIR TO REMOVE EXCESS WATER, THEN WORK THROUGH THE HAIR IN SECTIONS, LIFTING THE ROOTS UP AND AWAY FROM THE SCALP WITH A VOLUMIZING BRUSH TO GIVE EXTRA BODY TO THE HAIR AS IT DRIES.

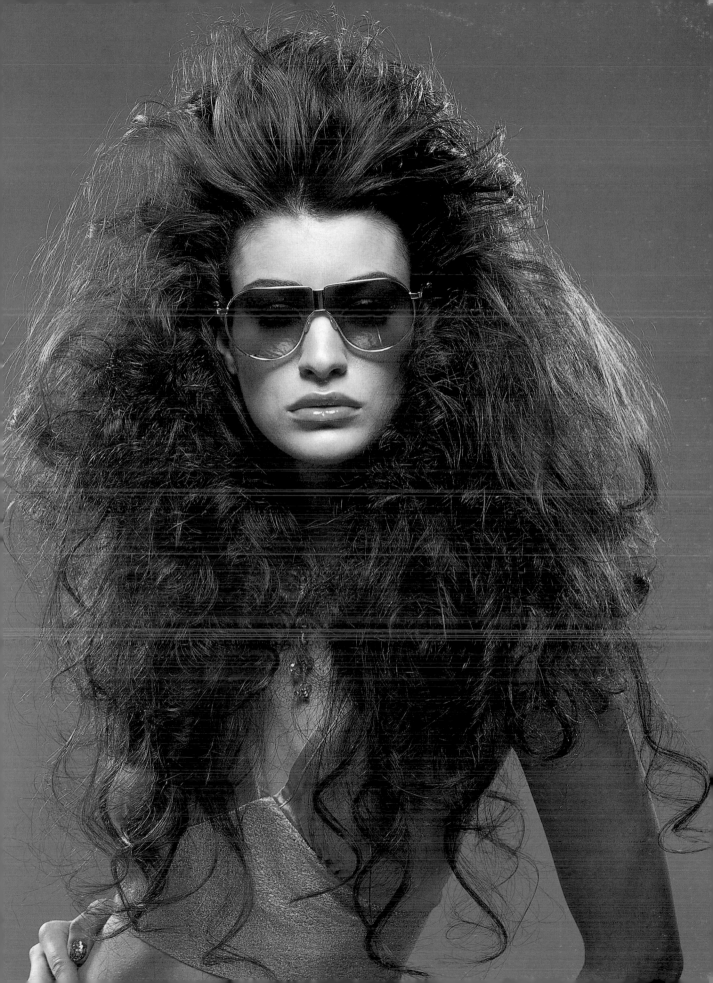

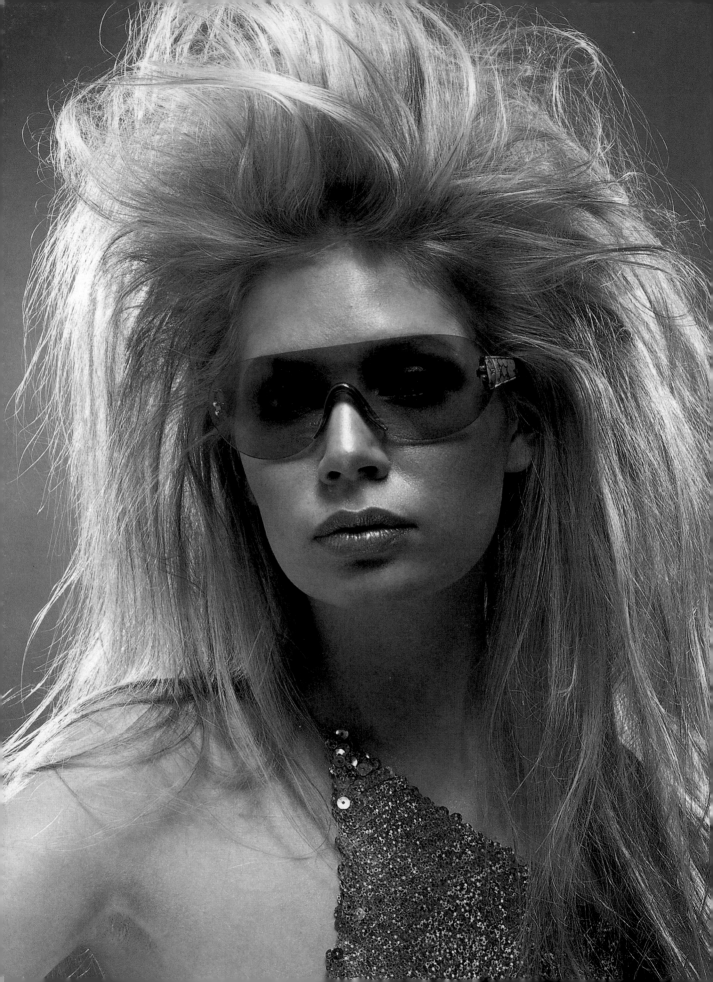

va-va-voom

A less curly — but equally glam — version of big, big hair. This is pure rock-chick-meets-European-princess.

you need
Hairdryer with diffuser • blow-drying primer • blow-drying spray • large velcro rollers • hair-spray • natural-bristle brush • light shine spray

1 Start by blow-drying the hair using a blow-drying primer to give body and "guts".

2 When the hair is 90 percent dry, spritz it evenly with blow-drying spray.

3 Using large velcro rollers, wind medium-sized sections of hair straight down onto the base of each section. Make sure that you wind the hair in the desired direction, otherwise it will be difficult to style.

4 Dry the hair using either a portable hood dryer or a diffuser. Make sure the hair is 100 percent dry, then let it cool right down.

5 Starting at the bottom and working up, take out the rollers, making sure that you do not tangle the hair.

6 Spray the hair with hairspray, then gently backbrush the root area to create lift.

7 Finish by smoothing a bristle brush over the surface of the hair and spray using a light shine spray.

accessorize it

The severity of this sleek style is counteracted by the pretty hair pins, which add instant sexiness and softness.

you need
Hairdryer • light-hold mousse • paddle brush • straightening iron • blow-drying spray • pretty hair pins • wax

HAIR SNIP
TAKE A HAIRPIECE AWAY WITH YOU TO ADD INSTANT LENGTH AND VOLUME TO YOUR LOCKS. THIS CAN BE ATTACHED AT THE BACK OF THE HEAD TO GIVE THE ILLUSION OF LENGTH, AND THE JOIN CAN EASILY BE DISGUISED WITH YOUR CHOSEN ACCESSORIES.

1 Start by blow drying hair smooth using a light-hold mousse and a paddle brush.

2 Starting at the nape, straighten the hair section by section using the straightening irons. Spritz each section with blow-drying spray first to protect the hair.

3 Tuck the front sections behind the ear and hold them in place with your chosen accessories.

4 Finish the ends with wax to add texture.

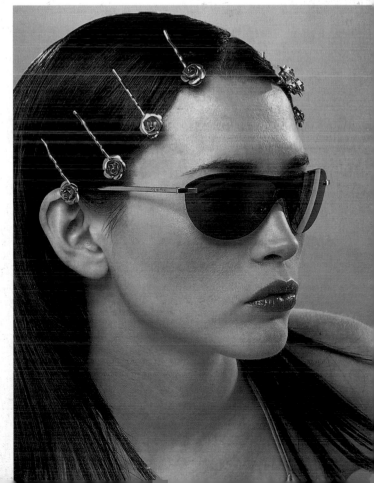

The pressure of keeping their relationship quiet at work, along with the normal demands of a fast-paced job in TV, has made Laura and John decide to take a break. They are both passionate about wildlife and quickly agree on a ten-day trek in the jungles of Sumatra to see orangutans in their natural habitat. It's far from a relaxing vacation but they both know they'll come back having had an adventure. Laura looks at the clothes and make-up laid out on her bed and sighs as she lifts up her compact backpack.

Despite her tomboy attitude she can't seem to organize her belongings into vital, possible and unnecessary items. It's early days in her relationship with John and while she won't need high heels or a hairdryer, she wants to look attractive and effortlessly cool. She'll be carrying her backpack from one camp to the next, so she needs to make sure it's as light as possible. A make-up bag full of products is a definite no: it seems to weigh a ton. She gets tough and singles out four T-shirts, two pairs of shorts, a

... laura's hair-raising dilemma

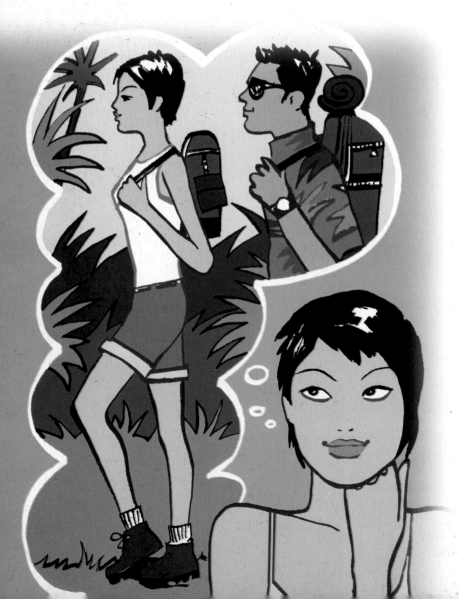

swimsuit, trekking boots and sandals. She faces the question of cosmetics. A light, frequent-wash shampoo and leave-in conditioner with UV protection are a must. She'll be lucky to find a bucket of water to wash with along the trail and she needs to protect her hair from the damaging rays of the sun. Her cropped hair will dry quickly in the heat, but the humidity will play havoc with her hair and she doesn't want to face John with a bad case of cotton-wool hair. A small bottle of anti-frizz serum should do the trick — she can use it sparingly to give texture to her hair, weigh it down a little, hold her style and stop the ends from frizzing. Sunscreen, after-sun cream with insect repellent, mascara, toothpaste, a tooth-brush and an all-over face and body cleanser all make it into her make-up bag. A wide-toothed comb will help keep tangled hair at bay. She's managed cut her packing in half.

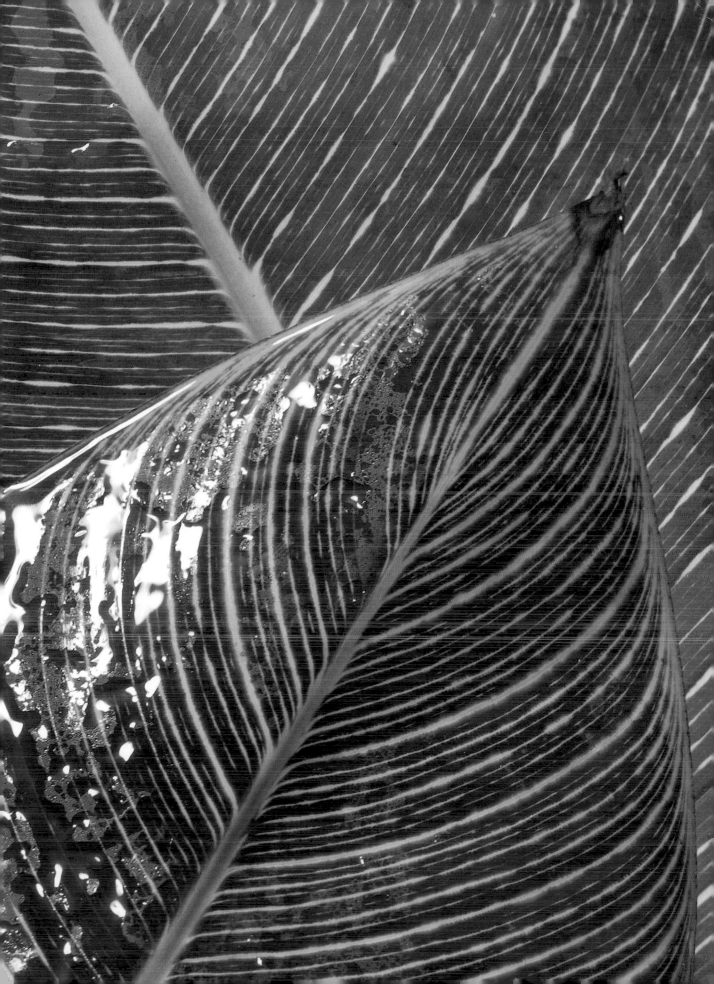

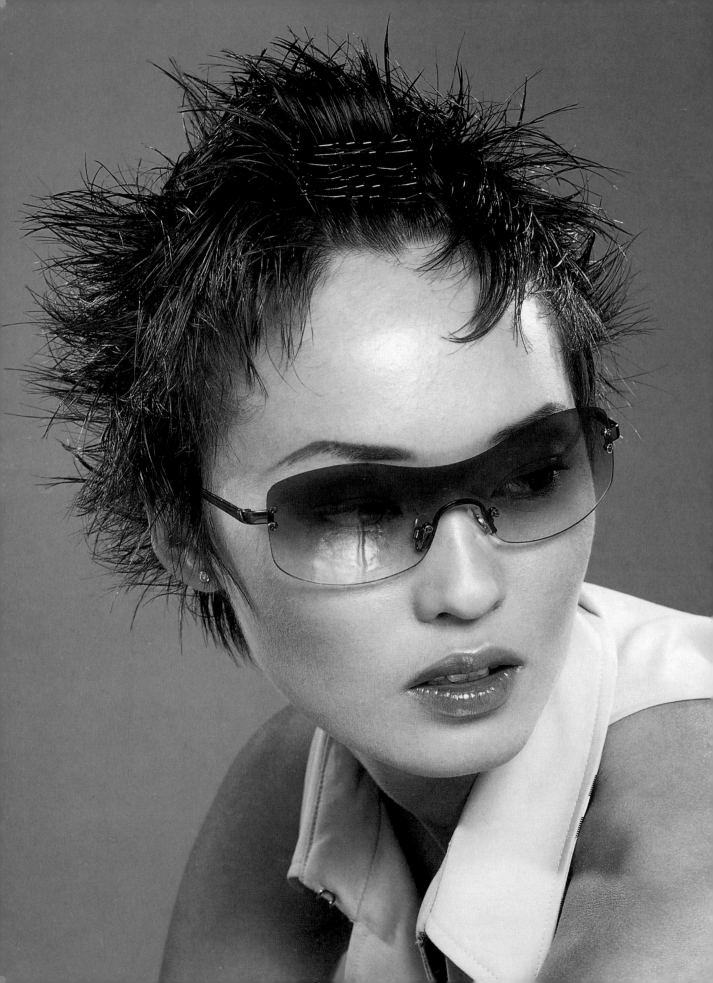

backpack girl

Freedom is a knapsack on your back and a guidebook in your hand. Your vacation is far from luxurious, but whether you're trekking in a jungle or camping on a beach, you'll be having the time of your life. You have to carry your bag on your back, so everything you pack must be useful.

hair solution

Take your favorite products in travel sizes to cut down on space and weight. You need a gentle, daily shampoo to rinse your hair quickly — your bathroom facilities will probably be basic. Use a leave-in conditioner to protect your hair from the sun. Take only the styling products you need to create a low-maintenance, casual look. Hair serums will help prevent frizz if you're in a humid climate and the easiest quick fix will be to tie your hair back. Clips and accessories will give instant glamour.

vacation tool kit

- Gentle daily-wash shampoo
- Leave-in conditioner (with UV filter)
- Hair serum and hair wax (to perk up a short hairstyle)
- SOS glamour kit: hair clips, accessories and snag-free elastic hair bands

short 'n' sweet

You do need a textured haircut to create this funky style, but it's easy to maintain when you don't have much time.

you need
Hairdryer • light gel spray • firm-hold wax • hair clips

1 Dry your hair using a light gel spray to give lift at the roots.

2 When your hair is dry, mould it into shape, then work in a firm-hold wax to create texture.

3 Comb the bangs back from the face and secure it with hair clips.

dreadlocks

Dreadlocks look cool, but they can be difficult to comb out, so be certain you like the look before you commit.

you need
Fine-tooth comb • light-hold hairspray • wax

1 Take a one-inch section of hair and gently twist it from roots to ends, then spritz it with light-hold hairspray.

2 Using a fine-tooth comb, gently backcomb along the length of the hair.

3 Run wax over the surface of the dreadlock to prevent it from unraveling.

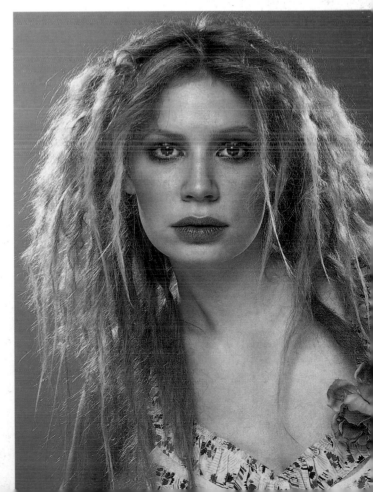

fresh-air queen

Whether you're walking, mountain biking or horse riding through the hills, your ideal vacation is always in the countryside. Glamour is not top of your list, but practicality is key for your activities. In the evenings you go for a natural look, making the most of your hair with an easy-to-style cut that holds its shape with minimum effort.

hair solutions

Depending on your destination, you're likely to be exposed to sun, wind or rain all day, so protect your hair with a leave-in conditioner. Keeping your hair out of the way will be essential. Use styling wax or an extra-hold gel on short hair to work it back from the face and tie longer hair back. A little hairspray will hold down those loose strands. Gently style your hair in the evenings with the help of a mousse — it'll make your post-shampoo styling quicker and help hold your hairstyle longer.

vacation tool kit

- Daily-wash shampoo
- Leave-in conditioner (with UV filter)
- Wax, styling gel or mousse and hairspray
- Snag-free bands or clips (to keep hair under control)
- Wide-tooth comb (to keep tangles at bay)

country curls

Just wear braids by day and unravel them for evening curls.

you need

Comb • styling spray • snag-free bands • clip

1 First shampoo and towel-dry your hair; then comb out any tangles and spritz with styling spray.

2 Section the hair into two-inch square sections and braid them tightly from roots to ends. Fasten with bands and dry the hair in the sun or with a hairdryer, then unravel the braids. Clip up the top section of the hair and add a flower.

twist and shout

These easy-to-do twists create a relaxed, fresh look.

you need

Hairdryer • blow-drying primer • hairpins • wax

1 Dry the hair using a blow-drying primer spray for extra lift and hold. Twist the top section of hair onto your crown and secure it with pins, letting strands fall out for added texture.

2 Twist the back section up and pin it as before, again leaving strands to fan out.

3 Finish by using wax on the ends to add definition.

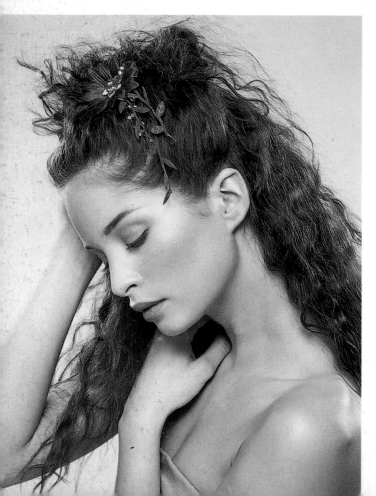

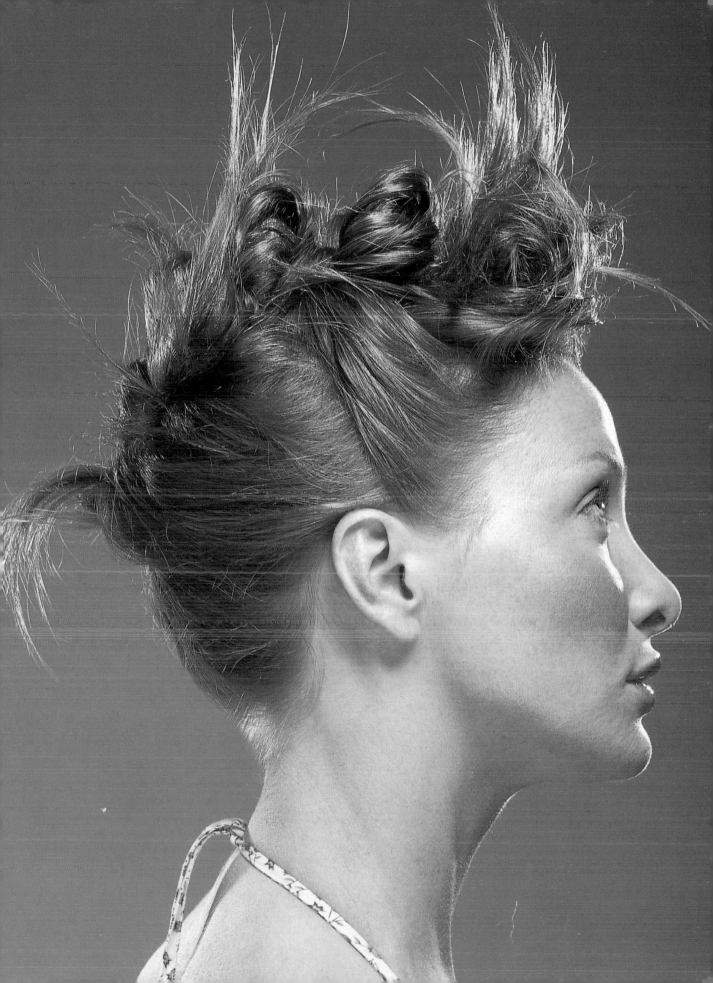

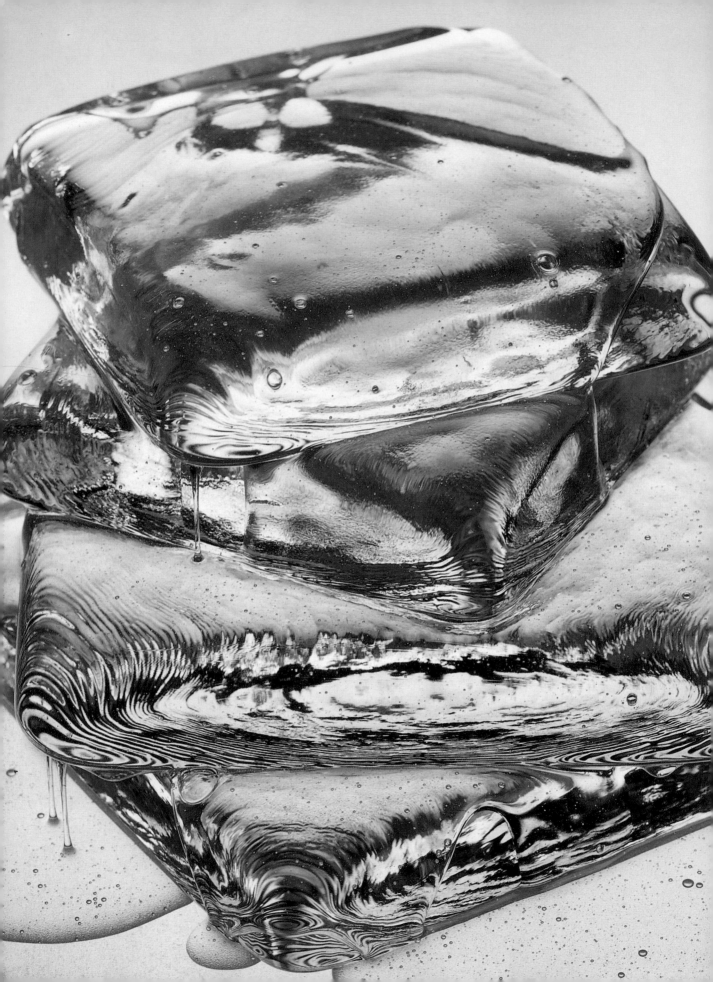

Chrissie and Jaz stumble onto the beach, hiding the signs of their hangovers behind dark sunglasses. Having clubbed through the night until 6 am, they haven't had much sleep and they hardly have the energy to do more than put on their bikinis and walk the short distance from their beds to the beach. They spot two free lounge chairs and, with a sudden burst of energy, run down the beach to grab them.

Jaz and Chrissie are having a fantastic time. The night before they'd made an extra effort to show off their newly acquired golden tans by wearing matching micro miniskirts and sparkly lycra tops which they'd bought specially for their vacation. (They knew they'd attract more attention if they wore identical outfits.) Jaz had decided to straighten her hair to a glossy sheen by spritzing on some anti-frizz serum and carefully running the straightening iron

along each section from the roots to the ends. She'd then pulled back the top and secured it with a sparkly rhinestone clip. Chrissie had scraped her hair back into a high ponytail and secured a platinum-blonde hairpiece to its base, covering the join with a strand of her own hair. The length of hair down her back almost reached her waist and she looked fantastic. "Aren't you ready yet?" she'd called to Jaz, "We've got some partying to do!"

Chrissie and Jaz party on...

"I'm done for the day," laughs Chrissie, as she spreads her towel across the lounge chair, flops down and closes her eyes. Jaz quietly begins her daily ritual of sun protection. She smooths sunscreen all over her body and then squeezes a blob of leave-in hair conditioner onto the palm of her hand and mixes some sunscreen into it. She works the mixture over her scalp and around her hairline. "You are ridiculous Jaz," teases Chrissie. "I can't believe you bother doing that every morning." "Just protecting myself from the sun," replies Jaz, as she combs her hair back into a loose ponytail. "You ought to wear a hat, with your blonde hair and fair skin," she warns, uncharacteristically sensible. "This vacation is about being wild and crazy, Jaz," says Chrissie. "I don't remember you playing it safe last night…"

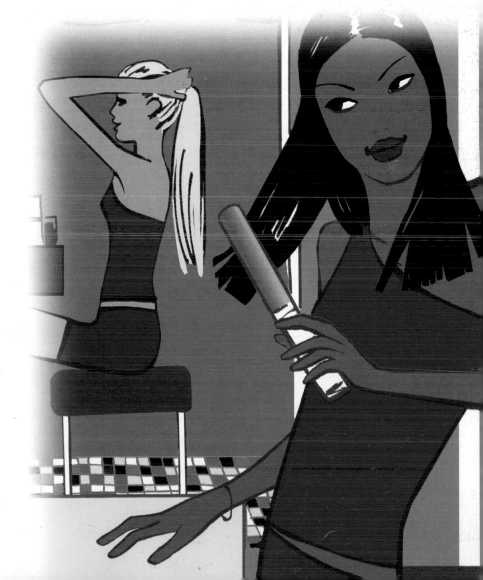

club bunny

You can be found dancing the night away from dusk until dawn and then sleeping off your hangover in the sun by day. This type of vacation is really going to put your hair to the test. You'll be exposing it to the sun's rays during the day and smoky environments by night. And not only that — you'll also be subjecting it to heavy-duty styling to create glamorous looks with a high wow-factor.

hair solutions

As well as giving your hair a daily cleanse and detox, you also need to condition it on a daily basis to keep it from drying out during your high hair-maintenance vacation. Your focus is going to be on creating sassy, funky styles for the evening, so make sure you pack your favorite strong-hold styling products to give extra staying power. A rich, conditioning hair mask will help keep your hair moisturized, so that you don't return home with dried-out, stressed tresses — use it at least twice a week on your trip.

vacation tool kit

- Detoxifying shampoo
- Leave-in conditioner (with UV filter)
- Hair mask
- Extra-hold styling products: mousse, hairspray, wax and stying lotion (depending on your hairstyle)
- Selection of pins and clips for stylish updos
- Snag-free elastics (for beach hair during the day)
- Glitzy hair accessories for instant glamour, such as flowers, butterflies, feathers and gemstones

funky hair

Funky hair is what every club bunny needs. The idea is to look hip, sexy and effortlessly cool. This disheveled look is easiest to create on short and medium-length layered styles. You just need plenty of firm-hold mousse to make sure your style lasts as long as you do.

you need

Firm-hold mousse • hairdryer (with diffuser) • several plastic hair combs • shine enhancing spray

1 Generously apply firm-hold mousse, making sure hair is completely covered.

2 Gently blow-dry hair until it is 80 percent dry using a diffuser or the slow setting on your hairdryer.

3 When the hair is 80 percent dry, place combs firmly into the hair as needed, positioning them so that hair fans out in different directions.

4 Once you are happy with the shape of your hair, continue drying until hair is completely dry; this will ensure it stays up all night.

5 Finish with a good spritz of shine enhancing spray, which to make your hair extra shiny.

tips for club bunnies

Use plenty of products to give your hair substance and hold — there is nothing worse than a collapsed hairdo halfway through the night.

Use snag-free elastic bands and bobby pins — these will hold the hair in place without damaging it.

If you have very long or thick hair, try to keep it tied back. This will keep you cool and prevent your hair from getting sweaty and collapsing when you're dancing.

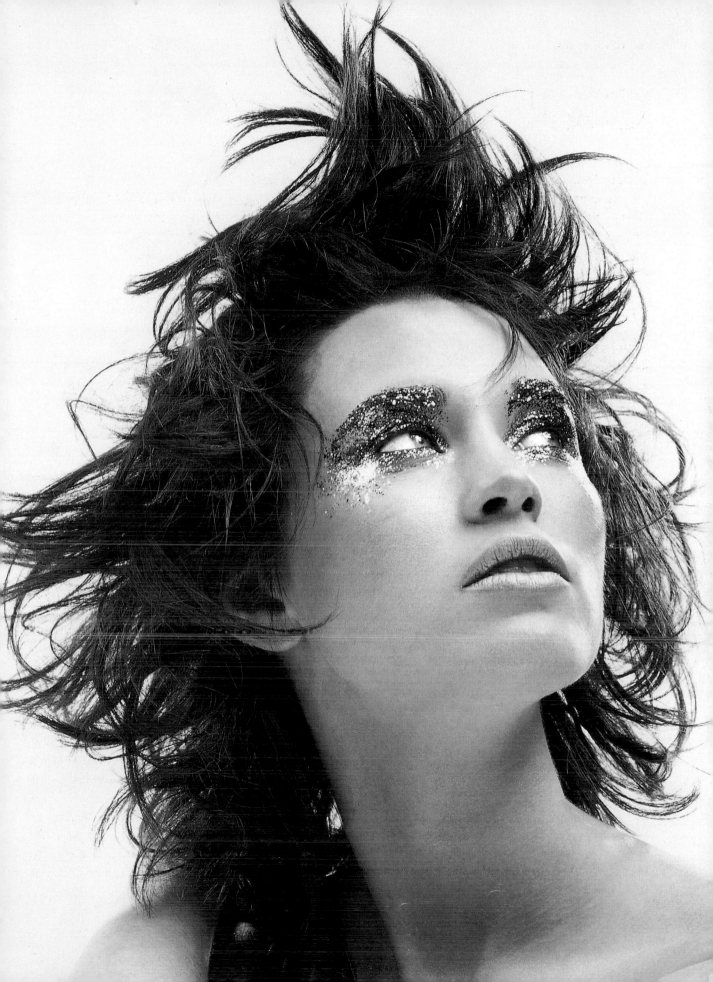

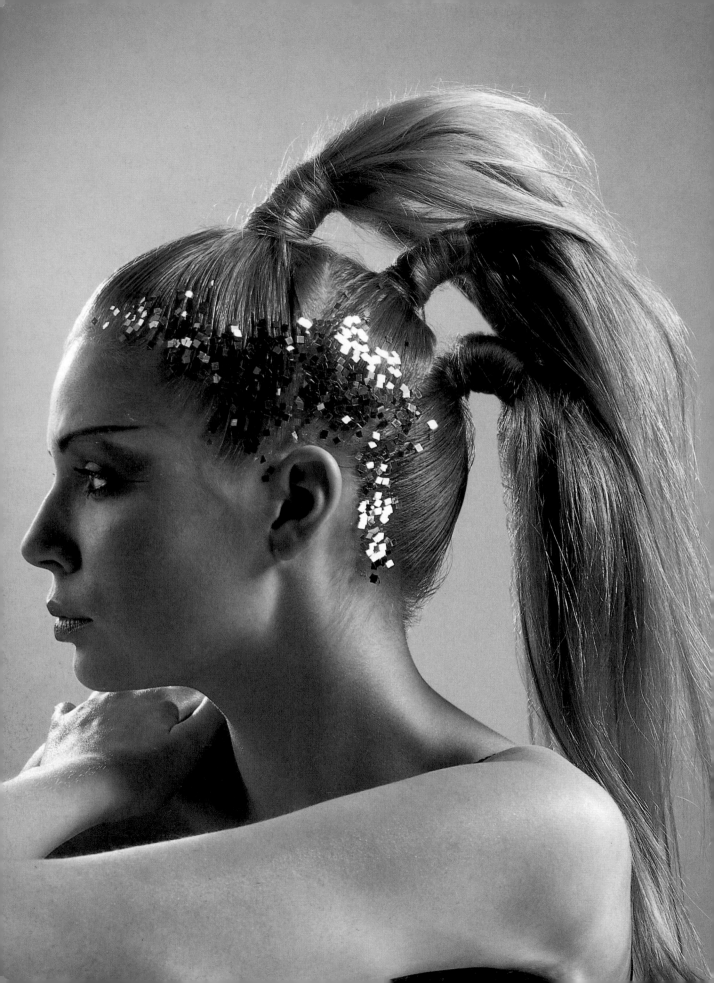

high pony

This is a sleek, high-glamour look that will look great and help keep you cool when you are dancing.

you need
Hairdryer • light-hold mousse • paddle brush • straightening iron • comb • three snag-free bands • hairpins • glitter and gel (optional)

1 Blow-dry the hair smooth using light-hold mousse and a paddle brush. Then straighten the hair section by section using the straightening iron.

2 Divide the hair into three horizontal sections, securing each with a snag-free elastic. Then wrap a strand of hair around the base of each bunch to disguise the band and secure it with hairpins.

3 Backcomb the base of each ponytail to make it stand away from the head and, for extra drama, use gel to stick chunky glitter along one side of the head.

chopstick twists

This excellent hairstyle is great for a big night out, and surprisingly quick to achieve (see overleaf).

you need
Hair clips • firm-hold hairspray • chopsticks

1 Taking a one-inch square section of hair, twist it tightly from ends to roots, letting the hair wind down on itself.

2 Wind the ends of the hair tightly around the base and secure it with a hair clip.

3 Continue by winding sections of hair all over. When you have twisted all the sections, apply firm-hold hairspray.

4 Accessorize the twists with chopsticks (as shown here), or with flowers, feathers or beads.

ponytail tips
Make sure ponytails are firmly secured to prevent them from slipping or loosening. Hold them in place with snag-free elastics or wet string, which contracts as it dries, holding the hair even more tightly.

To give a neat, slick finish, wrap a small section of hair around the ponytail base to cover and disguise the hair band. Secure the section of hair in place using a bobby pin.

Use chunky glitter to accessorize your hairstyle. This can be fixed in place by applying a little strong-hold gel to the desired area before adding the glitter. Finish with a strong-hold non-aerosol hairspray.

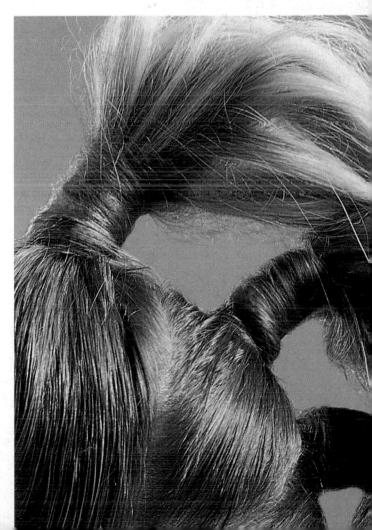

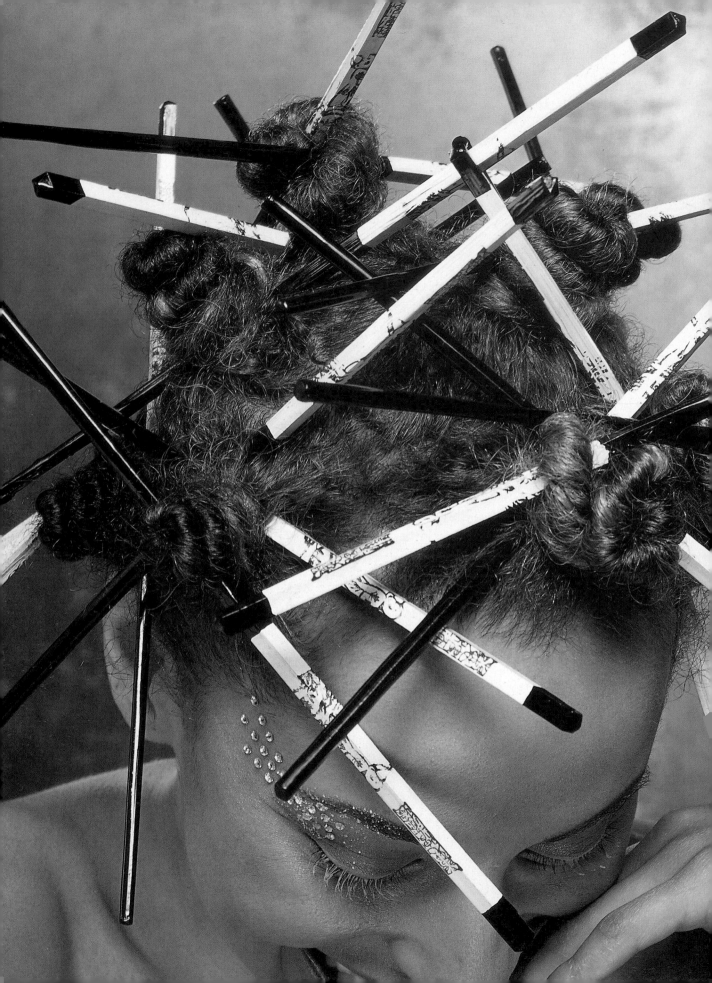

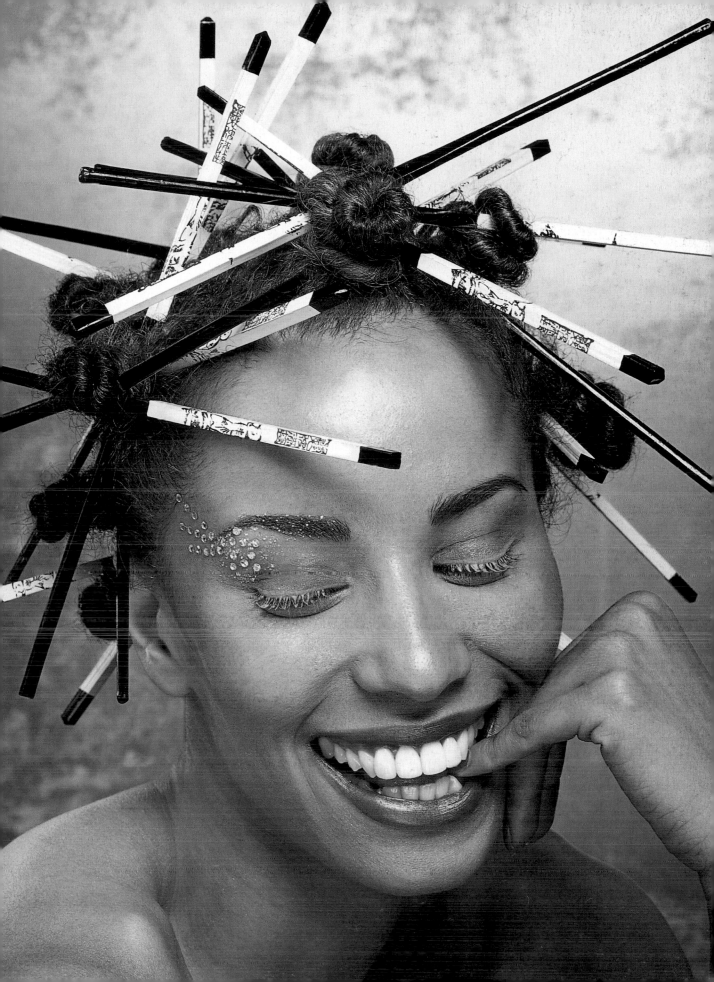

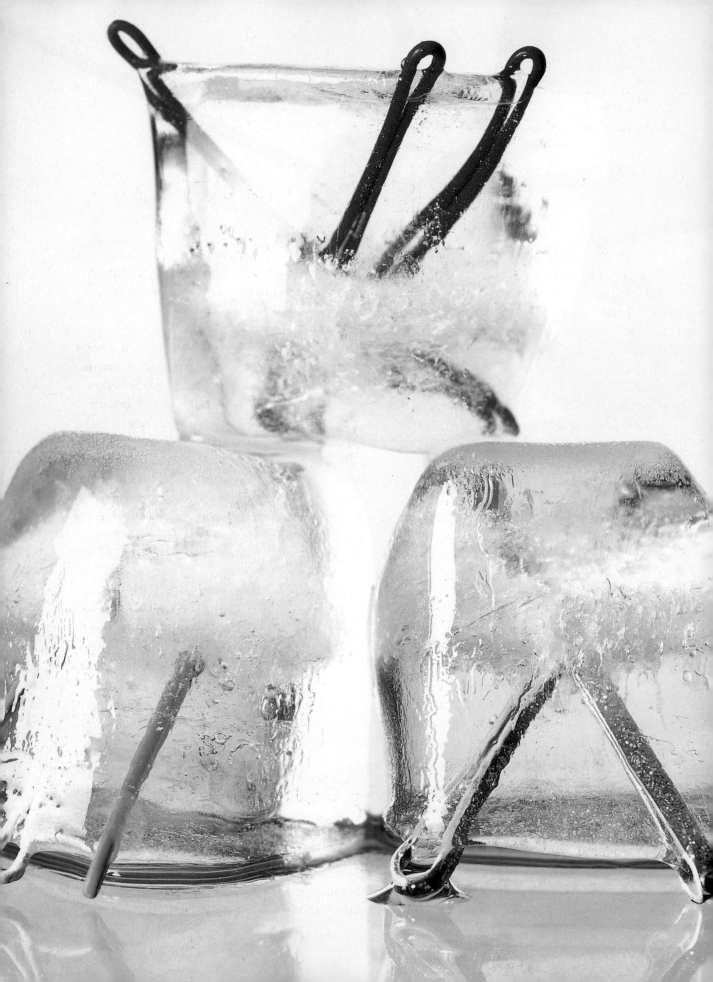

vacation hair quick fixes

1 Take a bottle of fresh tap water with you to the beach to rinse the salt out of your hair throughout the day. Remember to do this, and then to reapply leave-in conditioner (with a UV filter) or sun-protection spray to your hair (and sunscreen to your face and body) after every dip.

2 Keep a travel-sized bottle of leave-in conditioner or a travel-sized can of hairspray in your backpack or beach bag at all times in case of emergencies. You can use either one of these products to seal the ends of your hair or slick down stray ends for a quick style fix.

3 Keep a thick, cotton-covered hair band handy to tie back your hair for on-the-spot grooming. As an extra precaution, smooth a little conditioner over the band to help prevent snagging or tearing your hair when you remove the band later on.

4 This is a great quick fix for naturally curly hair. After washing your hair, apply a firm-hold styling mousse evenly through your hair. Taking one small section of hair at a time, twist each one from the roots to the ends. Continue until your entire head is covered in twists of hair. Then dry it slowly using a diffuser on your hairdryer, being careful not to disturb the twists of hair while you dry them. When your hair is dry, unwind the twists and you'll be left with a head full of spiral locks.

5 Apply sun-protection lotion to your hair as often as you would apply it to your face and body. The golden rule is to reapply. One spritz in the morning does not give day-long protection.

6 If it all gets too much, simply push your hair back from your face and hold it in place with your sunglasses. Wearing your sunglasses as if they were a hair band is a stylish — and fail-safe — quick fix.

7 If you have short hair, take styling wax with you on vacation. You can use it to rework your hairstyle into funky chunks in an instant if you get caught in the rain or are suffering the consequences of a humid climate.

8 Tie back long hair at the nape of your neck, rather than scrunching it up on the top of your head while you are out and about. This way you will avoid exposing the ends of your hair to the sun (important even on a cloudy day when the UV rays will still be strong), thereby preventing them from becoming dry and brittle.

9 Sunscreen body lotions and oils can be used on your hair (in small amounts only) to protect your scalp from the sun. Apply a few drops through your hair and work it onto your scalp by massaging with your fingertips. Don't forget to apply sunscreen to your ears, as they will be exposed to the sun, especially if you tie your hair back.

10 Give yourself a cool sporty look and slick back those loose ends with a wet-look sun-protection gel containing a UV filter (go for the no-hold type). This will give your hair extra protection if you are swimming and sunbathing; it works well on long hair if it is being tied back, as well as on short hair, and can be reapplied regularly during the day to keep up the sun-protection factor.

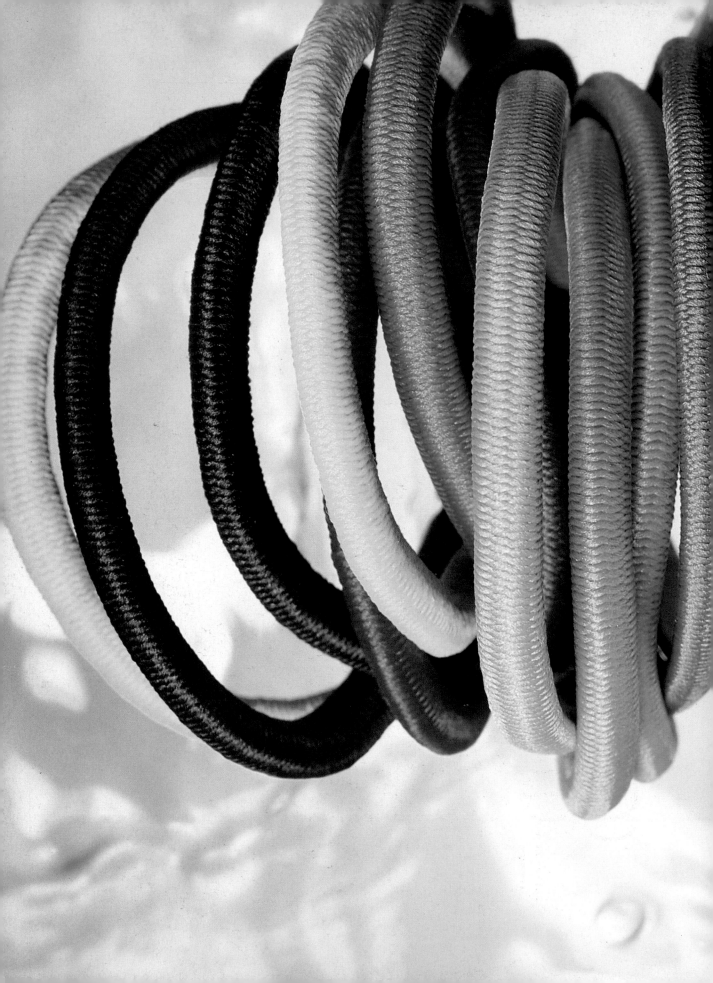

get back
into shape

exotic experiences

On her third morning, Kate woke in her tiny room at the ashram in Kerala. It was only 6 am and yet she felt completely awake and healthier than she had in ages. Her daily routine of yoga classes, meditation and cleansing Ayurvedic treatments were doing the trick. She felt more confident about herself. Her vegetarian diet and daily exercise regime had given her that sought-after smooth stomach. She knew she looked good, despite the fact that she hadn't bothered to put on even a stroke of mascara since she'd arrived. The only thing that didn't agree with the Indian climate was her hair: it had frizzed into bouncy ringlets and there was little Kate could do about it. She surprised herself by not caring in the least.

Stretching happily, Kate jumped out of bed and threw on some linen drawstring trousers and a white, fitted T-shirt. She grabbed a towel, slipped on her flip-flops and set off for her morning yoga lesson. "Good morning," said a voice behind her. It was Luke, a tall, suntanned guy who was living at the ashram for six months' training to become a yoga teacher. "Did you sleep well?" he asked Kate. "Fantastically," she replied. "I haven't felt this rested in ages. I won't know myself after two weeks here." "I thought I'd join your class this morning," said Luke.

"Great," said Kate, trying to contain her delight. She hadn't met anyone like Luke before; he was calm, intelligent and genuine to everyone he met. She was fascinated to find out more about him, what had drawn him to the ashram and why he wanted to become a yoga teacher. Perhaps breakfast after their yoga class would give them the chance to chat.

Polly was sitting on the hotel balcony at a table covered with a crisp linen tablecloth, enjoying a breakfast of fresh pineapple and papaya while gazing out over a sparkling, turquoise bay. Simon had just taken a shower and walked out onto the balcony wrapped up in a white terry robe. He looked wonderful, and Polly had never felt happier. New York, her city job and Harry all seemed a world away. "I've organized a day out on a speed boat for us, we're leaving at 10:30 so there's no need to rush," he said as he stroked her hair. "Then tonight we're having dinner at a rather special seafood restaurant one of the other guests recommended to me. It's in the next bay along from the hotel, looking out over a deserted beach."

Back in their minimalist hotel room after a sun-drenched day on the boat, Polly washed the salt and sunscreen out of her hair and thought about what she was going to wear for dinner. She wanted to look chic but relaxed, so she pulled a turquoise dress out of the wardrobe and slipped on some high-heel mules. Her golden skin looked fantastic against the turquoise of her dress. She spritzed a little volumizing spray through her hair, relieved that she had remembered to buy some mini-sized hair products in the airport before the flight. Polly then blow-dried her hair with a curling brush to put some volume into her blonde locks, before twisting her hair up into a casual but so chic chignon. She pinned her hair into place and looked at herself in the mirror. A dash of bronzing powder across her cheeks, a little sparkly eye-shadow, mascara and soft pink lip gloss were all she needed to enhance her healthy glow. She was ready for her evening with Simon.

After a short drive along the coastline, Polly and Simon were seated at a secluded table looking out over the golden sand. Simon ordered a bottle of Champagne, raised his glass to toast their evening and then reached across the table for Polly's hand. "Polly," he said, looking serious, "I've got something I want to talk to you about…"

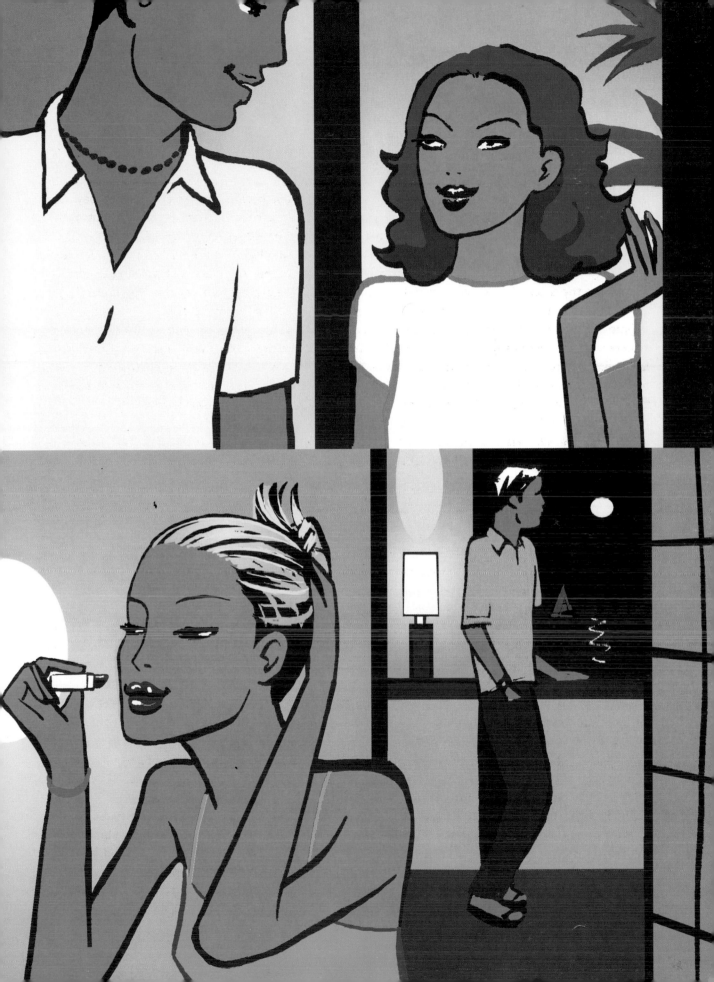

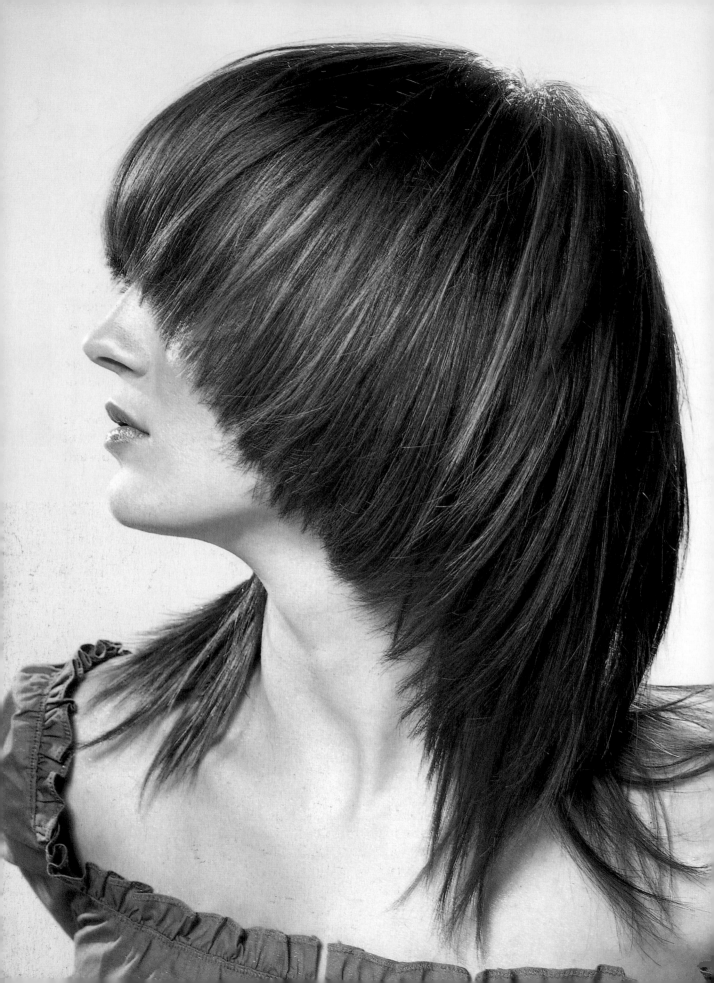

SOS hair repair

If you are concerned in any way about your hair once you get back from your vacation, go to your hair salon for a consultation. This is normally free of charge and gives you the chance to talk about the condition, cut and color of your hair with your stylist and colorist so that they can suggest the best plan of action for post-vacation haircare.

cut

The quickest way to get vacation hair back into condition is to cut out all the dry, split ends that leave it looking dull. Once hair has been cut back into shape, it will look sleek and shiny without much extra effort. Remember to book an appointment before you go away, so that you can dash into the salon when you return. If your hair is dry and damaged, your stylist may have to cut up to half an inch to get it back into condition. But if you've spent time conditioning your hair while you were away and it's in good shape on your return, your stylist can just cut the split ends without taking any length off your hair.

color

Once you are back from vacation, continue to treat your hair with conditioning treatments. This will even out porosity, maintain the condition and ensure that your next color treatment takes evenly. Give your hair a weekly detoxifying shampoo to remove the build-up of chlorine and salt water on the hair shaft. Have a good look at your color once you get home. You may love the sun-kissed highlights around your face and on the tips of your hair, so take a photograph of it. That way, your colorist has a reference and can re-create the look if you want vacation glamour put back into your hair at a later date. If your hair has gone too light, your colorist can add some deeper lowlights or apply a color gloss to tone down the overall color, make it look more natural or take it back to the color it was before your trip.

vacation tips for colored hair

A great way to start a hair-repair regime is with a scalp and head massage, as it stimulates the secretion of natural, moisturizing oils.

Use a cleansing detoxifying shampoo, which leaves the hair ultra-clean and revitalized, then apply a deep-conditioning treatment to replace moisture and even out the porosity of the hair.

Color glossing treatments rejuvenate hair color, and add shine and condition, without drying out hair.

There are products that help prevent color fade, so splash out on these before you go away — it'll be cheaper than a repair job when you return.

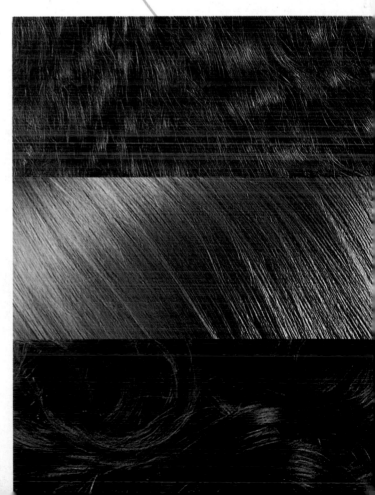

Back from their vacation, Jaz and Chrissie are feeling far from refreshed and rejuvenated. They have partied through the night and sunned themselves on the beach all day long for the entire week, and are now well and truly in need of a post-vacation overhaul. They're sitting in the kitchen assessing the damage. Chrissie has overdone the sunbathing and she's suffering the consequences — she's burned her scalp, her hair looks dry and brittle, and she's beginning to peel around her hairline. Jaz is worried about split ends. Despite her careful attempts to protect her hair, all the heat from the sun, together with her nightly hairstyling regime has left the ends dry. "Let's finish off our vacation with a pampering session," says Jaz.

"We've spent so much already, a little extra on a trip to the salon won't hurt," agrees Chrissie. "Great tans, girls," says Charles as he greets them at the salon. "But your hair is in distress!" "Do whatever you can," sighs Jaz, as the girls sit down in front of the mirrors for their consultations. Charles decides that both girls need to have an intensive deep-conditioning

...jaz's and chrissie's bad-hair day

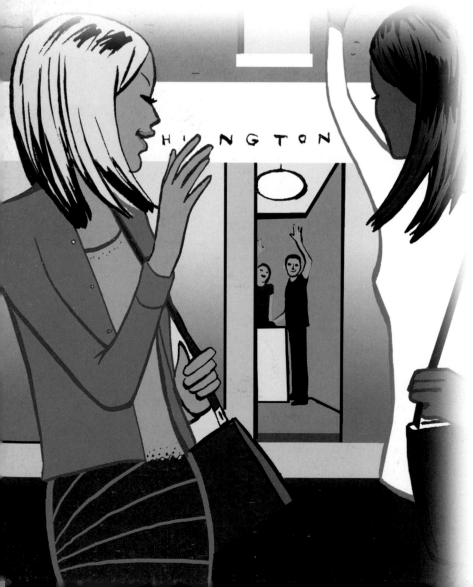

treatment to put the moisture back into their hair and revitalize the condition. Then he cuts just the ends off Jaz's hair to get rid of all the split ends without losing the length. Chrissie finds that she needs to have a bit more taken off her hair as the ends have got so dry. "You need to have some honey-blonde tints put through your hair Chrissie," says her colorist, Carolyn. "Your hair's been bleached by the sun and it's too hard on your skin tone," she advises. "I'm in your hands," says Chrissie.

Three hours later, Jaz and Chrissie leave the salon feeling more rested than they have in the whole of the last week. Their hair is looking sleek, shiny and full of body. "We should do this more often," says Chrissie as they head for a designer clothes store for a bit of window shopping. "I think I could just about get used to it," laughs Jaz.

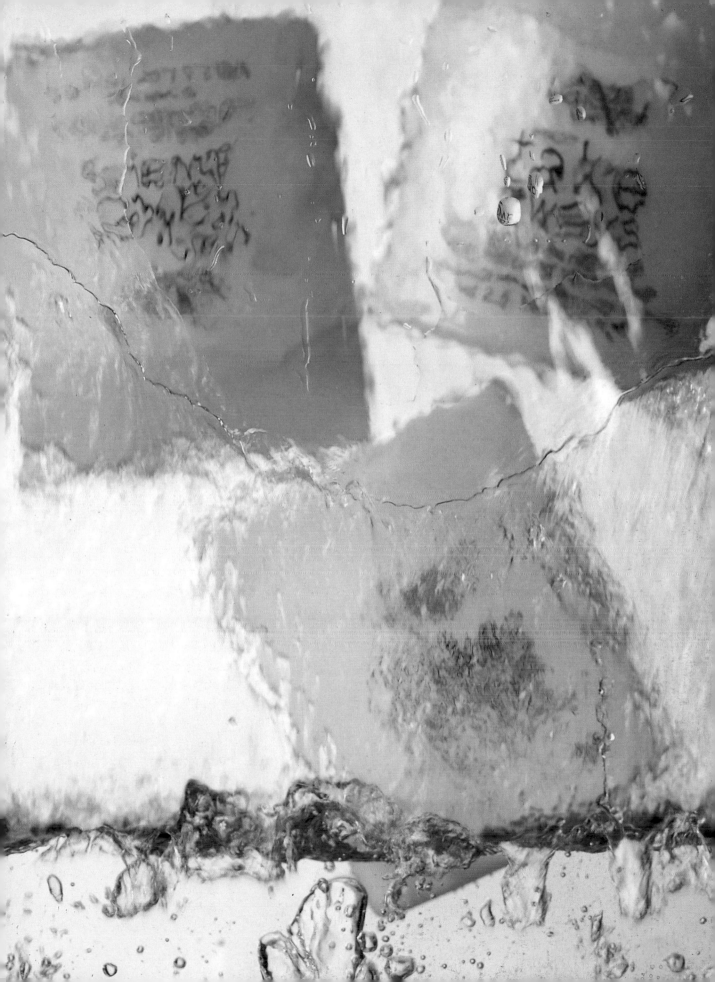

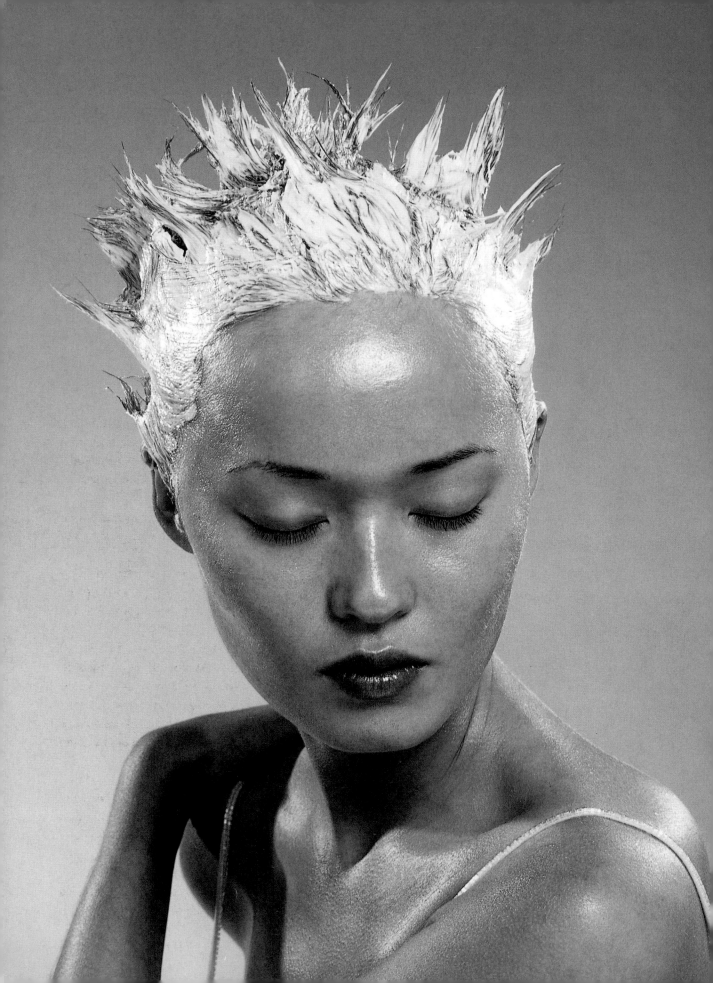

hair treats

There are a number of really effective treatments you can use to replenish the moisture levels of dehydrated hair, encourage growth, improve strength and flexibility and restore shine and gloss. You can book a treatment at your salon on your return, do it at home, or, even better, while you are on vacation to help maintain condition and prevent damage from occurring.

scalp treatment

As its name suggests, this treatment stimulates and revitalizes the skin of the scalp for better, stronger hair growth. It is usually made up of soothing and moisturizing ingredients that help to prevent itching, flaking and discomfort. It encourages the growth of new hair by nourishing the roots and it also conditions the hair shaft. Scalp treatments are good for all hair types, particularly if the scalp is burnt or dry after a vacation.

conditioning mask

Designed to be left on the hair for between three and 20 minutes, a conditioning mask will hydrate the hair shaft with moisturizing ingredients and nourish the hair and scalp without causing heaviness. Conditioning masks are designed to work most effectively on the damaged or dehydrated areas of the hair, leaving it nourished and protected. This is a good treatment to use during your vacation and on your return, whatever your hair type.

deep-conditioning treatment

More intensive than a conditioning mask, this hair treatment literally gets to the root of the problem by nourishing the scalp as well as the hair itself. It targets damaged areas and delivers intensive moisture exactly where it's needed. This extra rich treatment is best for extremely dry and parched hair.

hair detox

A deep-cleansing shampoo that removes the build-up of dirt, styling products and pollutants from the hair, without stripping it or leaving it dry. This is especially useful if your hair is looking dull after a vacation or for color-treated hair that might need a revitalizing boost.

nutrition

Diet plays a huge part in the health of our hair, and vacations are a great time to eat well and boost the body's vitality with good nutrition. The sure-fire way to make your hair limp and thin is to skip meals or eat badly. So what do you need to eat?

diet tips

Do not crash diet before you go away, as this puts strain on the system and deprives your body of essential nutrients — the first to suffer will be your hair.

A balanced wholefood diet, with essential fats, plenty of carbohydrates, protein and fresh fruit and vegetables keeps your hair healthy and shiny.

The best sources of essential fats are oily fish, such as sardines and salmon, and vegetable oils, such as olive and linseed (flax); these help to keep the skin and hair in good condition.

Eat plenty of carbohydrates such as brown rice, wholewheat pasta and lentils.

Fresh fruit, vegetables and salads provide antioxidant vitamins, which help prevent premature ageing in the body and the hair.

Since the hair is made up of protein, you need to keep your protein levels high in your diet. Fish, chicken, meat and eggs all provide the best proteins, although other sources such as nuts, cereals, milk and cheese will also supplement your intake.

hair supplements

A good daily multivitamin gives you the balance of vitamins and minerals that your body and hair need to keep them in optimum condition. The condition of your hair is boosted by all the B vitamins, gamma-linolenic acid (GLA), fish oil, linseed (flax) oil, antioxidant vitamins including beta-carotene, vitamins C and E, and the minerals selenium and zinc.

Back at home again, Kate decides to spend spend the last few hours of her vacation relaxing. She has a long shower and then applies a conditioning hair mask to her hair, twists a small towel into a turban on her head and wraps herself up in her dressing gown. Kate makes a cup of tea and then, feeling wonderfully relaxed, she settles down on the couch to watch a video.

Next morning, Kate wakes early and performs her new ritual of yoga stretches before breakfast. Getting ready for work, she takes a good look at herself in the mirror. Her lightly tanned, glowing skin needs little make-up, so she sticks to mascara and a touch of bronzer. Her curly hair is looking glossy and healthy with flattering golden streaks from the sun. She decides to leave it natural and

simply works some styling cream through the ends to give the curls extra definition. Work, and most importantly Matthew, will have to take her as they find her. If two weeks at the yoga retreat have taught her anything, it's to have the confidence to be herself. Her Miss-Get-Ahead-At-Work act has got her nowhere — perhaps her new-found contentment and inner strength will do the trick.

...kate returns home from India

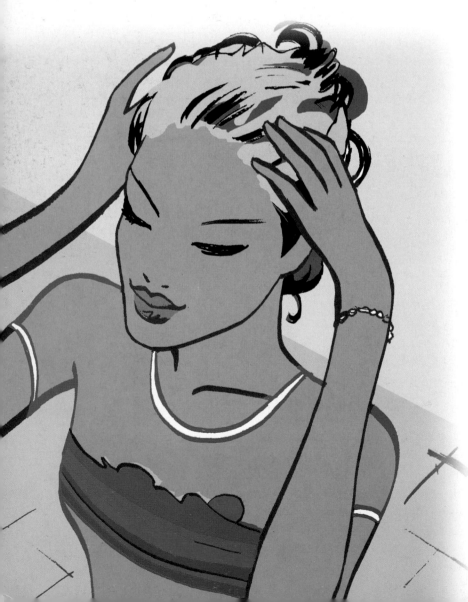

An hour later she walks into the office, makes herself a cup of green tea and sits down at her desk to check her e-mail. Matthew walks past her desk and then stops suddenly. "Kate, I hardly recognized you," he gasps. His expression changes from surprise to pleasure. "You're looking fabulous — where did you go again?" he asks. "You'd know if you'd bothered to ask," thinks Kate to herself. "India," she replies brightly. "Well, it's obviously agreed with you," Matthew says, looking her up and down. Keeping his eyes fixed on Kate as he hands her some paperwork, he suggests they go out for lunch so he can fill her in on the latest marketing project. "Sure," Kate replies calmly. She turns back to her computer, and there in her e-mail inbox is a message from Luke. "Got the job at The Yoga Centre in the Village. Will be back in two months. Missing you," it said.

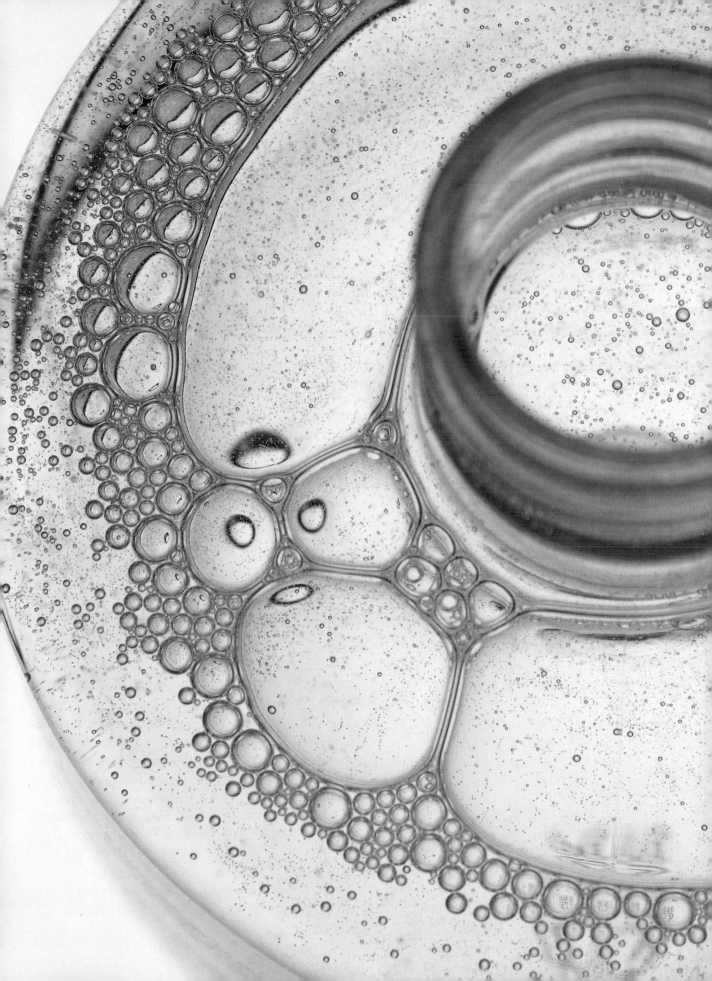

hair doctor

my blonde hair looks distinctly green after my vacation. Is there anything I can do?

The reason your hair can go green is because of the blue dye that is used to show up the chlorine in swimming pools (chlorine is, in fact, clear). Highlights make your hair more porous than usual and so the blue dye can penetrate the hair shaft and react with the highlighting chemicals in your hair. Try using a deep cleansing shampoo designed to thoroughly but gently clean hair. Or, try applying concentrated tomato juice or tomato ketchup to the hair, as the red coloring should neutralize any green in your hair. If the green tinge to your hair will not budge, you need to go to a hair salon where the stylist will "deep cleanse" your hair with a mild pre-lightening agent to lift out the color. Your colorist will then freshen up your original color.

my hair seems dull, lackluster and flat after my week away. Why is it looking so bad?

It is possible that your hair has been beaten by the combination of sun damage, chlorine or salt and, if you have been using styling products that contain silica, a build-up of product on your hair. When you return from vacation, use a clarifying shampoo to remove deep deposits of dirt and the build-up of styling products. Then book yourself into your salon and ask your stylist to trim off all the split ends — the result is immediate. Your hair will look sharp, clean and sleek. Your stylist may also recommend that you have a revitalizing hair treatment while you are in the salon, but the combination of simple cut and condition should do the trick.

my scalp is dry and flaky after my vacation. Do I have dandruff?

It's more than likely that you have burnt your scalp in the sun while you were away and the skin on your scalp is peeling. Dandruff tends to be more common among people who have oily hair, not a dry scalp. So if you have post-vacation flakes, visit your hair salon for an intensive deep-conditioning treatment that includes a scalp treatment to feed the hair as well as soothe and rehydrate the scalp. Don't rush for the nearest anti-dandruff shampoo unless the problem persists well after your return. If, after a few weeks, you still see flakes in your hairline, try using an anti-dandruff shampoo every other day. When lathered up, remember to leave the shampoo on for a few minutes to allow the ingredients to work, moisturizing and exfoliating the scalp. Alternate anti-dandruff shampoo with your usual shampoo until the problem clears.

if I wash my hair every day on vacation, will it be more oily when I return home?

It is one of the big haircare myths that washing your hair every day will make it oilier. Using a gentle, daily shampoo will not leave your hair more oily or stimulate the sebum glands on your scalp to produce more oil. More importantly, washing out the cocktail of haircare products, salt and chlorine that usually comes with vacations and putting the moisture back into your hair at the end of each day with a good conditioner leaves your hair shiny, well conditioned and healthy.

the ends of my hair seem really dry. Can I use a product to repair my split ends?

Any product that is designed to treat split ends offers only a temporary, cosmetic solution. Split-end products and hairsprays simply hold the ends together until either the hair is brushed vigorously or washed. The only way to get rid of post-vacation split ends is to have them cut off. Your hairstylist can trim the ends without taking much length off your hair, provided that you have kept it in good condition while you were away.

if I use lemon on my hair while I sunbathe, is it a "natural" way to give me highlights?

Lemon juice may help to bleach hair in the sun as the juice is acidic (although how effective it is remains debatable). But be warned: straight lemon juice is extremely damaging to the hair. It will dry it out while you lie in the sun and your scalp may be left sore and sun-sensitive. The sun will fade your hair color in a hot climate and this bleaching action damages your hair as it weakens the structure of the cells and causes permanent damage. It's best to forget about lemon juice and leave it to your hair colorist to change your color and add highlights.

polly's big announcement

The girls were all back from their globe-trotting and, at Polly's request, were having a night in together. Her living room was filled with excited chatter as they caught up on each other's news. Polly had called from the office to say that she would have to work until 8:30 but that she would bring supper with her. She had to put in some extra time after her break in Jamaica with Simon in case anyone at her firm thought she wasn't taking her job seriously.

"I'm going to open a bottle of wine — does anyone want a glass while we wait for Polly?" asked Jaz.
"Yes, and grab some chips while you're at it," ordered Chrissie, who was curled up on the floor painting her toenails with iridescent pink varnish.
"So you survived the jungle and John?" she said sarcastically to Laura, who was showing Kate her photographs of river rafting and orangutan in the jungle's nature reserve.
"It was incredible," replied Laura, who was very happily reliving the trip. "John's thinking of moving into nature documentaries. We were both so taken with the wildlife and we want to raise awareness for the conservation work that needs to be done in the jungle," she said.
"So you'd actually consider living out there for months, with all those huge insects?" asked Chrissie, shuddering visibly.
"Well, I can see how you'd have a problem living without your high heels and your hairdryer," laughed Kate, "but Laura's pretty resourceful."

"I'm home," yelled Polly, as she headed for the kitchen with a bag full of Thai food. "Come and have some food while it's hot," she called to the girls.

"I've got green curry, rice and steamed vegetables," she said as they gathered round. They each grabbed a bowl of food and took it back into the sitting room. "Champagne?" asked Polly as she joined them with a large, chilled bottle and glasses. "This is overdoing it a bit isn't it?" said Laura.
"Well, it seems to me that we've got things to celebrate," said Polly, handing the girls a glass each. Polly raised her glass in the air. "Here's to Jaz's new job in the fashion world, and to Laura and John's new venture — let's hope it works out." The girls toasted their future as they drank.

"So let's hear about Jamaica and Simon," demanded Chrissie. An uncontrollable smile spread instantly across Polly's face.
"You really like him, don't you Polly?" asked Kate.
"He's just perfect. We had the most incredible time and the thing is, well, he's asked me to marry him," Polly burst out excitedly. There was a moment's stunned silence before the girls shrieked in unison. "Marry him?" gasped Laura. "Polly, that's so quick."
"I know it seems like a whirlwind romance," agreed Polly. "I've only known him for a few months but we both know it's right and we can't see the point in hanging around and waiting. I was hoping you would all be there for me — as my bridesmaids."
"Of course we will," answered Laura quickly.
"Now tell us about the ring — have you chosen a huge stone?" asked Chrissie, true to form.

The rest of the evening was filled with wedding talk as the girls debated what Polly should wear, laughed about hideous meringue dresses and discussed how they should have their hair. Life in Tribeca certainly has changed.

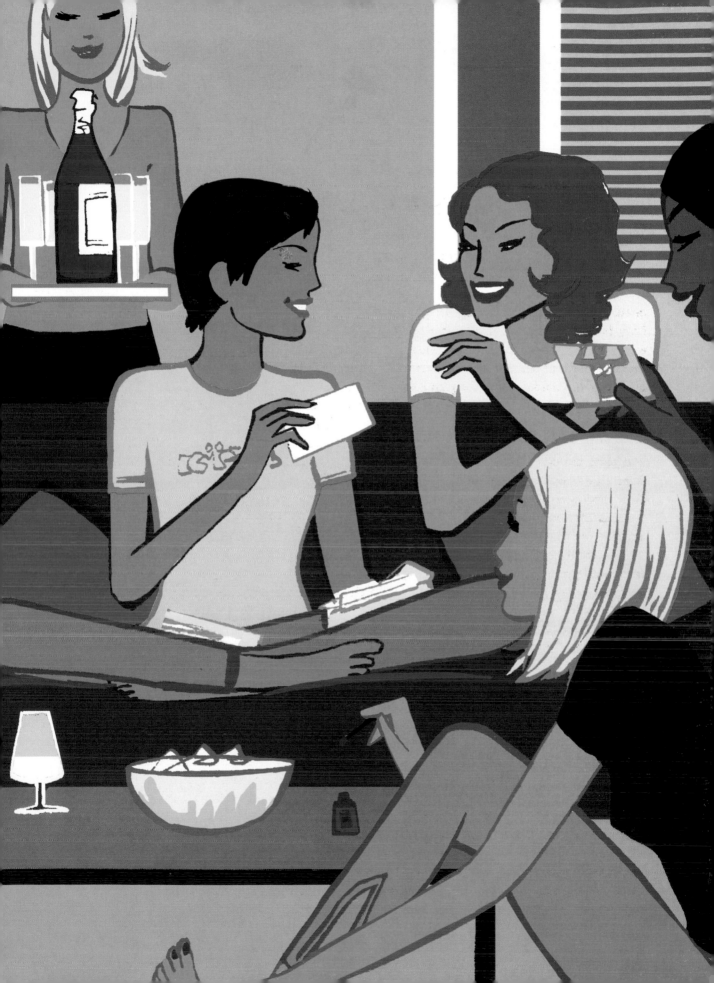

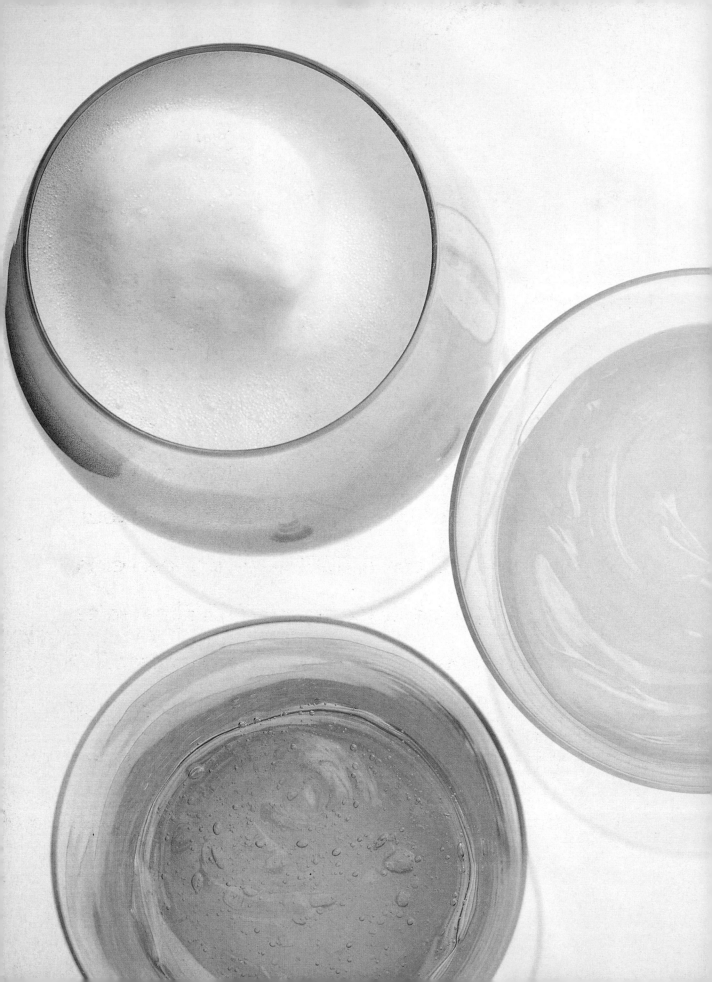

big day hair

Whatever your choice of **wedding**, think of your hair as your greatest **accessory**. Big Day Hair offers **advice** on identifying the look that best suits your **face**, dress and accessories, **tips** for getting your hair in peak **condition** before to the big day, **great** hairstyles for every type of wedding — from bohemian vintage, **classic** and country to **fashionista**, beach and **rock chic** and ideas for easy **transformations** for the **reception** and honeymoon.

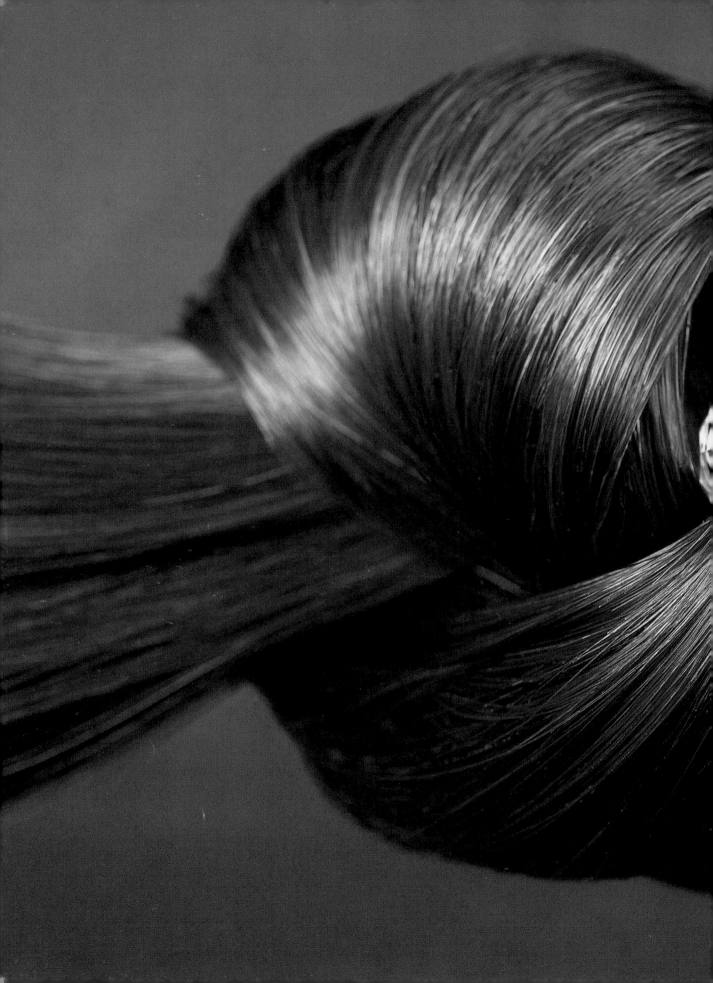

choose
your style

the girls digest polly's big news

"I think I need a drink," said Chrissie, the confirmed bachelorette of the group, in the light of Polly's announcement. "Luckily, we have some Champagne," beamed Polly, who couldn't contain her obvious glee. Jaz, Laura and Kate silently exchanged stunned glances, while they tried to take in the alarming fact that aliens may have abducted and replaced their dear friend, sensible "perfect" Polly. At last, incurably romantic Kate threw her arms around Polly. "Oh, I just knew it! This is so fabulous, you must be thrilled!" she squealed excitedly.

Laura, Polly's best friend from college, was a little less enthusiastic. "But, Polly, you've only known Simon for a few months, how can you be sure?" she asked, frowning. Polly had known that Laura would try to be the voice of reason. Even her own budding love affair with her long-term object of desire, John, didn't seem to have softened her stoic tomboy nature. "Look, I know you're only concerned for me," Polly said, flopping down onto the couch next to Laura and taking her hand, "but I know this is the right thing." She smiled happily. "We love each other. He's funny and kind, and he treats me really well." (This was a veiled reference to Polly's ex-boyfriend Harry, who had been more interested in his bank balance than in Polly.) "Well I think it's really wonderful," gushed Kate, tossing her head of wild red curls defiantly. This was unlike the normally shy Kate, who could usually be relied upon for a rather cautious response. Chrissie eyed her from head to toe, taking in her smooth honey-colored skin and her surprisingly svelte, toned thighs, revealed to their advantage by her cut-off denims. (At times, Kate had been known to overindulge in the broken rejects from her workplace, Crunch Cookies.) To top it off, she had allowed her hair to revert to its naturally curly state, and it was made even prettier by a smattering of sun-kissed golden highlights. Chrissie, as resident glamour puss, was not amused. "It's not like you to be so excitable, Kate. You didn't have a vacation romance, too, did you?" she purred, knowing full well about Kate's unrequited obsession with her boss, marketing director Matthew. But Kate remained unruffled, purring back, "Oh, this isn't about me, Chrissie, this is about Pol." Chrissie bit back her fury — why did she feel so angry?

Polly turned to Jaz, who was the only one of her friends who had yet to express an opinion. "Well, what do you think?" She enquired nervously. "I think you're not taking this seriously enough at all," Jaz responded sternly. "Don't you realize, Polly," she continued, her smile spreading as she caught the look on Polly's crestfallen face, "that this is the most important dress you're ever going to buy?"

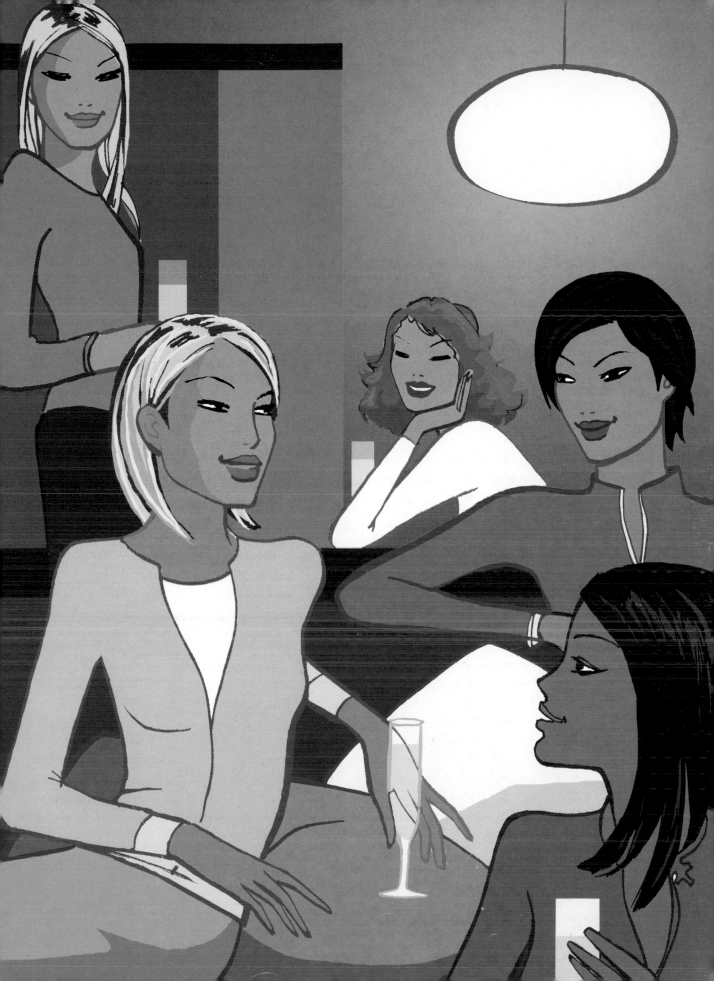

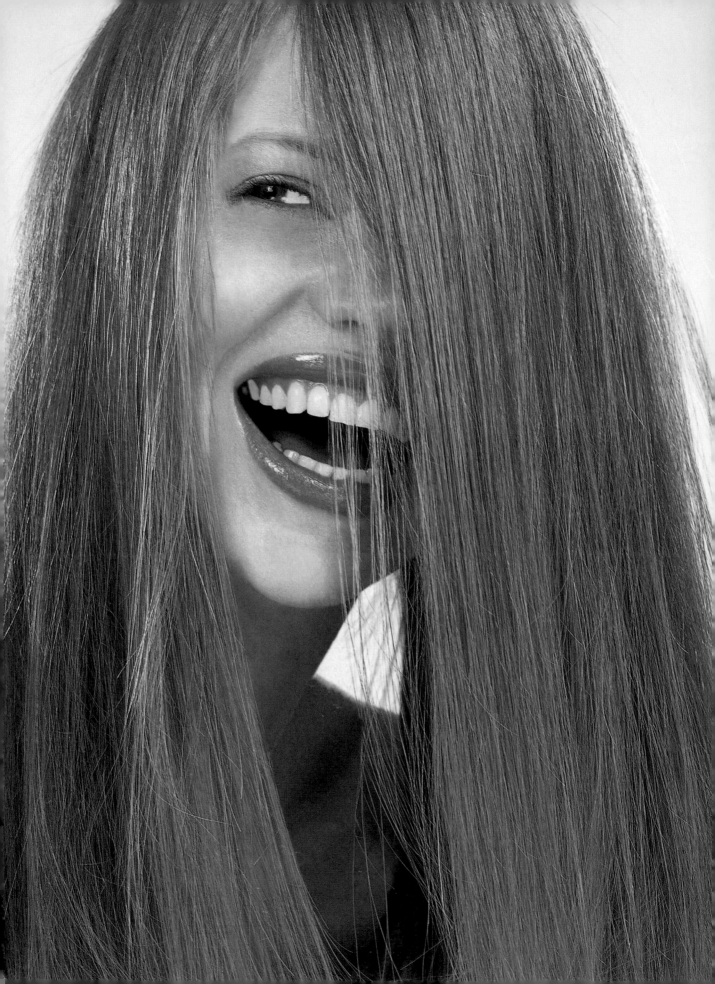

finding a look

Forget everything you know about what suits you. Whether you live in high heels and pretty cardigans or running shoes and denim, the chances are that the way you want to look on your wedding day will be completely unrelated to the way you look in your everyday life. And every variable will affect the hairstyle that you choose. Start by considering the following few elements.

dress style

Have you pictured yourself in something simple and floaty or a huge, structured confection that would be the envy of Cinderella? The way you imagine your dress to be and what style actually suits you may be two entirely different things, so take a close friend or family member shopping with you, and try on many different styles. You will be surprised.

body shape and height

We are all shaped differently, and the satin bias-cut dress of our dreams might not have been part of Mother Nature's plan when she made us. As a result, you may look fabulous enhancing your tiny waist with a fitted bodice and hiding your less tiny hips under a full skirt. This means you may need a hairstyle with more body or height to create a balanced silhouette.

neckline

Your hairstyle and dress need to work together. A low scooping neckline can look wonderfully romantic with loose tendrils of hair, whereas a chic bob with a sleek slash neck is exceptionally elegant. If you have a low back on your dress, you can draw attention to this feature by wearing your hair swept up and away from your neck. Take a photograph or sketch of your dress with you to your hairdresser so you can consider which hairstyles will make the most of its features.

tiaras and veils

Although it is not uncommon to have both a tiara and a veil, most brides choose to wear either one or the other. And, as weddings have become more informal, a few simple flowers dotted through the hair are also a popular alternative to both of these options. A long veil or heavy tiara will need to be held securely in place, and this will influence your choice of hairstyle. If you can, take your tiara (or at least a photograph of it) with you when you go for a consultation with your hairdresser, so that he or she can work out exactly what will need to be done.

face shape

You probably know what suits you by now, and this is not usually the time that women opt for a drastic change in their look. (It's nice if he recognizes you when you walk down the aisle.) However, unless you are a very high-maintenance girl and do your weekly shopping wearing a tiara, you probably won't know how it affects the proportions of your face. A petite heart-shaped face may look better with a simple beaded tiara, rather than drowned by a grand crown and full veil. So it's back to dressing up — try on many styles and see if your reality matches your fantasy.

jewelry

One of the "Something old, something new" categories is often fulfilled with jewelry. So, whether you choose a string of antique pearls from your grandmother or a funky, dramatic choker from one of your bridesmaids, it needs consideration at this stage, too. A tiara, veil, earrings, choker and high collar can quickly become very fussy. Don't let your look become cluttered — less is always more (even with diamonds).

HAIR SNIP
WHEN CHOOSING ACCESSORIES FOR YOUR HAIR, WHETHER IT IS FRESH FLOWERS OR AN ANTIQUE BROOCH, MAKE SURE IT BALANCES WITH THE REST OF YOUR OUTFIT — SOMETIMES LESS IS MORE.

In beauty and fashion matters, Jaz is regarded as the oracle, so Polly invites her along to her appointment with her trusted stylist Charles. For the last few years, he has kept her wavy locks blonder and straighter than nature ever intended them to be.

Despite her impulsive decision to get married, Polly's cautious nature has reasserted itself and she pulls from her bag a neat file of pictures from bridal magazines. At the same time, Jaz produces a jumble of catwalk photos, slides from hair shows (borrowed from Aristo PR) and pages torn out of *Gloss* magazine. Charles grins and tells the girls that they need to go back to basics. Polly's hair has a natural wave, which she usually straightens and smooths with a styling lotion. The sun has lightened it to a uniform, creamy blonde that works well with her tan, but makes her fine hair seem thin. They agree that she should have caramel lowlights to make her hair look thicker.

Next, they look at pictures of the dress. Polly has chosen a close-fitting, full-length dress in off-white duchesse satin. Chic and elegant, it has a high neck, three-quarter length sleeves and a low, scooped back. For protection from the elements,

...polly's consultation with charles

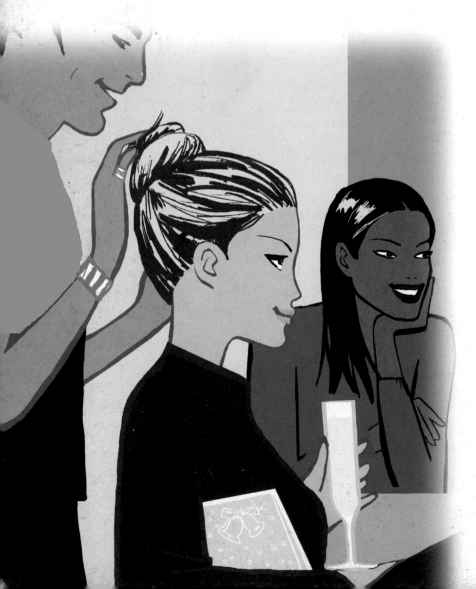

she's chosen a fitted high-collar jacket. Charles believes that such a formal dress deserves a formal updo. The hair should be swept up to draw attention to the dramatic plunging dress and show off her slender, tanned back. The next consideration is the jacket, the high collar of which will skim the back of her neck. Charles thinks that to avoid looking fussy, her hairstyle must be simple and clean (which rules out Jaz's pictures of a half-up, half-down do with wispy tendrils and rhinestone clips). After much wrangling (veil too much with the jacket, jewelery too fussy for the neckline), they settle on a classic chignon, with a tiara and simple diamond earrings. A slightly despondent Jaz (doesn't Polly know that matrimony is fashionable?) is cheered when Polly escorts her out of the salon, telling her it's time to select the bridesmaids' dresses.

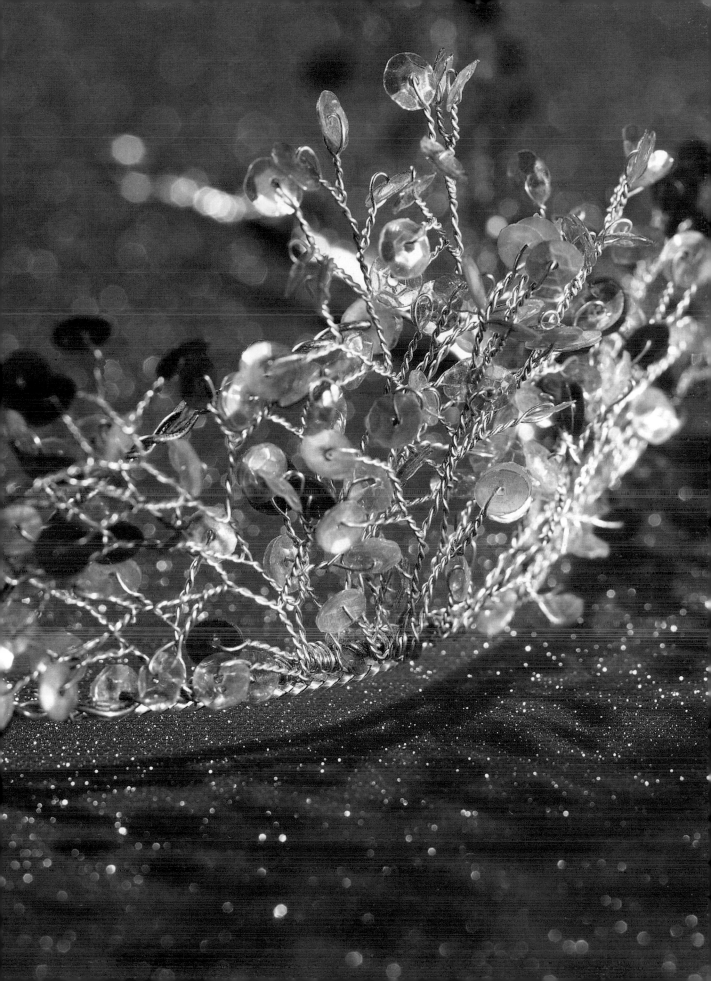

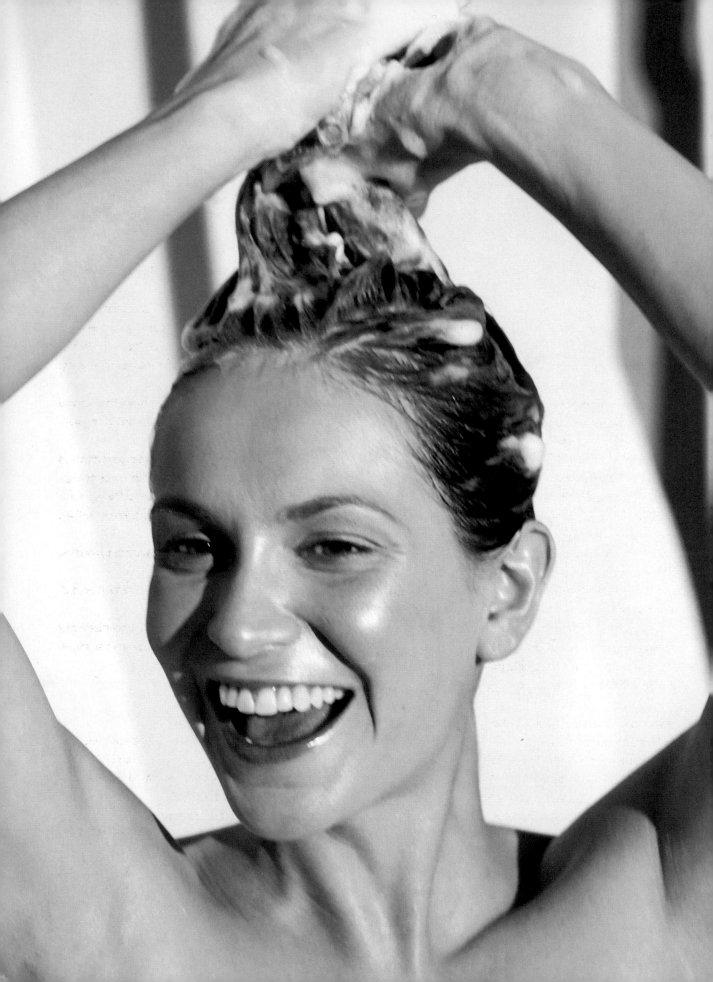

condition

The next consideration is the condition of your hair. A head of strong, beautifully conditioned hair always attracts the eye (and compliments). You can tackle this in two ways — from the inside and the outside.

inside

It makes sense that what we put into our bodies affects how well we look and feel, and the quality of our diet is reflected in the state of our hair. Although you can use good-quality shampoos and styling agents to enhance the cosmetic appearance of your hair, you can improve its condition drastically by giving it the nourishment it needs from inside. Hair needs iron, zinc, protein and vitamins A, C and B_{12}. While a good, varied diet that includes all of these should be enough for healthy hair, a significant deficiency in some of them (such as zinc or vitamin B_{12}) can be linked to hair loss. As well as standard vitamin pills, there are also specific supplements designed to promote healthy hair, skin and nails. Dehydration can have a disastrous effect on the condition of the hair, so make sure that you drink at least eight glasses of water every day.

Another important issue for many brides is weight loss. Shedding extra pounds quickly may be tempting, but if you do not diet sensibly, you deprive your hair — and the rest of your body — of essential nutrients. When under stress (and crash dieting is an attack on the system), the body shuts down the delivery of nutrients to all non-essential organs, and the first to suffer are hair and nails. The results of crash dieting can take up to three months to show in your hair and also appear in your skin. Even with such an important deadline looming, there is no substitute for a sensible exercise and dieting routine.

warning

If you are concerned about a supplement, consult your pharmacist. If you experience problems, see your doctor.

Stress, anxiety and sleeplessness can all take their toll on the condition of the hair. Here are a few of the many excellent herbal remedies and supplements that can help:

Calcium and magnesium are often depleted through stress and are needed to help control anxiety and fear.

Camomile tea is soothing and can be great for keeping nervousness at bay; it is a good alternative to regular tea, which contains caffeine — a known stimulant that can heighten feelings of anxiety.

Kava kava promotes a feeling of wellbeing and is very good for soothing tension.

Lavender is a relaxing essential oil. Dilute a few drops in water or vegetable oil and massage it into your scalp. The massage helps increase the blood flow to the scalp and bring nutrients to the hair follicle.

Mimulus helps alleviate fears over impending events.

Valerian can be used as a relaxant or sleeping aid.

White chestnut stops those constant organizational worries from keeping you awake at night.

outside

If you have serious concerns, visit a trichologist; hair loss, flaky scalp or dandruff may be signs of a diet deficiency, which can be easily remedied. However, if the bad condition of your hair is due to overprocessing or an ill-advised color experiment, your hairdresser should be able to help restore your crowning glory. See your hairdresser as soon as possible to give them the opportunity to organize an effective treatment plan. Although treatments have their limitations, a lot can be done to salvage beleaguered hair.

salon solutions

regular trims

Be realistic, and don't scrimp on trims just because you want to change your style. If you have only two months until the big day and always imagined having undulating waves to the small of your back, obviously you will have to accept defeat if you are currently sporting a gamine crop (unless you want to go for the full wig option — which is not usually a wise idea if you don't want it to be the topic of conversation all day). Hair grows at an average rate of half an inch per month, and making the classic mistake of scrapping regular trims won't help — split ends will keep on splitting up the hair shaft and look awful. The only permanent remedy is cutting them off.

intense moisture mask

This cream-based conditioning treatment is designed to work on the hair in much the same way as a facial moisturizer works on the skin. Once the cream has been spread evenly through the hair, heat is applied, in the form of hot towels or a dryer, to open the hair shaft and allow conditioning agents to penetrate it fully.

express destress

Tailor-made to tackle your specific hair problems, this treatment often incorporates a scalp and shoulder massage. This helps increase the blood flow (and therefore the delivery of nutrients) to the hair shaft, as well as relieving stress, a serious contributor to dull hair.

intense strengthening mask

Ideal for those who have seriously abused their hair, this liquid-form protein-based moisturizer is designed to give a boost to weak, damaged hair. Your hairdresser may suggest a series of these treatments, as the effects are cumulative. For best results, a shine enhancing conditioner is applied at the final stage.

shine-on color treatment

Color is a great way of bringing condition and body to the hair. Even if you are happy with your natural color, a rinse in the same tone can bring extra shine. Derived from vegetable extracts, shine-on colors are excellent for rehydrating dry hair and bringing "oomph" back to hair that has already been dyed but has lost its original sheen. On fine hair, the color can plump up the hair shaft and add much-needed volume. To provide maximum depth to flat hair, two colors are used, one on the top section and one underneath.

It is very important to remember that even some of the gentlest of chemical treatments can dehydrate the hair, therefore it might need a little more TLC than normal. Choose a shampoo, conditioner and styling products that are designed to help maintain your color and reduce any discoloring or fading.

scalp energizer

A healthy scalp usually means healthy hair, but even those without scalp problems can benefit from this treatment. The exfoliating action leaves the scalp exceptionally clean, while the increased blood flow delivers extra nutrients and oxygen to the hair, improving its condition.

home help

A great way to get your bridesmaids to help with the invitations, guest list or any other wedding chore, is to have a big girls' night in, under the pretense of some pre-nuptial pampering. You could even make them a monthly event, which will do your hair and organizational skills the world of good.

Most salon treatments can be simplified for home use, and there are many great effective treatments available from your salon. Take a few tips from the professionals, and use hot towels and plastic caps to encourage the hair shaft to open and to maximize the effectiveness of your chosen products.

HAIR SNIP
REMEMBER, ALWAYS RINSE YOUR HAIR THOROUGHLY — AND FINISHING WITH AN ICE-COLD RINSE WILL GIVE MAXIMUM SHINE.

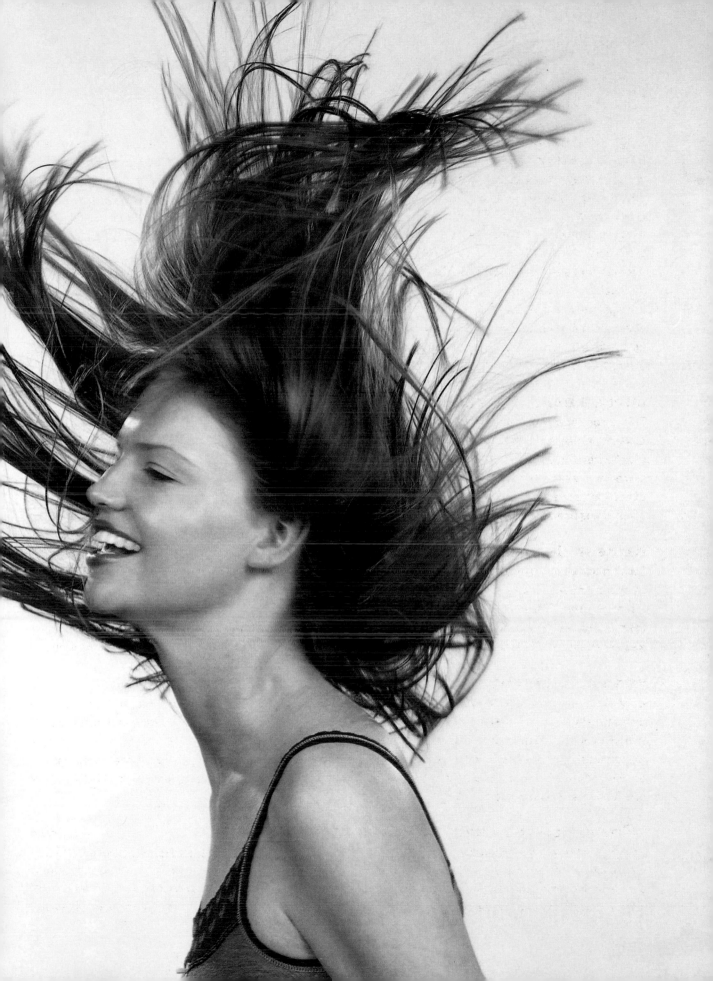

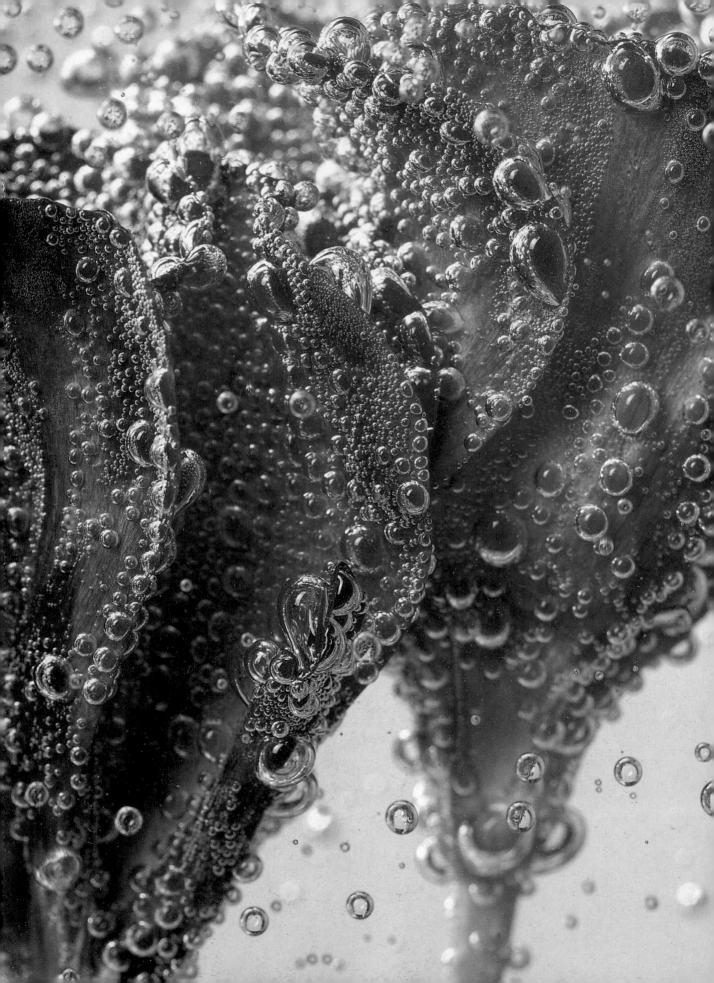

Laura knows that she has changed since meeting John, much more so than she'd like to admit. After spending such a long time hoping to get his attention, things are moving pretty fast. She's even had to acknowledge that her growing interest in her appearance is earlier in the year from a low-maintenance crop to a slightly longer bangs and light flick-outs at the nape, is thrilled to get a second chance to reinvent Laura. In two and a half months, hair will grow over one inch. As Laura's current style is already beginning to grow out, her stylist suggests letting the bangs grow out and having it cut over to one side. The rest of her hair will be allowed to grow into a sleek, slightly layered short bob — feminine, but still right for Laura's usual uniform of T-shirt and combat boots.

...laura goes for another restyle

less to do with sharing a place with looks-obsessed Chrissie and Jaz, and more to do with catching John's attention.

After the initial shock, Laura has become more supportive of what she considers to be Polly's impulsive decision to marry Simon — despite the fact it might leave them all homeless. It may also have something to do with flattery — Polly has asked her to be Maid of Honour (although Laura sometimes wonders whether Polly reached this decision largely because of her organizational skills, especially considering the lack of help she's had from the others with planning the hen night).

Laura's decided to see her stylist about growing her short hair, hoping that a slightly longer style will seem less severe next to Polly's sleek updo. Her hairdresser, who helped her restyle her hair

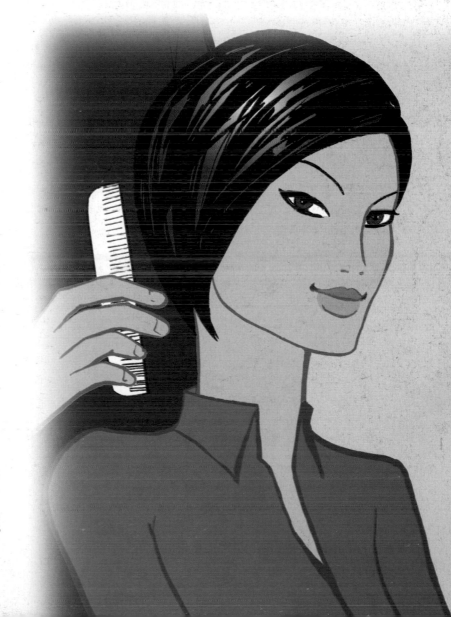

wedding wisdom

As soon as a girl accepts a proposal, everyone has an opinion. Hopefully these tips should help you keep focused on what you want.

1 Start cheating. Don't be despondent if you think your hair doesn't naturally have the qualities you want. This is the most special of occasions and your style doesn't have to be practical or able to function in the real world — just as long as you can make it last the day. There are many tricks of the trade to help you create the illusion that you want: hairpieces can add volume, straighteners can make hair ultra-sleek and a well-placed veil can make even short hair appear long. Your hairdresser could be your greatest ally.

2 If you are wearing a long veil, keep your hairstyle as simple as possible.

3 Don't be tempted to go for a radical restyle — it's you he has asked to marry and it's you he wants to see at the altar.

4 How will you get to the church? Whether it's a horse-drawn carriage or a scooter, tell your stylist so that he or she can disaster-proof you!

5 Remember to have long hair trimmed before the big day — even just an inch of growth could make the style you have settled on impossible to achieve.

6 Always have a full trial run with your veil and/or tiara before the big day.

7 If you are not happy with what your hairdresser has done, say so. He or she would rather start again than have it ruin your day.

8 Your dress, veil, flowers, tiara, hair and even shoes should all create a cohesive look — give your stylist as much visual reference as you can to help you achieve that.

9 There's no need to change hairdressers if you have a good rapport with your current one. He or she knows your hair and how to get the best from it. Do make sure, though, that they feel comfortable doing it. (Your favorite colorist, for example, may not be the person for the job!)

10 Don't get an attack of "wedding ringlets". If your style is simple, don't let others bully you into a look you don't feel comfortable with just because they perceive it as being more glamorous.

11 Short hair can look just as feminine as longer styles, and if you know that it suits you, you're better off sticking with what you've got.

12 Some subtle highlights around the face are a great way to lift the complexion and draw attention to the face.

13 Make sure you give plenty of notice if you want a particular stylist to do your hair on the morning of the wedding.

14 Using every styling product on the market to try and keep your hair in place will only make it look dirty and weighed down. Select products carefully and have a trial run to see how much you really need.

15 Work with your hair type if you can — will your long, straight hair really stay in curls all day?

16 Take a camera to the hairdresser's with you. You will be surprised how something that looks good in real life doesn't always look great in photographs. This will also give you some reference material to show to your family and friends.

17 You must start planning your hairstyle approximately three months in advance. This means that you will have the time to get your hair into top condition, with two or three conditioning treatments at your salon, and have two trial runs of the actual style. Having trial runs will make sure you get the style right so that you feel more positive about the day.

countdown

In an ideal world, brides would begin thinking about their haircare regime at least nine months before the wedding. This would allow ample time to improve the condition of the hair with treatments and any necessary changes to diet and lifestyle before even choosing a hairstyle. This is especially important if you suffer from alopecia (hair loss) or seborheic dermatitis (a condition that results in a flaky scalp); these are often caused by a dietary deficiency and can be treated by a trichologist (see page 239). Likewise, if your hair is in poor condition due to chemical processing or overstyling, make an appointment to see your hairdresser as soon as you can to allow time to implement an effective treatment program.

Ultimately, your hairdo and the accessories you choose should reflect your style and personality in the same way as your choice of dress. So, while it is a good idea to gather inspiration from magazines, don't force yourself to adopt a look that is not really "you". Try not to change yourself too much, but make the most of what you've got and maximize your good points. Always take a photo or sketch of your dress and a swatch of fabric to your first hair consultation and ask your hairdresser's advice on accessories and flowers. You might like to try out a few different hairstyles before settling on the right one, and always have a full trial run — complete with accessories, veil and tiara — in advance of the big day. Take someone with you whose advice you trust for an honest second opinion. Use the table below to help you plan ahead.

pre-wedding hair tips

Are you using the right haircare products for your hair type? For example, if your hair is fine and limp, this may be due to your conditioner being too heavy. Assess the condition of your hair and look at your current haircare regime.

Collect pictures for your scrapbook of hairstyles and colors that you like from all sources, not just from wedding magazines.

Do take polaroids of your hair rehearsals — otherwise it will be impossible for you or your hairdresser to remember every detail.

Even if results seem slow to emerge, stick with your treatment plan. The effects are cumulative and the end result will be worth it.

In the period leading up to your wedding, try and give your hair a break from intensive styling methods whenever possible.

Florists can provide blooms all year round now, but find out which will be in season on the big day. It's a sweet reminder of your wedding to see the flowers you wore in your hair in bloom for your anniversary in years to come.

6 months	5 months	4 months	3 months	2 months	1 month
See your hair-dresser to discuss your plans and book all your appointments.	Experiment with various color options so you can achieve the optimum look.	Collect a scrapbook of style options and discuss these with your stylist.	Begin weekly conditioning treatments.	Order the flowers for your hair. Have your first trial run at the salon.	Have a second trial run with your veil/tiara. Reconfirm your final cut and color.

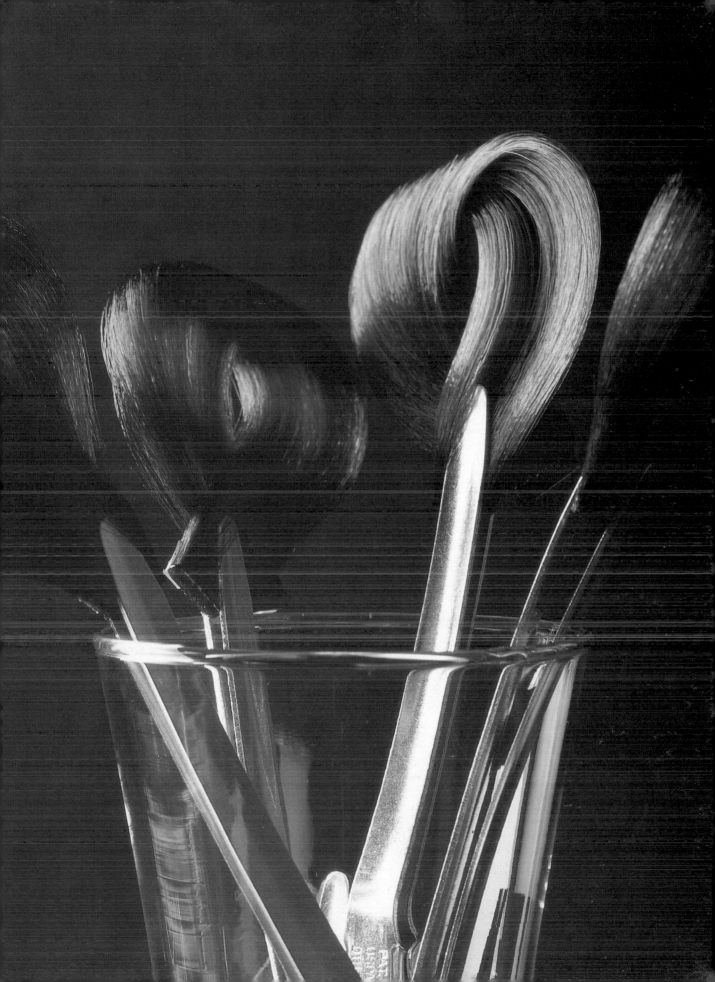

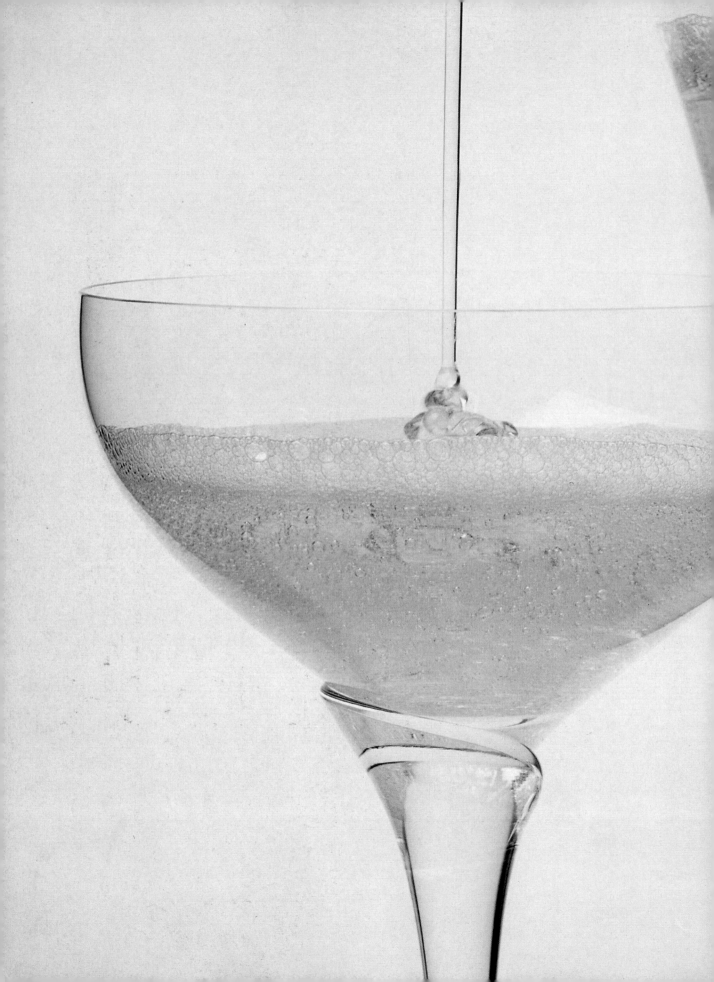

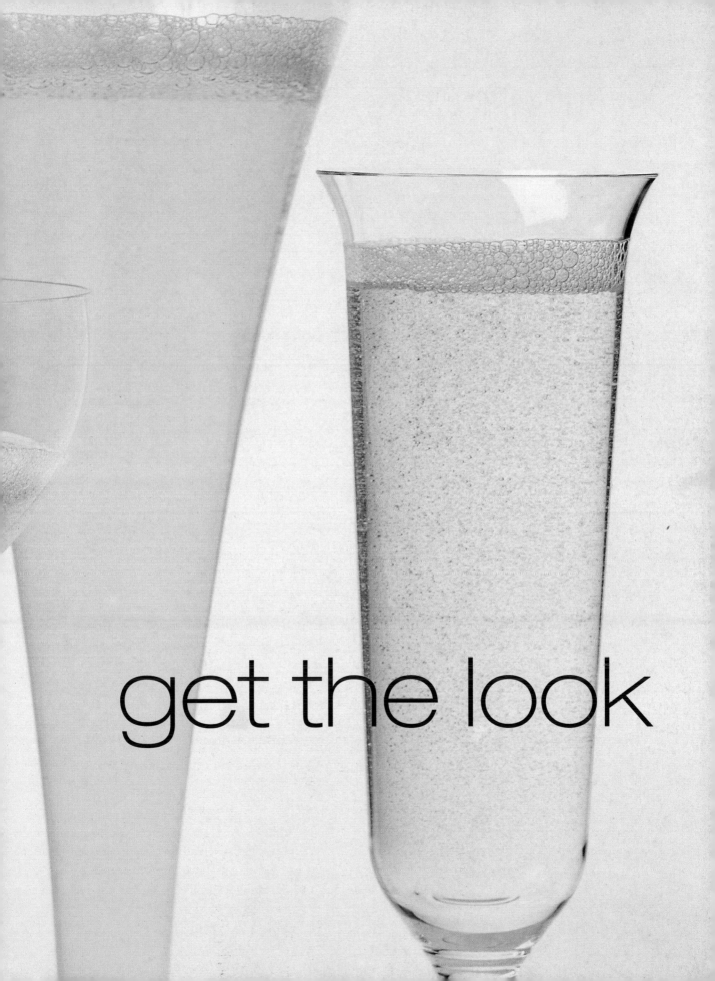

get the look

wedding fever

Every surface of Polly's formerly immaculate condo was covered with wedding magazines, invitations, lists and scraps of fabric.

"I would have thought," said Chrissie, pinching a piece of Laura's toast and munching it cautiously through her regular Saturday morning face pack, "that you would have approached this wedding with your usual degree of organization." Laura and Kate exchanged glances. Chrissie was becoming unbearable, always ready with a sharp word or criticism.

"You try organizing a wedding in only two months," sighed Polly, oblivious to Chrissie's critical tone. "Now, let's get on with the business in hand — your outfits."

Jaz started to wriggle on her chair, never more excited than when talking about clothes. "Well, girls, we chose the fabric last week and I think you are just going to love it!" she squealed. The girls held their breath collectively — why on earth was Polly letting Jaz choose their dresses? Did she really want them tripping down the aisle in leopard skin and neon fishnets? Jaz pulled out two swatches of fabric, silk georgette in pale pink and lilac. So far, so elegant. Surely there had to be a catch.

"We thought," said Polly, enjoying their surprise, "or rather Jaz did, that these two colors would suit all your hair and skin tones."

"And," added Jaz excitedly, "that we would have each dress in the color you choose with a contrasting detail. For example, Laura, with your dark hair, you'd look lovely in lilac with a split revealing the pink; and Kate, you'd suit pink with a draped neck lined with lilac."

Chrissie was impressed and slightly annoyed — maybe Jaz knew more about fashion than just trends. "So we don't all have to look the same?" she asked — she hated the thought of resembling anyone else.

"Well, within reason," cautioned Polly. "But since you're all different shapes, as well as such different characters, it makes sense to let you all have an input and make the most of your best features."

"And what about our hair?" asked Chrissie, who had long believed that her straight, blonde, shiny hair was the secret to all her powers. She had been praying that Polly wouldn't expect her to hide it all away in a childish corn row or, worse, an attack of dreaded "wedding ringlets".

"Well, I want you all to incorporate some little pink roses into your style in some way, but how is entirely up to you. Just nothing too crazy," Polly said, eyeing Jaz's latest tie-dyed style.

"What about your hair?" asked Kate. Polly beamed, "Well, I'm not giving too much away, but I saw Charles last week and we have a plan — I'm getting it cut and colored the week before, and in the mean time I'm having treatments every two weeks to improve the condition." She paused to pop a slab of buttery, white muffin into her mouth. Kate looked startled. "But don't you know that what you put into your body is just as important to your hair's condition as what you treat it with externally? By the time you get married all the stress of the planning, late nights and takeout food will start showing in your hair." Polly sipped her coffee guiltily — Kate was right, she had been pushing herself extra hard at work to get things finished so she could go on a long honeymoon. Simon was still in Miami, so all the planning was left mainly to her. On top of that, she still hadn't told the girls that she wasn't moving to Miami to be with Simon, but that he would be transferring to New York. That meant that they would want the condo for themselves — and the girls would have to move out. She was definitely a woman under pressure.

"There's nothing like a convert for giving unsolicited advice," said Chrissie, referring to Kate's recent transformation from cookie-muncher to abs-cruncher. Sensing Kate's and Chrissie's rivalry, Laura stepped in. "Don't forget, everyone, that I expect you all to be ready to hit the bars running next Saturday for one of Polly's last nights of freedom." She wrapped an arm around each of the girls' shoulders, "and I expect all of Polly's friends to be very friendly."

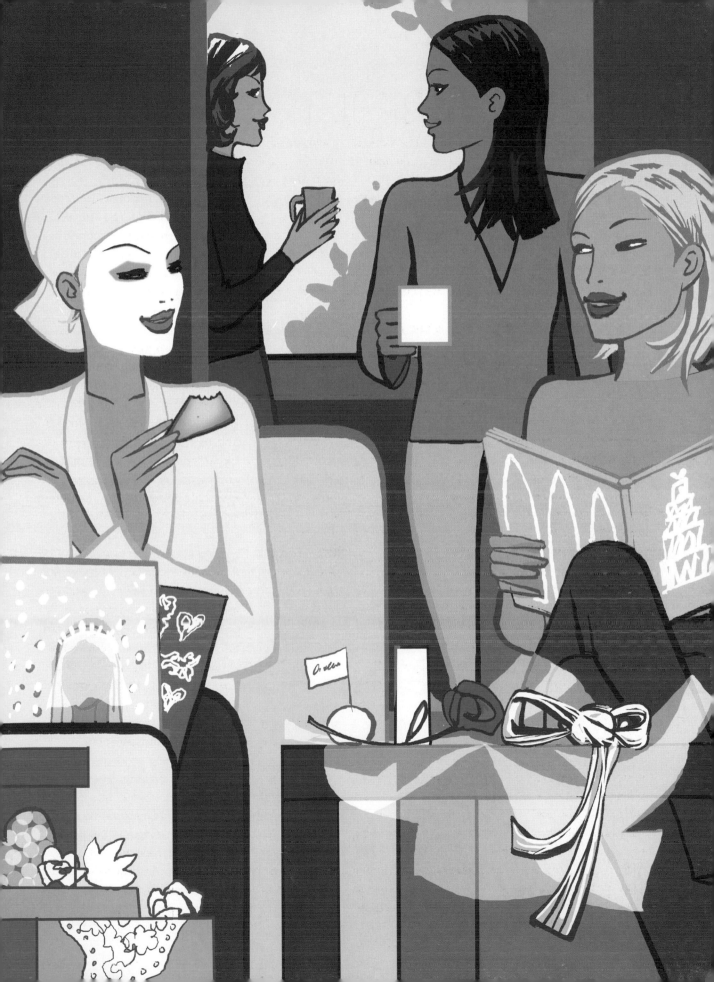

bohemian vintage

This girl is never happier than when rummaging through antique shops and flea markets, searching for vintage dresses, silk gloves and beaded purses. At the end of her bed she keeps an old pine trunk, overflowing with diaphanous slips, pretty scraps of antique lace, and romantic Victorian nightgowns. For her wedding day, she'd team a snugly fitting Edwardian bodice with a full tulle skirt, and wear a romantic amethyst choker.

hair solutions

If you have long hair, you could opt for a half-up, half-down do, with your hair half obscuring your crown, but with delicate tendrils framing your face. Mid-length hair can create the illusion of length when it is pulled back under a two-tier lace veil. Short hair can be softened with light-hold wax and decorated with beaded clips or ornaments, such as butterflies.

LEFT AND RIGHT

The hair is curled using a light blow-dry spray to give flexibility and movement. Three bun rings are pinned together and placed on the crown of the head. The hair is wrapped around the rings, pinned securely in place and finished with firm-hold hairspray. A natural-colored cord is wound around the hair and fastened behind the ear. If you want to dress the hair further, add an ornate hair pin on one side of the head, and hold it in place using fine pins.

OVERLEAF

To create this romantic look, you can employ either the classic technique of braiding damp hair and leaving it to dry before you unraveling the braids, or the modern technique of using a hot waving iron. Use a shine enhancing spray to finish and simply dress the style with a fine necklace or hair ornament pinned around the forehead.

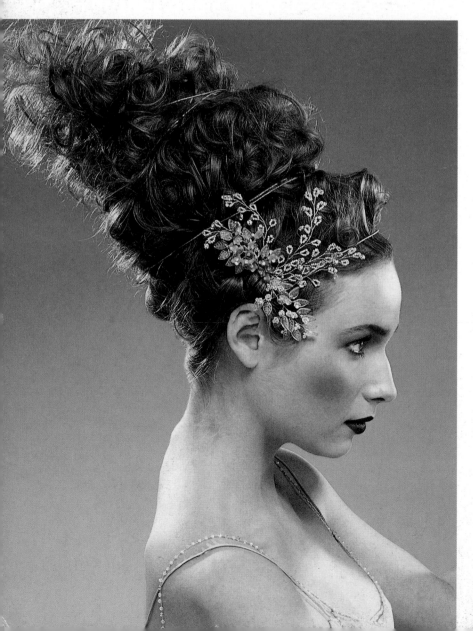

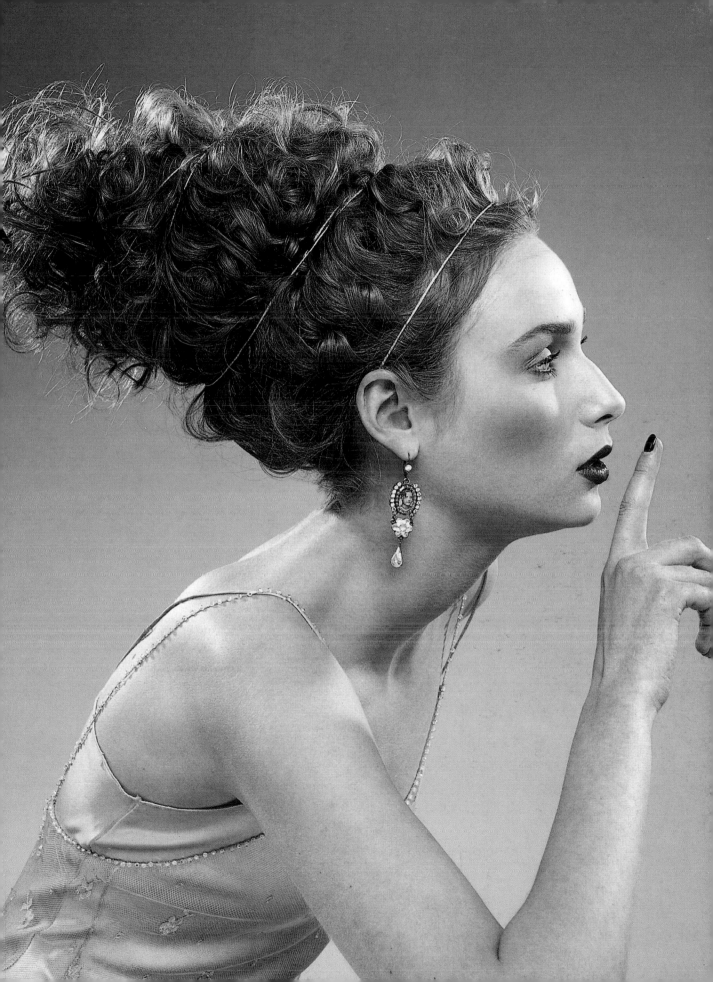

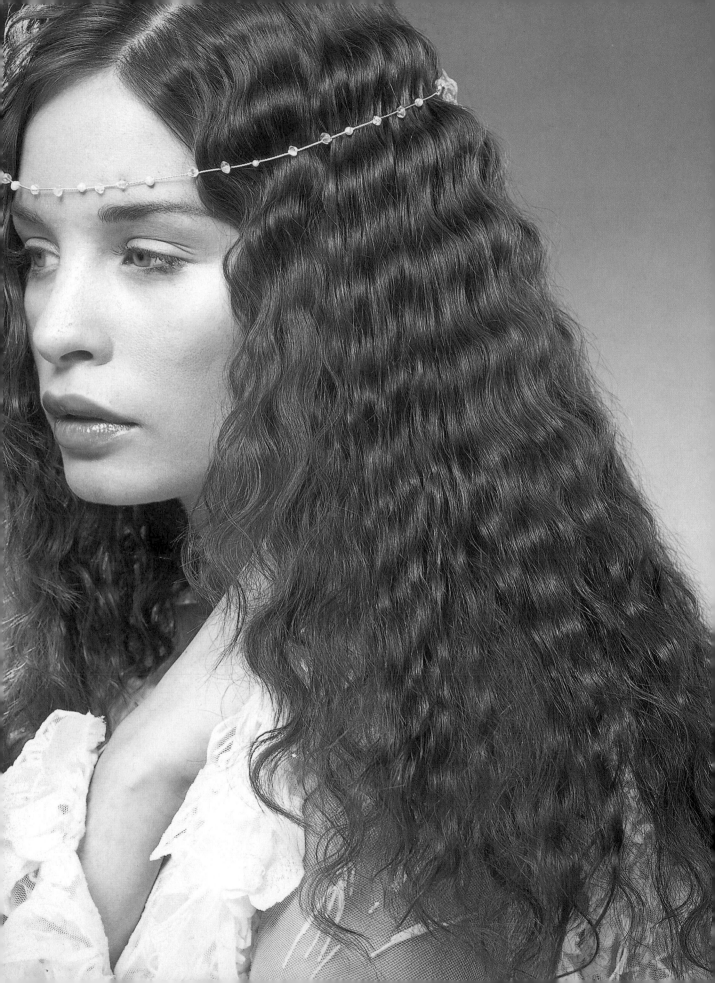

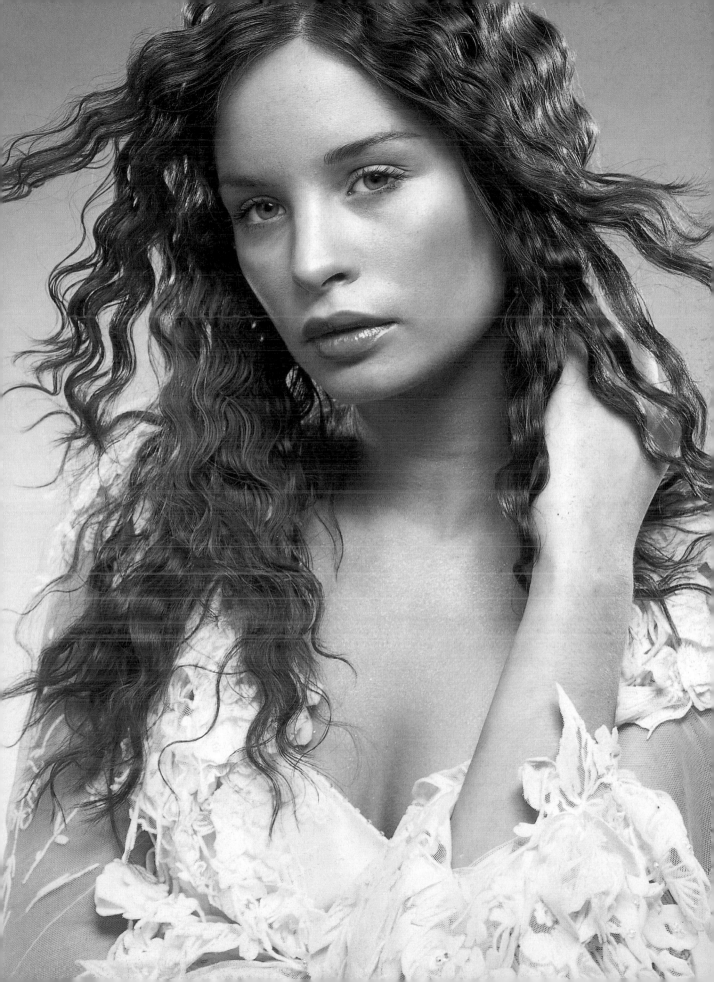

country

The girl who goes for the country style loves all things pretty and natural, and that includes her look. Her dress will be a simple, feminine home-made affair; she'll carry a bouquet of wild flowers and wear a garland in her hair.

hair solutions

Keep your hair unstructured and, if it's long, flowing loose over your shoulders. Flowers are the obvious choice for decoration, but keep them simple, small and dotted throughout the hair. Alternatively, take two sections of hair from the front and braid them, incorporating fine ribbons in shades of bright and baby pink; secure the back with a band and conceal it by wrapping a length of ribbon around it. A wild flower garland creates a feminine look for short hair.

BELOW AND RIGHT

The hair is sectioned into narrow segments, working forwards from the centre of the crown, twisted into tight knots and secured along the hairline with bobby pins. The ends of the hair are left loose for a natural, romantic finish. For a dramatic look, decorate the knots with feathers that match your outfit.

OVERLEAF

Sections of the hair are sprayed using a fine-hold hairspray, and various sizes of curling irons are used to create romantic ringlets. These can be left *au naturel* for a stronger look (left), or the curls can be broken up with fingers for a Lady Godiva look (right). Finish with a shine-enhancing spray or styling lotion to add curl definition. Various accessories can be used — from natural blooms to tiaras and strands of beads.

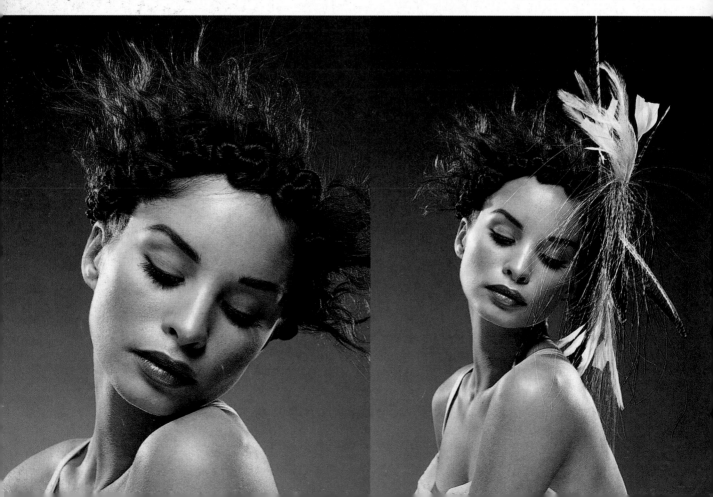

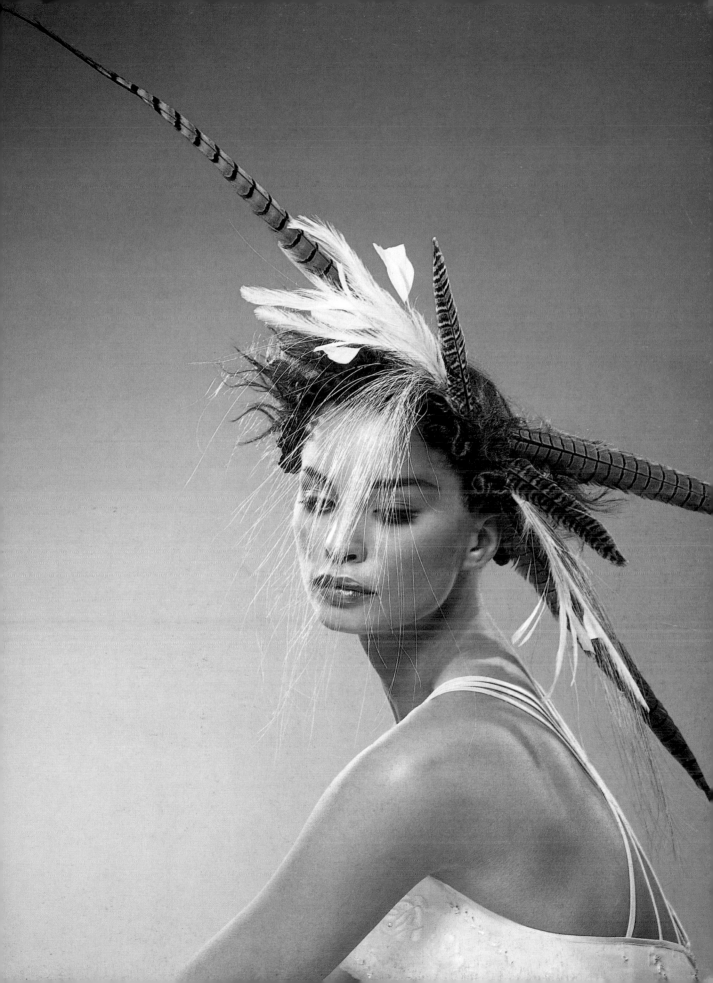

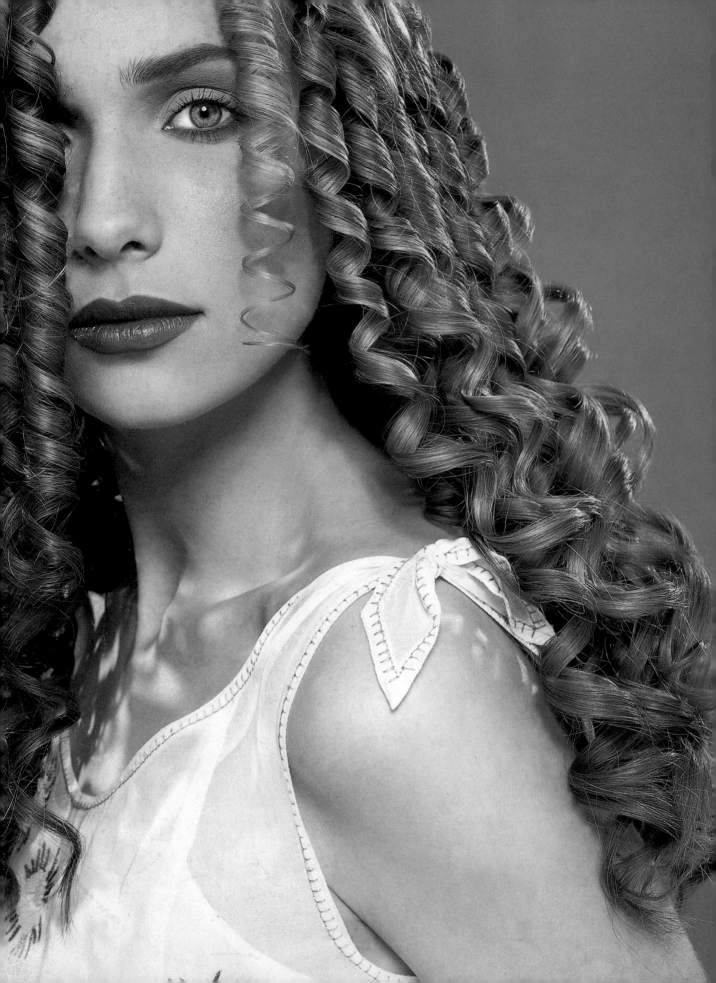

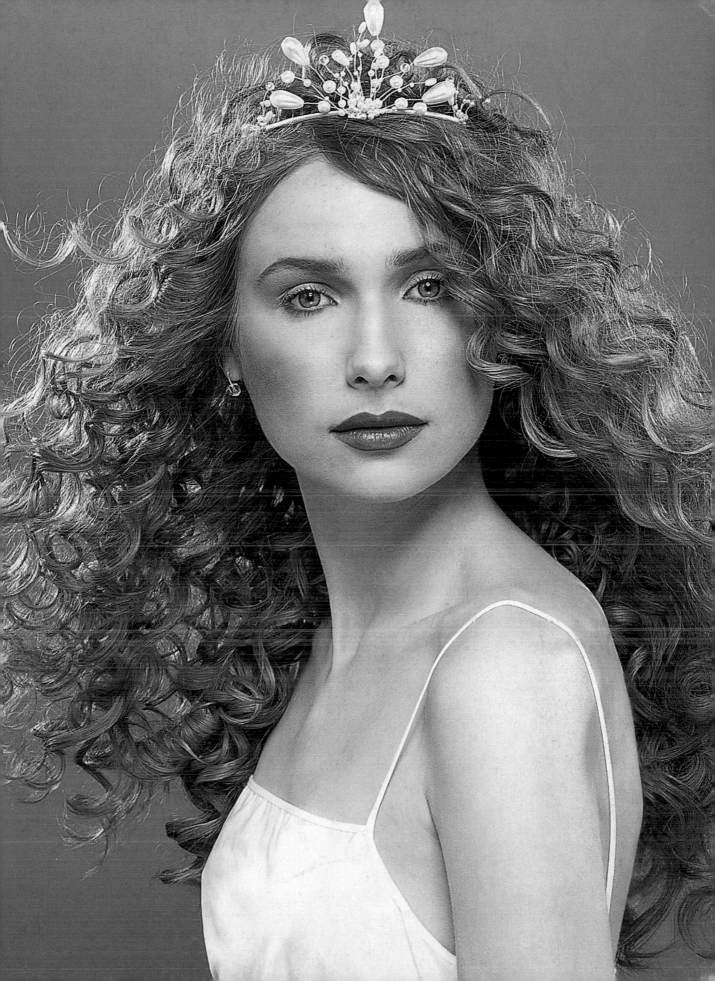

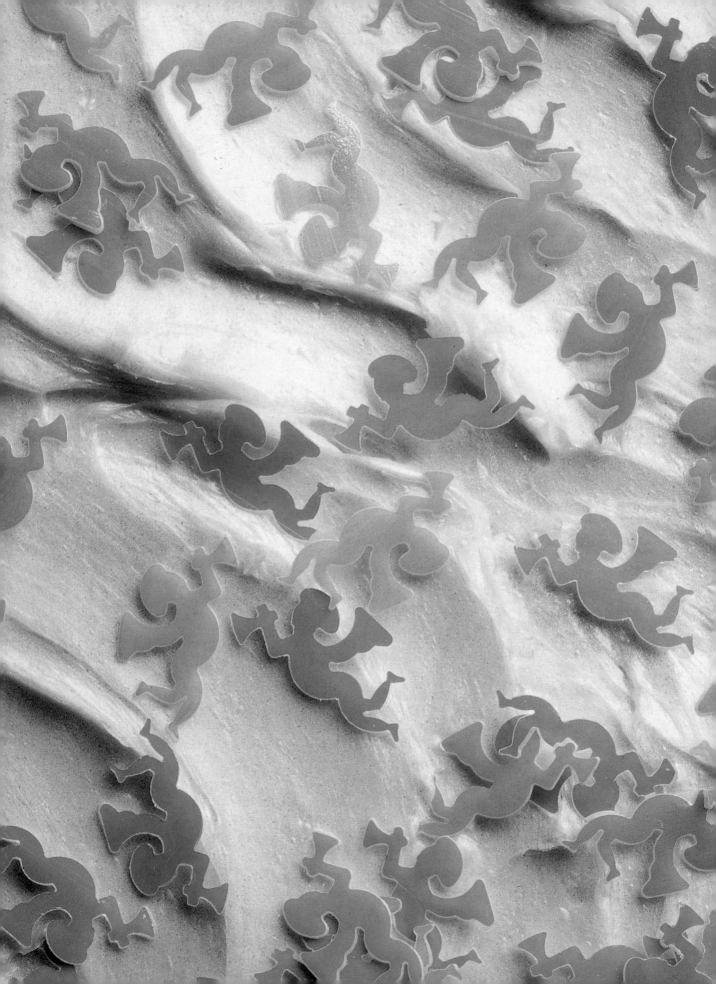

"**Grown up?**" exclaims Jaz's stylist, Zoe. She's been doing Jaz's hair since she was a junior stylist and has tried out all of her trendiest looks on her. Jaz nods firmly. Her job at Astrid PR is everything she had hoped it would be, but she's started to think that she's being overlooked for promotion. Her cutting-edge look is great when she's dealing with designers or at the shows, but when it comes to important meetings she's often left behind. Is it because Astrid feels she can't deal with the business side of things? Or just that she can't get them to take her seriously in her present incarnation? Either way, she's ready for a change.

"I want to go for a classic, straight bob with bangs," says Jaz. Zoe raises an eyebrow. "Aha, the power bob. Trouble at work?" she asks. "First of all, Jaz, you need to look like you, and that is so not your style. Secondly, it will drown your face.

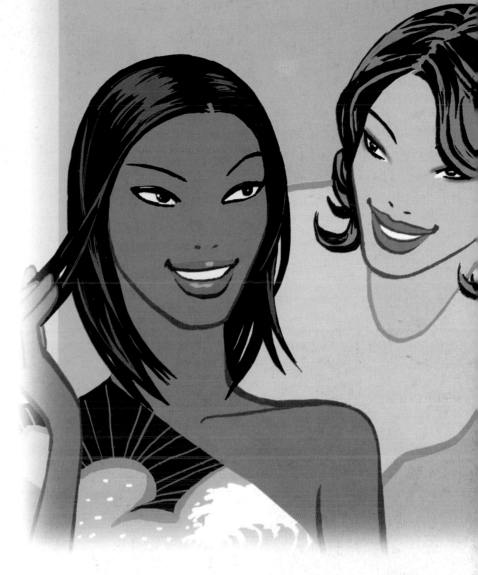

...jaz goes for a grown-up look

just look at your face shape. "Zoe is right; Jaz's slim heart-shaped face couldn't carry off such a look. "Why don't we meet halfway?" Zoe suggests, "and dye it back to its natural black, then cut it into a long bob, sloping down at the front and without bangs. If we razor the ends, you can stop it from hanging in a single, heavy chunk. That way you have lots of versatility when you're not being Mrs Business

Woman." "Sounds like you and I are changing places," giggles Kate, slipping into the chair next to Jaz. "Kate! What are you doing here?" asks Jaz, slightly unnerved to be caught dicing with conformity. "I'm getting back to my roots, literally," says Kate. "My highlights from the vacation are growing out, so I'm having a vegetable color put on to bring back my normal red color." Jaz eyes her old school friend in the

mirror. She looks great; she hasn't used her straightening iron since her vacation, letting her natural curl reassert itself with a vengeance. She seems so much more confident and relaxed than the girl who went away. "Is there something you're not telling me?" Jaz asks. Kate smiles as Zoe leads Jaz away to wash her hair. "No," she says. "It's just that some things are better left alone."

urbanite

Everything in her life is luxurious but with a thoroughly modern edge. She's a high-maintenance girl whose wardrobe is filled with elegant, well-cut clothes and whose look is one of understated glamour. Naturally, her wedding outfit is no exception. She'll be wearing an exquisitely cut white pant suit with a plunging neckline revealing a fair amount of bare *décolletage*. Jewelry will be simple and modern, and a flower-ball bouquet will be dangling from her slender wrist.

hair solutions

Short hair naturally complements this sharp look, while mid-length hair is best in a 1920s-style bob. Long hair is great sleet and straight with an extreme side part and a section pulled back into a feather headdress. Keep it simple, with the accent on impeccable condition.

LEFT AND RIGHT

For the textured look (right), the hair is tousled using wet-look gel to give a glossy, almost glass-like finish. The hair on the crown is styled using the fingers to give texture, height and a spiky finish. If you have short hair but want a longer look, use a three-quarter hairpiece to add length and interest around the face (left).

OVERLEAF LEFT

The hair is scrunch-dried using a blow-dry primer spray for volume and texture. It is swept back into a high ponytail, and backbrushed and sculpted into the required shape. The style is finished with a firm-hold hairspray and a necklace or bracelet pinned to the front of the "sculpture". Veil-type bangs are also an option.

OVERLEAF RIGHT

The hair is slicked back into a mid-height ponytail and set with hot rollers. The curls are broken up with the fingers and piled into a clear, natural hairnet, secured with fine pins. A feathered comb can be added to the side of the bun.

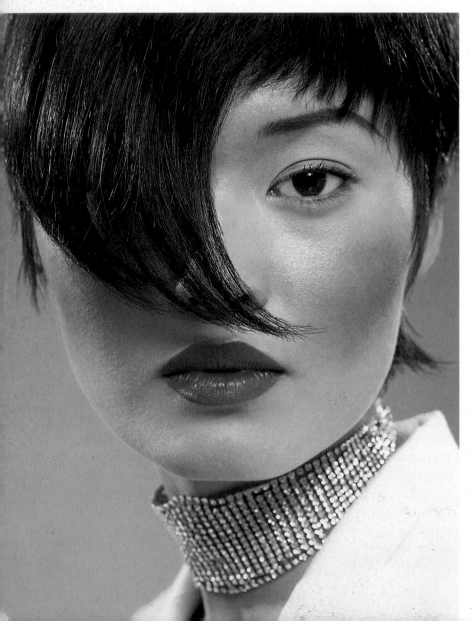

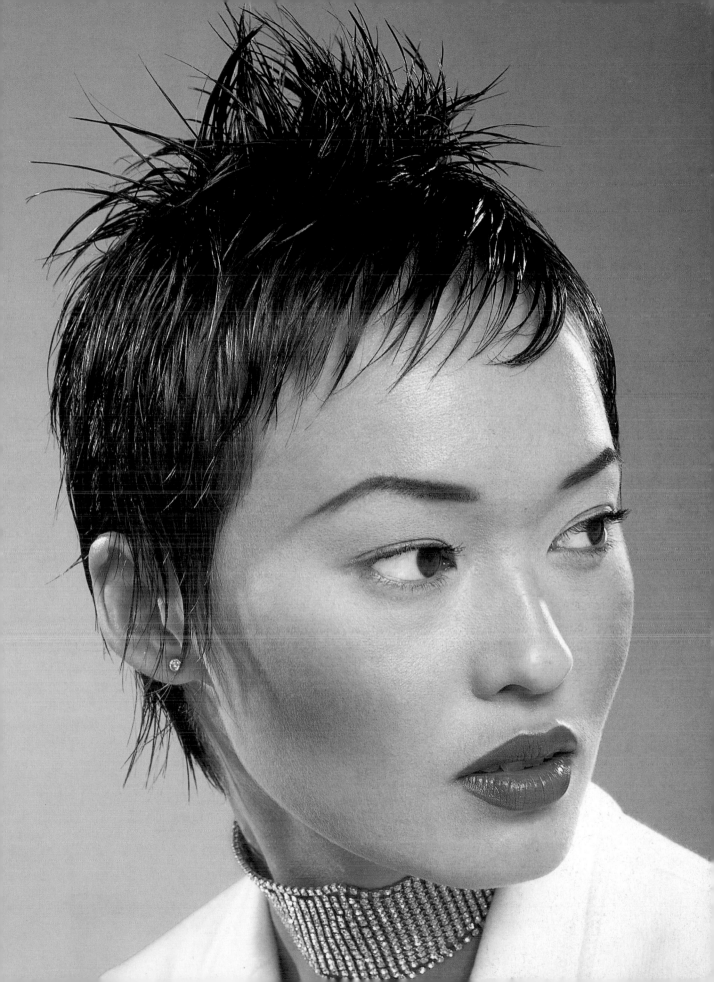

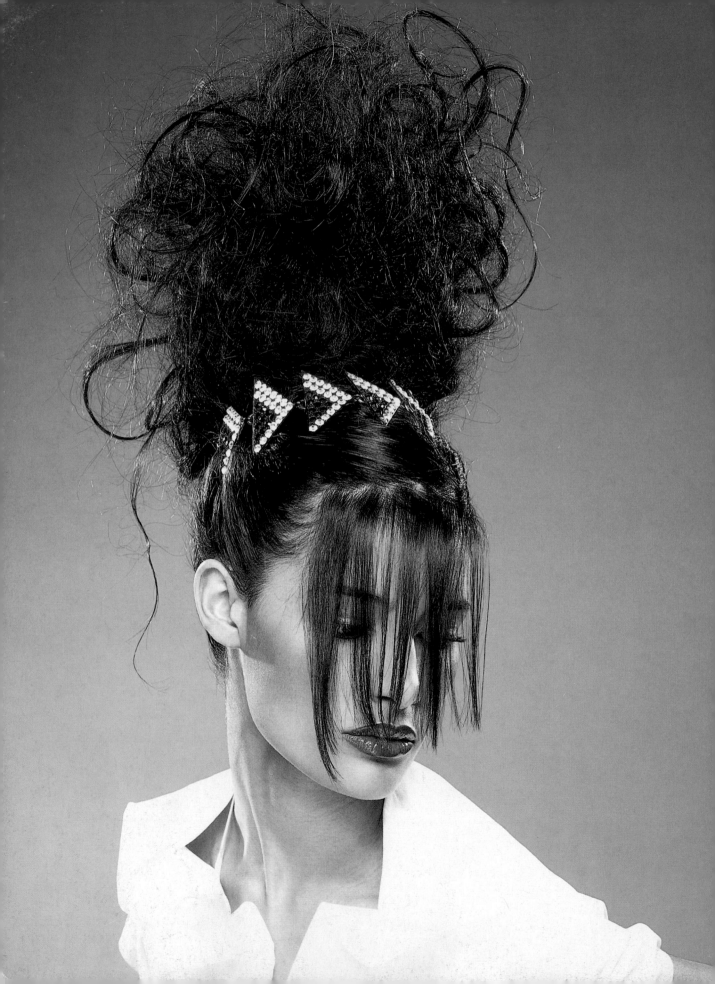

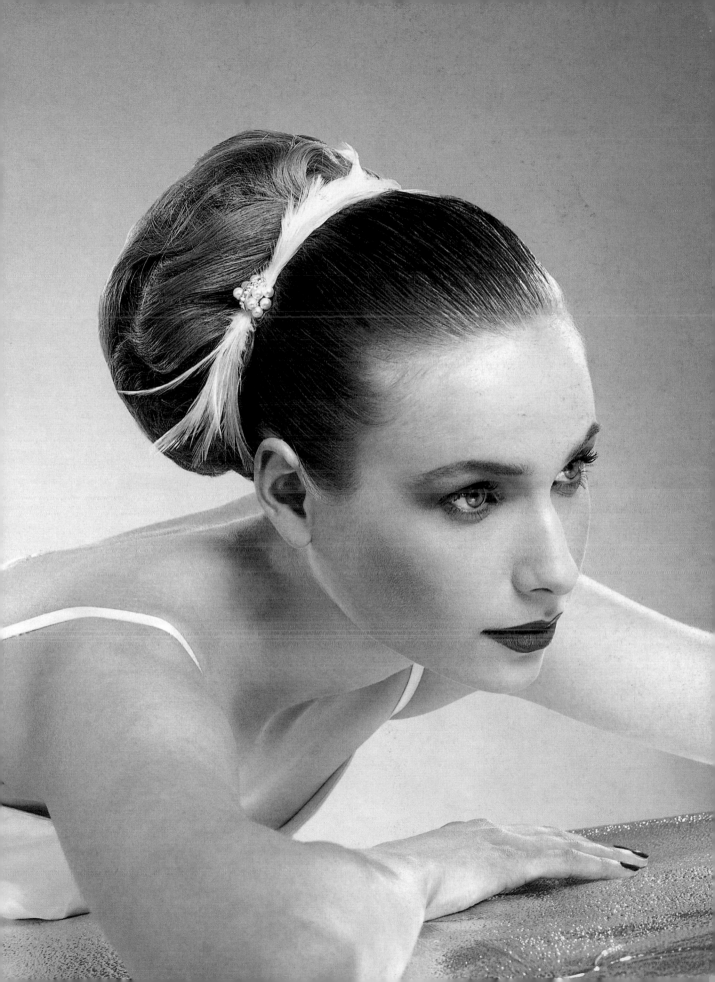

audrey

Her biggest style influence is, of course, Audrey Hepburn in *Breakfast at Tiffany's*. She always looks well groomed and classically elegant — her uniform is crisp linen shift dresses for summer and neat pencil skirts and fitted sweaters for winter. For her wedding, she'll be wearing a sleeveless column dress in off-white satin, and carrying either a tight bouquet of cream roses tied with pale blue ribbon or a single long-stemmed amaryllis or lily.

hair solutions

Smoothing your long hair into a neat chignon, with a subtle tiara and a satin-trimmed shoulder-length veil, is a perfectly classic look. Mid-length hair looks great accessorized with an Alice band and mini-veil, while vivid orchids and green tendrils secured behind one ear are ideal for short hair.

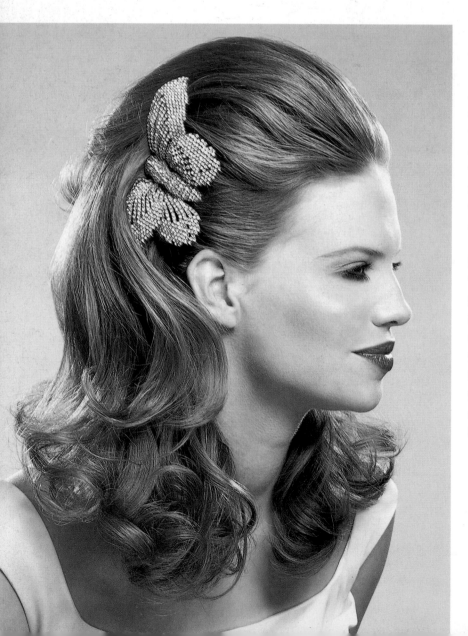

LEFT

The hair is set on medium-sized rollers using a fine flexible hold hair-spray and allowed to cool completely before gently removing them. The curls are broken up using a wide-tooth comb and the roots at the crown is backcombed. The sides are smoothed back and secured with bobby pins. A decorative comb completes the look.

RIGHT

The hair is swept up into a neat high ponytail in the center of the head. It is then set on hot rollers, which are removed when they are totally cool. The hair is pulled through two bun rings over which the curls are placed and pinned. A necklace can be pinned across the hairline for decoration.

HAIR SNIP

BALANCE IS ABSOLUTELY ESSENTIAL. DO NOT GO TOO BIG IF YOU ARE TALL, BUT TRY BIGGER HAIR IF YOU ARE ON THE SHORT SIDE — YOU NEVER KNOW, YOU MAY LOVE IT.

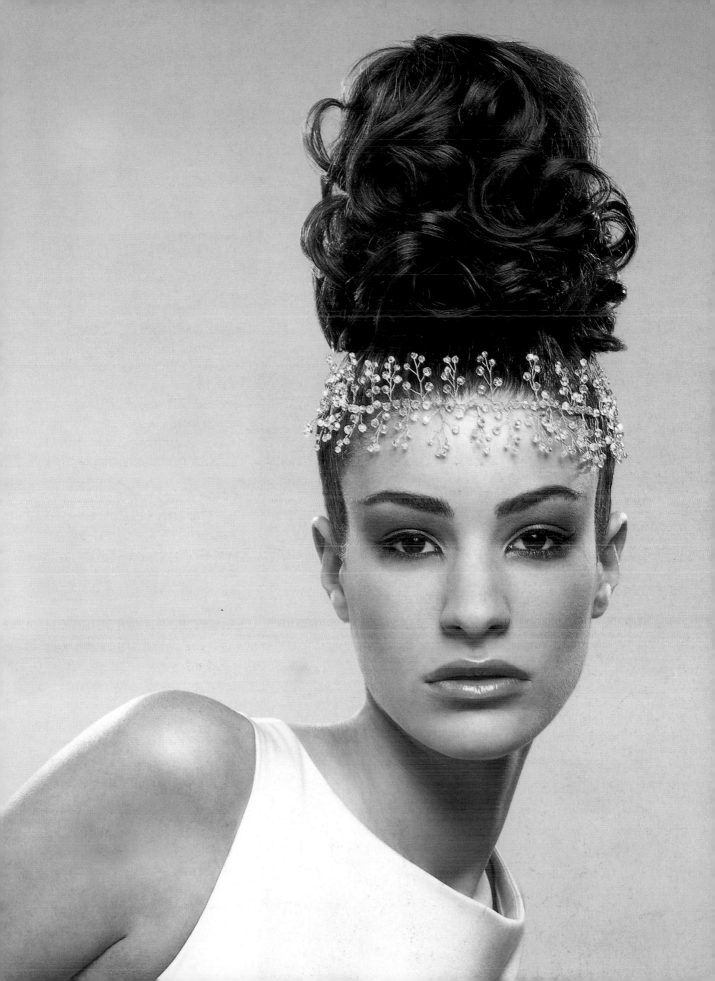

classic

"Refined good taste" are this girl's favorite words. She always looks immaculate, even on casual days. For work she wears beautifully tailored suits and relaxes at the weekend in smart but fashionable jeans or cords. She thrives on tradition and ceremony, and never more so than at her own wedding. Her elegant empire-line gown in duchesse satin is offset with a frothy white veil and a trailing bouquet of white flowers and green foliage for a timelessly stylish look.

hair solutions

This is perfect for those who want the quintessential bridal look of veil and tiara. A crown tiara is great on short hair, while long hair demands to be piled up high. For fine or mid-length hair, try adding a hairpiece.

LEFT AND RIGHT

Ultra-shiny hair is swept back and secured into a French braid using fine pins and hair clips. A small circular tiara is placed onto the crown, and a braided section of hair is positioned inside and held in place with hair pins and hairspray.

OVERLEAF LEFT

The root area of freshly blow-dried or set hair is backbrushed. The nape section is swept up to the crown and secured with bobby pins. The top section is brought over, wound down onto the mid-section and fastened with bobby pins to create a soft roll. Accessories or feathers can be added to the base of the roll.

OVERLEAF RIGHT

The hair is set on medium-sized rollers using a fine flexible hold hair-spray. When cool, the rollers are removed and the curls are broken up using a wide-tooth comb. Using fingers as a comb, the hair is shaped around the face in large sweeping waves. For gentle hold, hairspray is applied to the fingers and run through the hair.

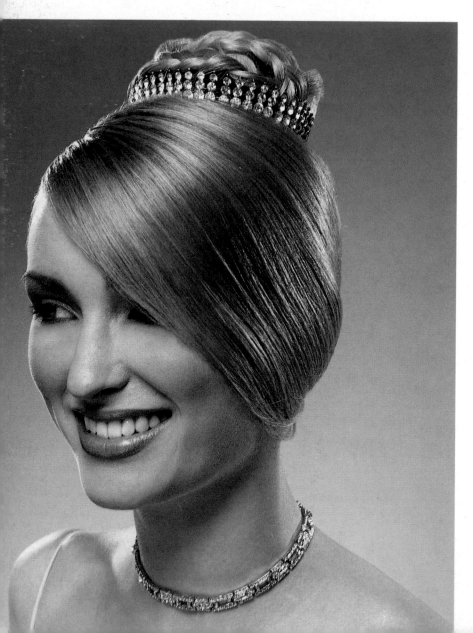

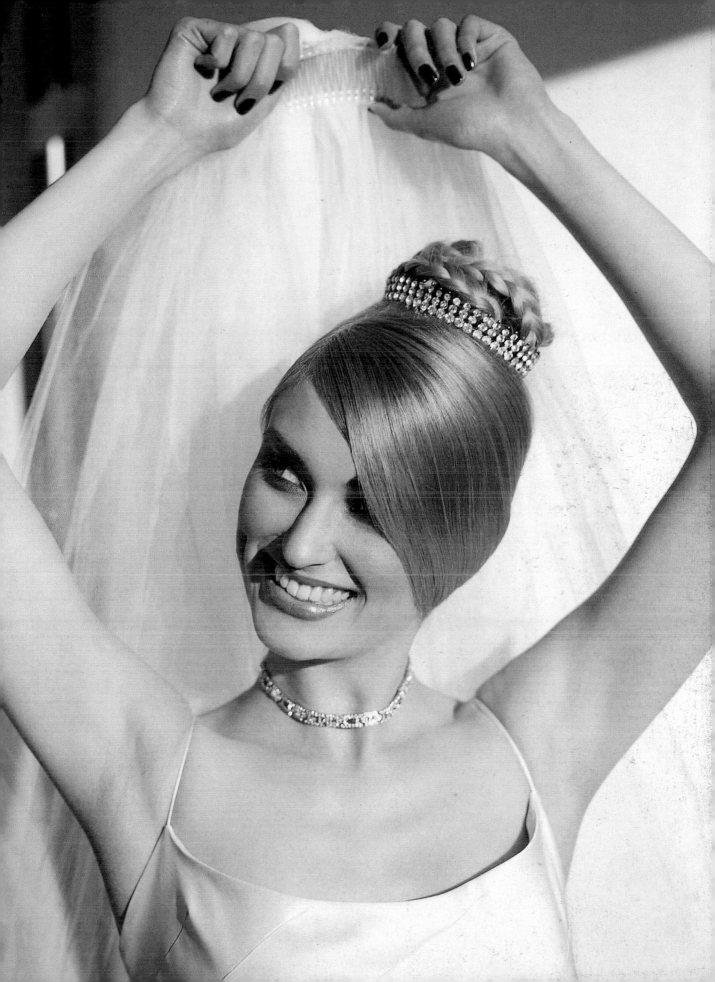

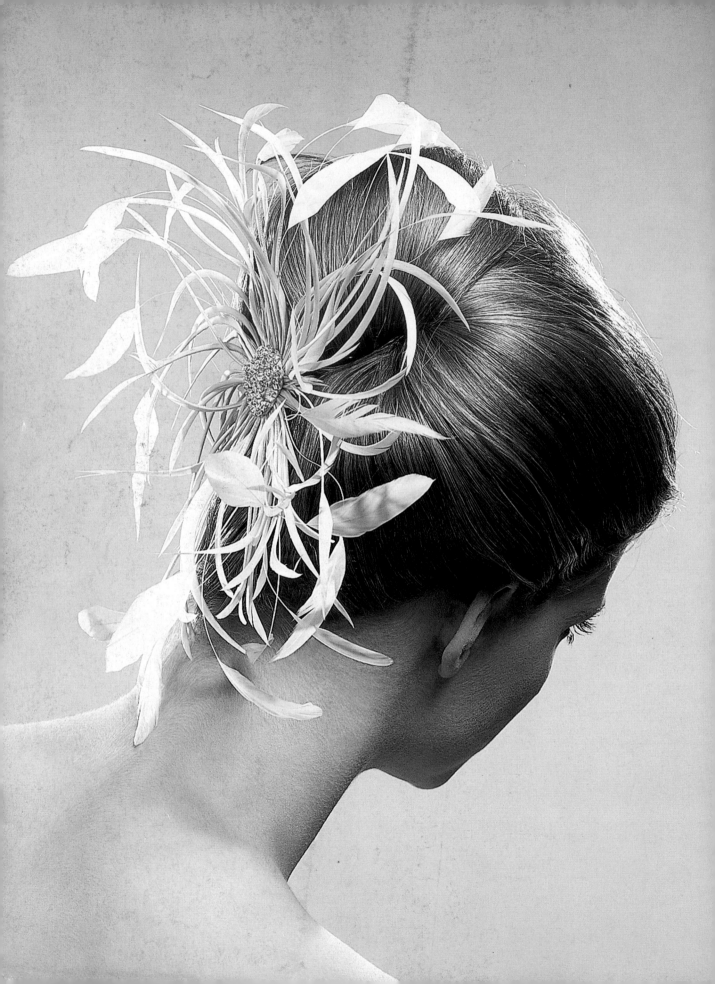

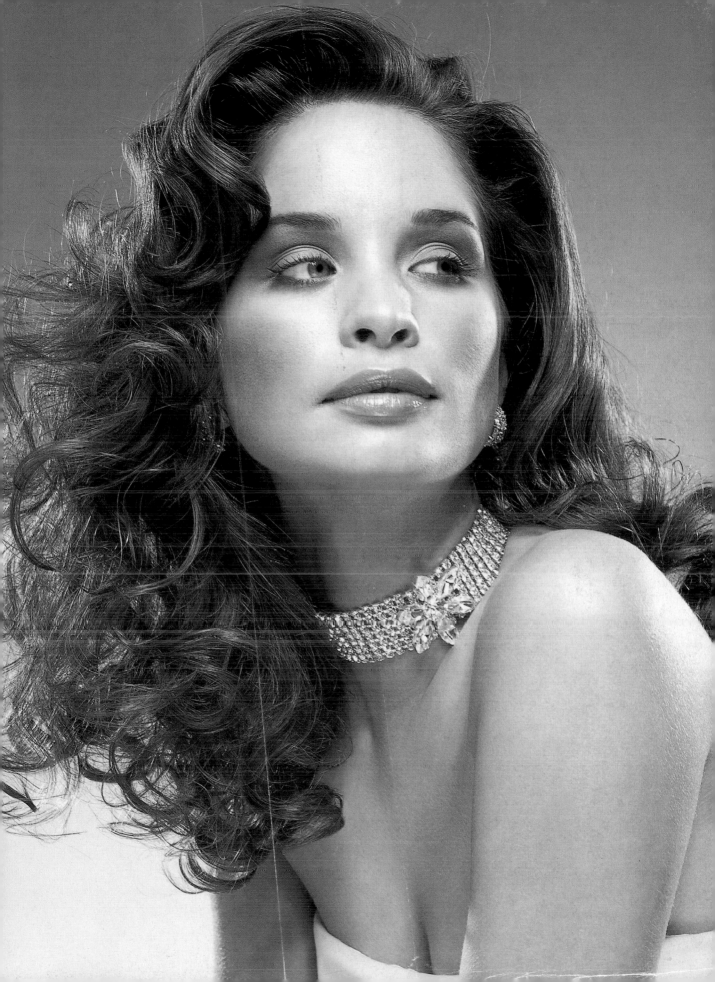

rock chick

This girl loves to play — and her wedding day will be no exception. Her usual uniform is skin-tight jeans, tiny ripped T-shirts, leather cuffs and high-heeled, snake-skin ankle boots. Her bridal version will comprise of a very short skirt, a slash-neck top and fishnets — all in snowy white. She won't carry flowers, but will finish off the look with a rhinestone collar and cuffs, smoky eyes and hair with serious attitude.

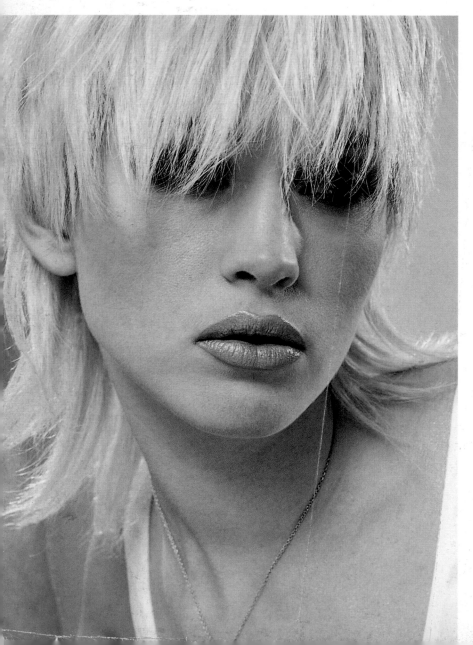

hair solutions

Regardless of length, the look here is big, big, big. Plenty of texture and backcombing will give long hair that super-sexy just-about-to-fall-into-bed-head look — but remember to use products only at the roots, or the hair will be weighed down. With shorter hair, try a tiara on a choppy, textured cut. On any length, don't forget height at the crown.

LEFT AND RIGHT

For a classic rock-chick look, hair is dyed "peroxide" blonde and cut dry using a razor to inject some attitude into this modern style. Wax is used to give a matte, chunky finish and a sparkling crystal tiara makes this look a little more feminine.

OVERLEAF LEFT

For an ultra-modern rock-chick look, hair is cut randomly using texturizing scissors and colored with a variety of red and bluish-black tones to create an edgy effect.

OVERLEAF RIGHT

The hair is blow-dried using blow-dry priming spray to give volume and create a tendril effect. It is then pulled up into ponytails along the center of the head in a mohican formation, then randomly placed and pinned to give a soft but edgy finish. Fake hairpieces can be added for extra drama if desired.

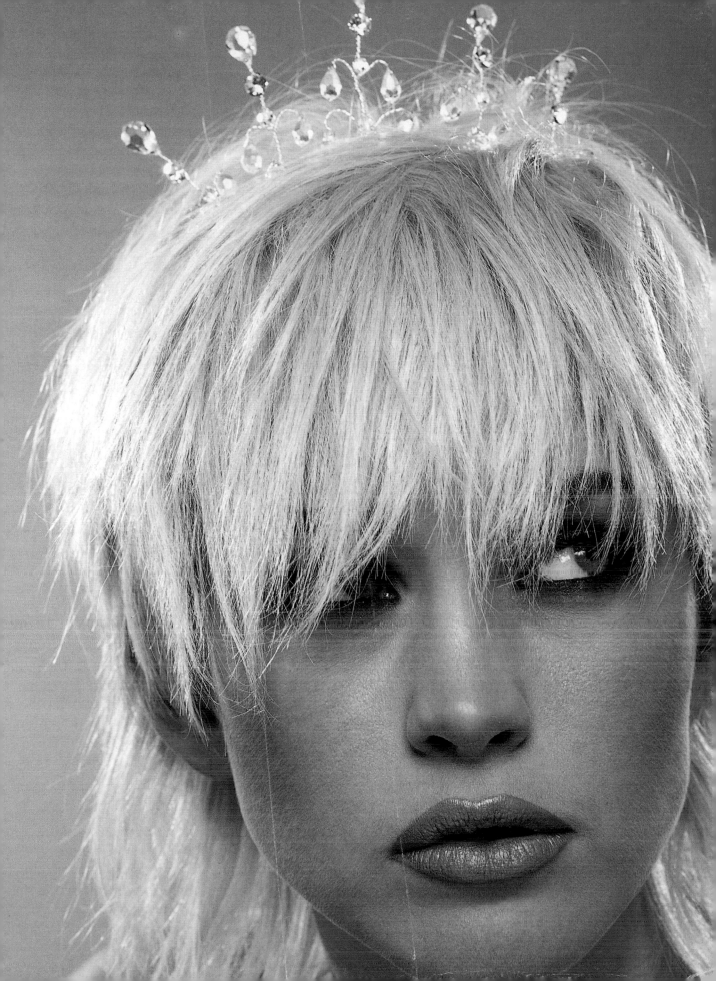

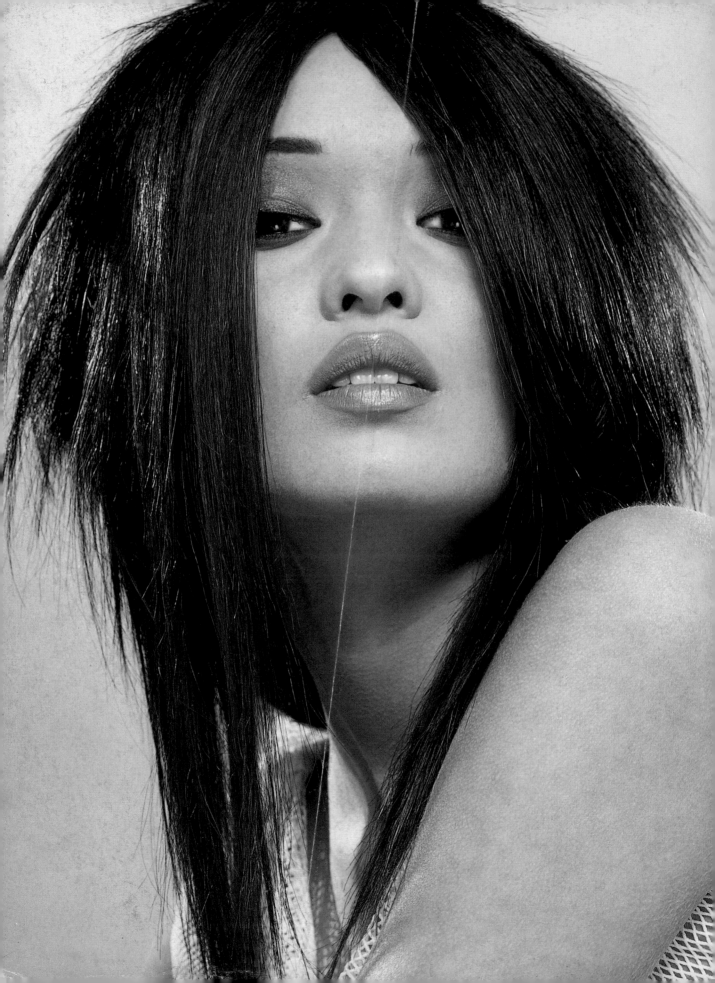

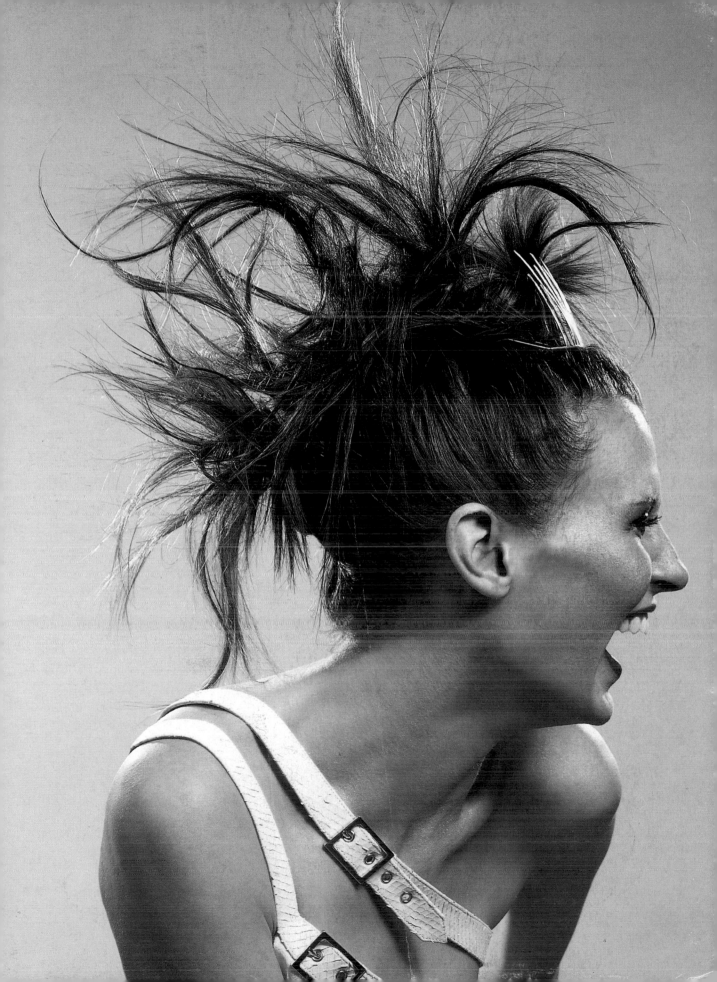

fashionista

Luckily, marriage is back in fashion and this bride-to-be has embraced it with as much enthusiasm as she always has for designer sales. Her dress will be *couture*, of course — a bright pink slip covered with transparent, spider-web lace. She'll be sashaying down the aisle as though it were a catwalk, wearing perilously high strappy slingbacks. Flowers are a wrist corsage or choker, consisting of a single orchid.

hair solutions

Whatever the length of your hair, its condition is vital, so make sure you book for some conditioning treatments well before the big day. On long hair, instead wearing of a traditional tiara, try pinning a necklace across the forehead over unstructured big hair. A shorter style can look stunning when the hair is textured and single diamanté studs are clipped into it. Medium-length hair looks feminine in a shaggy style — create the separation by twisting damp, moussed hair into bands and leaving it to dry. Beaded flower clips can be used to pull hair back and draw attention to the face.

LEFT

This is achieved with a "scrunching" technique, which provides a modern take on curly hair. The hair is drenched with mousse, scrunched down and pinned, then left to dry. The pins are removed and the hair is formed and shaped into the required style. A firm-hold hairspray sets and holds the style. Add a modern band or tiara to maximize the dramatic impact.

RIGHT

The hair is swept back into a twist, leaving the ends to splay out to one side of the head in a fan effect. Wax or pomade is used to give definition and texture to the ends. A theatrical necklace works well as a modern skull-cap.

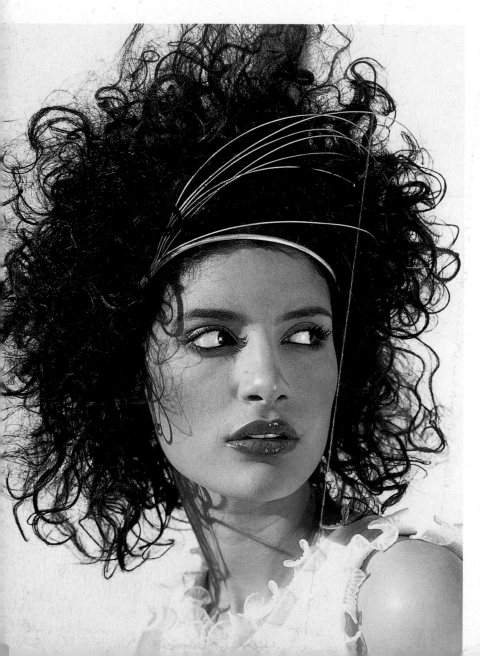

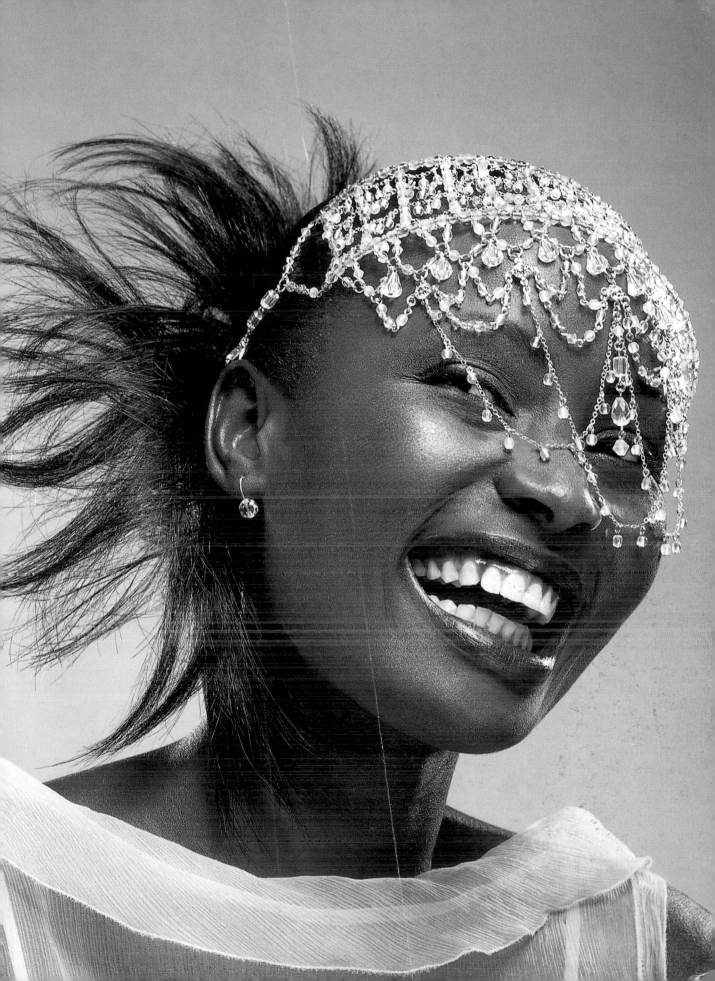

It's **Saturday night** and the girls are rushing around, brushes in hand, music blaring and empty wine bottles starting to gather on the kitchen table.

"Oh god, I look like a sheepdog," moans Laura, trying to tease her hair, which has reached the highly unpopular "difficult" stage, into some kind of style. Jaz pops her hair around the bathroom door.

"Want some help?" she offers, looking as if she's never had a bad-hair day in her life. She loves her new style so much that she's left it hanging loose, dressing it up with only a slick of blue hair mascara to enhance the natural shine. Luckily, her dressing table is still littered with every new beauty fix on the market. She grabs some hair clips with

subtle flowers fashioned from jade and ruby beads. Laura looks dubious as Jaz runs a little texturizing wax through her hair, pulling the shorter sections from the front and twisting them into ridges. Despite Laura's general aversion to all things feminine, she has to admit that Jaz has made a virtue of her hair's unruliness.

...the girls get ready to party

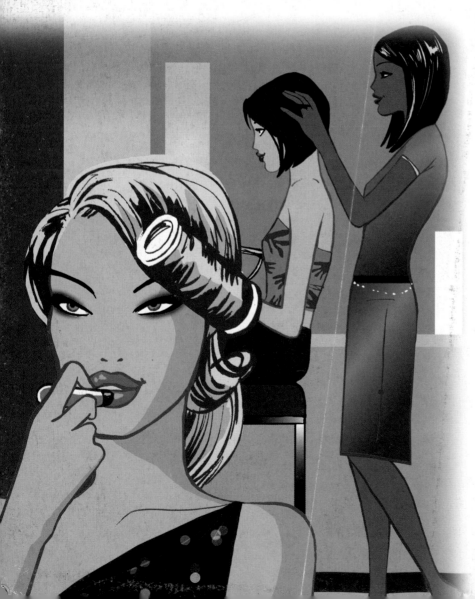

Chrissie limps past with one foot in a tiger-print mule, and spies the missing one poking out from underneath Jaz's bed. Remembering Laura's warning, she bites back her annoyance, only to catch a glimpse of Laura looking fabulous in casual jeans with her hair in a pretty half-updo. Determined not to be outdone by the house tomboy, she stomps back into her room to turn her braids into something a bit more glamorous.

Chrissie flicks through *Gloss* magazine until she finds a picture of her favorite glam "do" of the moment — the 1970s-inspired flick. She applies some volumizing mousse to the front section of her long hair, and then winds it around a huge Velcro roller. After a blast of hot air from her hairdryer and a spritz of hairspray, she leaves it to set and gets to work with the lip gloss.

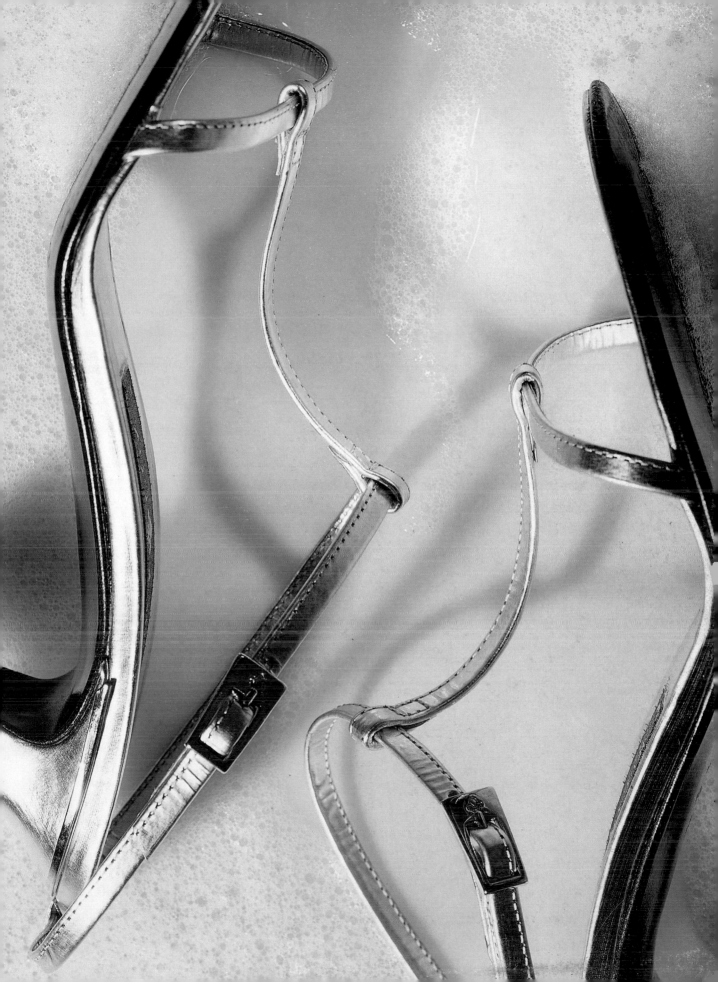

romantic

This girl is a true romantic. She loves nothing better than watching reruns of *Gone with the Wind* on rainy days — and it never fails to bring tears to her eyes. She's been planning her wedding day for as long as she can remember. Her dress will be fit for a princess — a beautiful full-skirted, tight-bodiced affair with the longest train she can find — and there will be flowers everywhere, in blush pink and cream.

hair solutions

Long hair will be worn loose and full with a gentle wave and fresh flowers woven into it at the crown. With mid-length hair, fresh tea roses in muted purples and pinks can be used to form a natural Alice band over the crown. You can create a dramatic short-hair look by smoothing hair away from the face with a beaded tiara.

LEFT AND RIGHT

This is a very modern take on the classic pin curl. Sections of hair, approximately two-inches square, are twisted around the fingers and pinned in place all over the head using bobby pins. Large, fresh flowers are interspersed between the curls.

OVERLEAF

Very straight, long hair is waved using a large-barreled curling iron to create gentle curles that are left loose to cascade down the back. For added interest, a natural flower garland is pinned in place in the center of the crown.

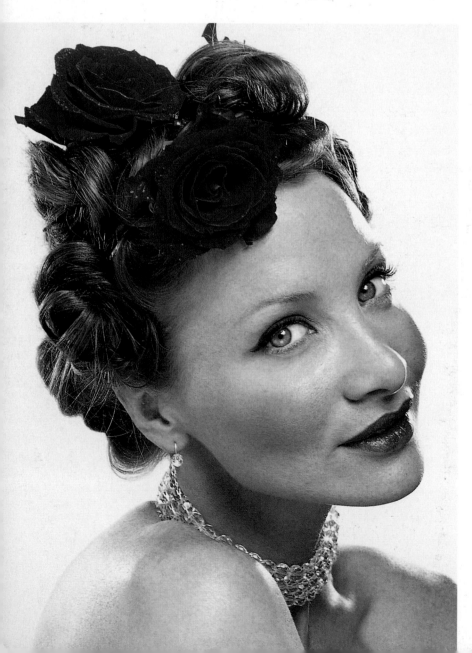

HAIR SNIP
IF YOU ARE USING FRESH FLOWERS IN YOUR HAIR, CAREFULLY SPRITZ THEM WITH WATER USING A VERY FINE SPRAY TO PREVENT THEM FROM DROOPING AND KEEP THEM FRESH ALL DAY LONG.

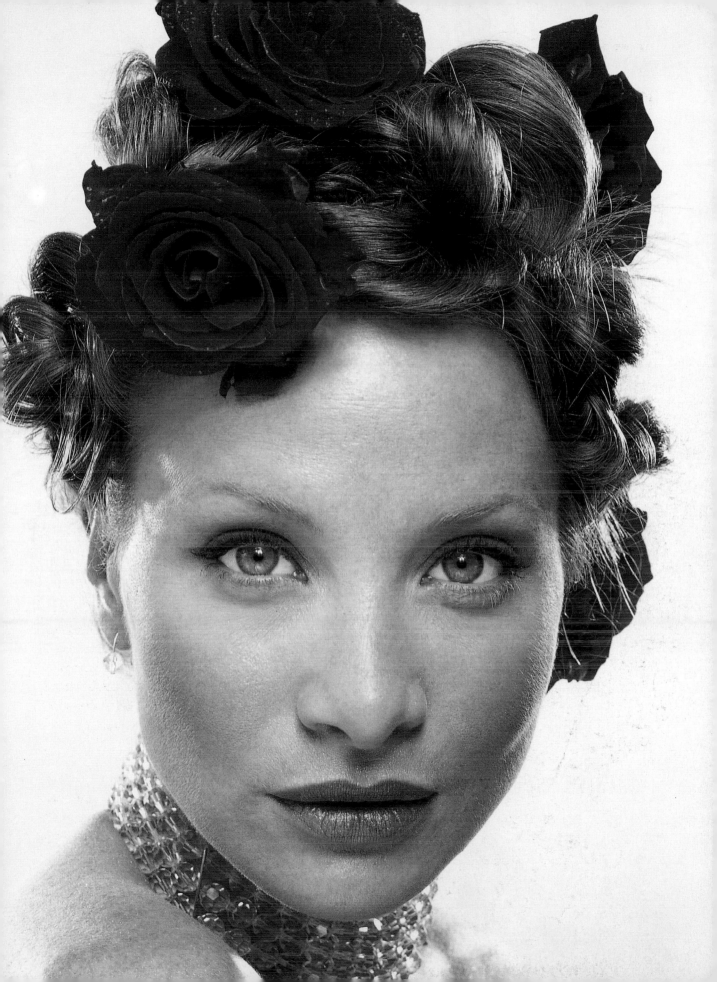

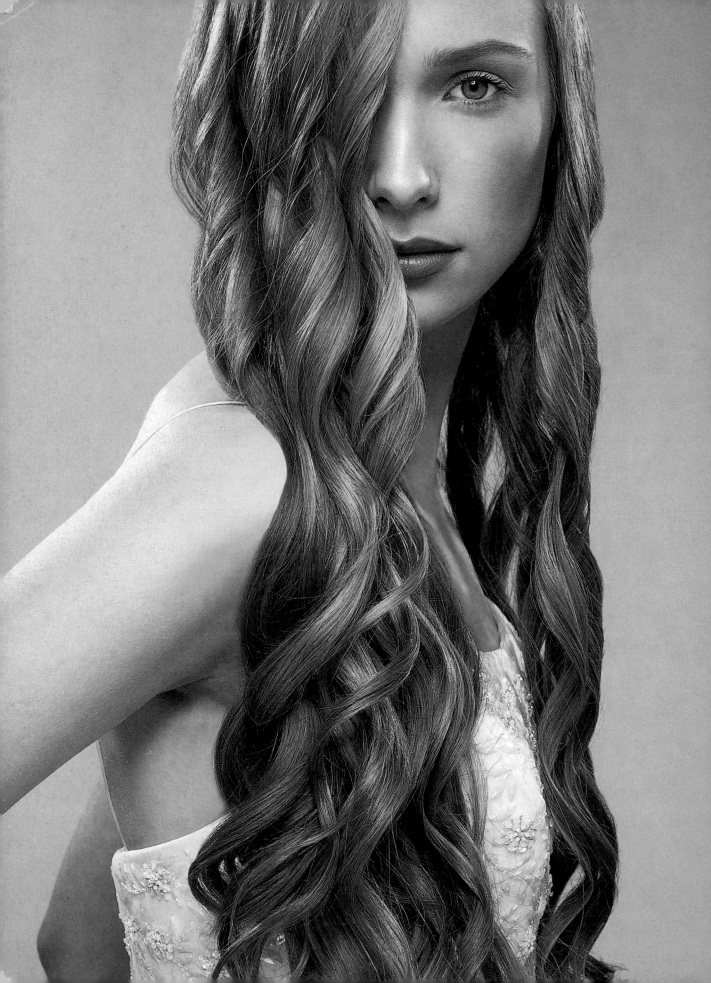

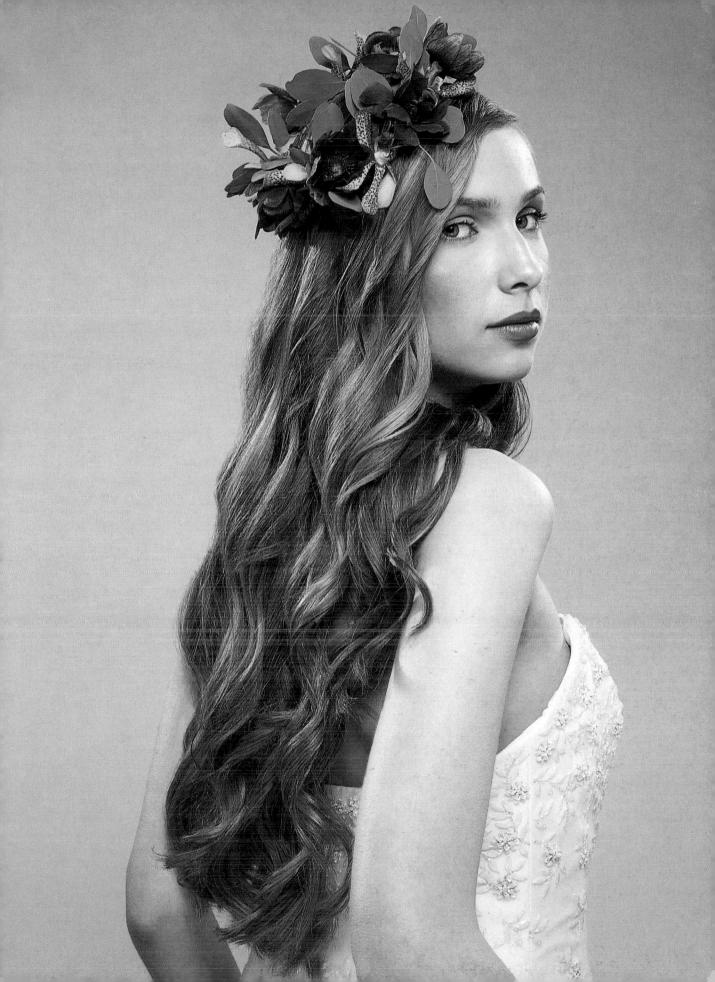

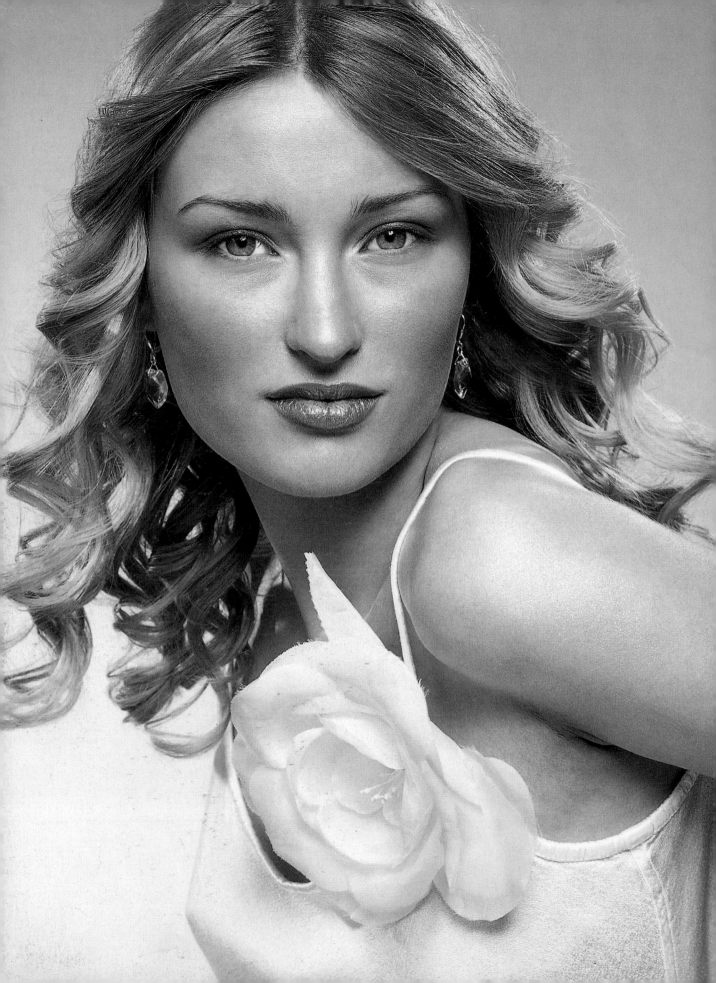

beach

This fun- and sun-loving girl is the ultimate beach babe, so it's no surprise that she wants a wedding by the ocean. She'll wear a strappy white dress or a string bikini and toe rings, with only her parasol to shield her from the rays.

hair solutions

Minimum fuss with maximum effect is the order of the day here. Whatever your hair length, running some hair oil through your locks will keep it protected from the sun and ocean air. Long hair looks great secured in a low bun off to one side at the nape of the neck. Pull some loose ends out to keep it playful. Veils and tiaras are pretty much out, but a big, exotic single bloom can look great tucked behind your ear.

LEFT AND BELOW LEFT

The hair is curled using a multi-sized curling iron to give loose romantic ringlets. An anti-humidity blow-dry spray is used to maximize the longevity of the style and also to minimize frizz. Alternatively, the curls can be broken up with a light styling lotion and a comb pulled through the top section and secured above the crown (below left).

BELOW

The hair is sectioned into 1-inch (2.5 cm) squares. Ribbons, chosen to match the outfit, are tied around the base of each section of hair and then wrapped around its length in a crisscross formation, keeping the tension all the way down, and tied securely at the ends of the hair. The ends of the ribbons can either be left to hang free, or snipped off for a tidier look.

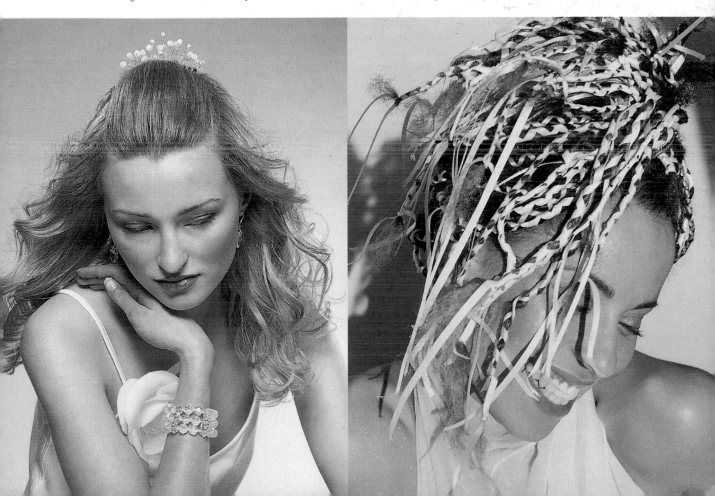

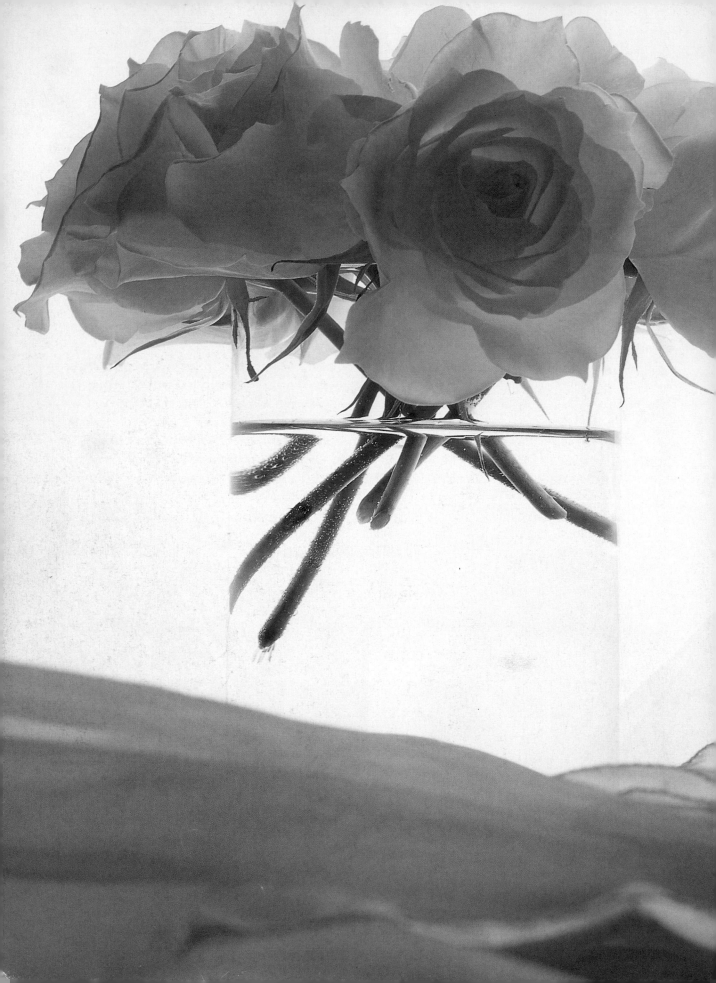

the big day

the big day dawns at last...

"You are so sly!" giggled Polly, as she accepted a glass of Champagne from Kate. Kate had finally let everyone in on her news — which explained her recent secrecy and absences from the condo.

"Well, I wanted to make sure that I'd been accepted before I told you," she said. "And also, the course I want to do, the only one that combines nutrition and physiotherapy, is based in Boston...which means I'll be moving out." Polly looked up from under the slab of backcombed bangs that currently flopped in front of her face. "I'm glad you've brought that up," she began, "because there's something I have to tell you all, too. We've decided to live in New York. It'll take at least three months to organize Simon's transfer, so there's plenty of time to make other arrangements." She looked imploringly at each of her friends.

"Oh, stop looking like Bambi," said Chrissie. "We're all big girls, you know, we'll be fine!" Laura nodded in agreement, but secretly wasn't so sure. Things between her and John had been strained recently, and she was concerned that maybe he was starting to lose interest in her. Instead of chatting and laughing away as usual, he seemed withdrawn and anxious.

"Polly, unless you to want to wear your crown around your neck it might be a good idea to keep your head still," chided Charles affectionately. He had come to Polly's home as a special treat for her big day. Keeping her silky, fine blonde hair in a chignon was going to take all his skill and a few industry tricks. He began by applying thickening spray to the hair and winding it onto large rollers to give as much height and body as possible. After drying the hair, he gave it a burst of hot then cold air to help hold the shape, and removed the rollers. Charles then scooped back the hair into a classic twist and attached the tiara, a delicate pearl affair, toward the front of the crown. After a fine spray of firm-hold hairspray, Charles stepped back to admire his work. It was the perfect look for Polly, elegant and simple but with enough grandeur to carry off her glamorous gown.

Despite her original concerns about allowing the girls to choose their own dresses and hairstyles, they all looked fantastic. Jaz had chosen a pink dress, tied on one shoulder with an asymmetrical hem. Her sleek black hair followed her hemline, parted to one side and secured with a cluster of pink roses attached to a sequined clip. She also wore a wrist band of roses. Polly had never seen Laura looking as feminine as she did in her long lilac shift dress with a low, draped back, her hair in a short bob with a band of pale pink roses against her dark hair. Kate had left her hair loose, with roses dotted through its tumbling curls. Her milky complexion was set off perfectly against the pink of her knee-length dress, which, as Jaz had advised had a slightly draped neck. Chrissie, whose natural instinct was to grab attention wherever she could, had chosen a flowing style in pink, with contrasting lilac ruffles and a split starting at mid-thigh. A large rose was pinned behind one ear, pulling back her thick blonde hair. The dress had caused Laura to scowl when Chrissie had pulled it off the hanger, but Polly loved it. It was exactly what she would have expected, and it was for their differences that she loved them.

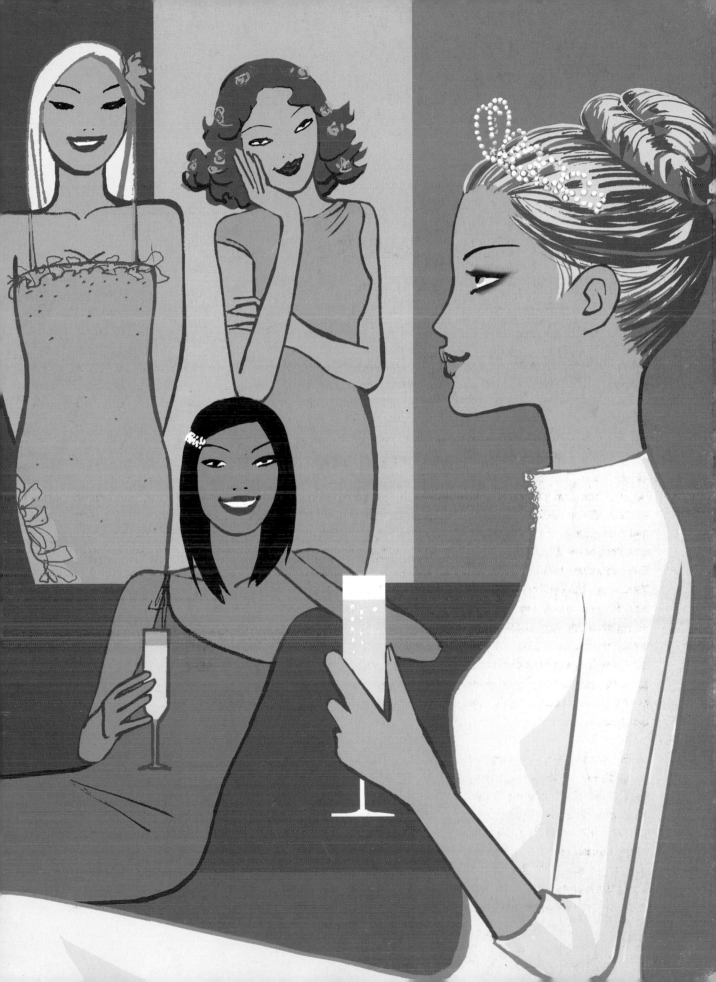

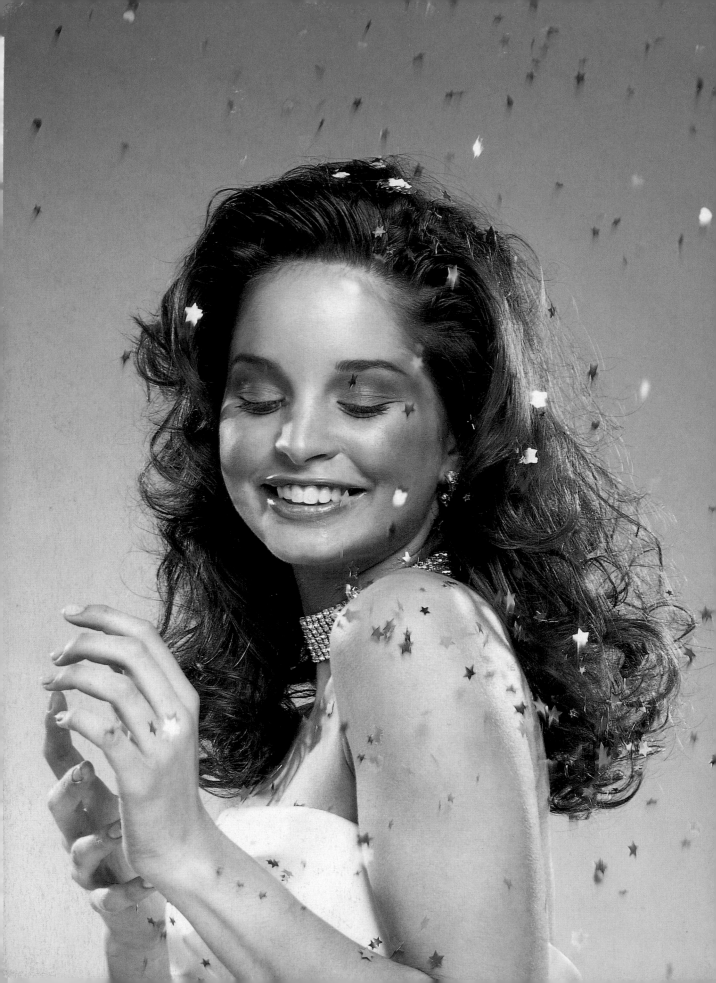

on the day

Due to all your hard work and preparation, your hair should now be in fabulous condition, ready and waiting to be transformed into your chosen style. Resist the urge to slather on conditioner for a last-minute boost, or fill your hair with extra product — it will only weigh it down. Stick to your tried-and-tested routine.

entourage

In the same way that you wouldn't leave your bridesmaids' dresses until the last minute, you should also consider in advance how their hairstyles will work with yours. Are you theming your looks and want them to have scaled-down versions of your style? Is this practical? Will they feel more comfortable in a style similar to their normal look?

A key thing to consider is the ages of your bridesmaids. Little girls are usually happy to take instruction, but adult bridesmaids will often have strong feelings about their look. It is sometimes better (and more harmonious) if bridesmaids are allowed to wear their hair — and dresses — in a more individual way (it is also highly unlikely that grown-up bridesmaids will have similar hairstyles). A great way to do this is by using flowers, small tiaras or hair accessories and allowing them to be interpreted in individual ways. Try to create an atmosphere that will allow your bridesmaids to tell you if they are uncomfortable. Ask them to keep a scrapbook of looks they like and try to find a compromise.

products

Although there is a whole array of hair products available to help you achieve your perfect look, they will be most effective if you use fewer of them in the right combination. Remember, the products you use every day may not be right for achieving a more elaborate hairstyle, so make sure you select the right ones.

mousse

This airy foam will thicken flyaway hair and give control with a natural appearance.

curl activator

Curly hair can sometimes suffer from lack of moisture, of which this product is packed full. Use it sparingly, though, so you can turn definition into a wet-look.

gel

Ideal for controling and volumizing short or fine hair, gel is a bride's best friend. Even if you've never used if before, consider using it for updos and to tame unruly wisps.

hairspray

The classic mistake for those needing staying power is to spray too much of this stylist's staple, rather than selecting the right holding strength. This will give your hair a hard look and dull its shine. Get the strength right in the first place and it will last.

styling cream

Some leave-in conditioners also double as a styling cream, which can create a smooth, flat finish. It can also be used on dry ends. Use it sparingly.

shine enhancers

This can be used to control frizz or enhance shine. It is a great way to make the hair look healthily polished, but don't use too much, since it can make hair look greasy.

wax and pomade

These range from a hard, shoe polish-like wax to a softer, creamy texture. Use these products to create excellent definition on short hair, and to separate strands and enhance the layers of long hair or bangs.

shine spray

This can be used on top of other products to restore gloss.

Ceremony over, guests greeted and speeches read, Polly slips away to spice up her look for the evening reception, taking the girls for company.
"I hope Simon's parents will recognize you when you return," giggles Laura, as Jaz produces powders and potions from her seemingly bottomless bag.
"Not that it matters," says Kate. "Now that you're Mrs Simon they

can hardly call off the wedding." Polly smiles serenely. Everything had been perfect. It had been a wonderful Indian-summer day; all of the people she loves had been around her, and watching Simon waiting for her at the end of the aisle had given her the best feeling she'd ever known.
"Can you turn into the light a bit Pol?" asks Jaz, removing Polly's tiara and unpinning her chignon

as Charles had shown her. She takes a large bristle brush and brushes out the hairspray, letting the hair bounce back in big, soft curls. Grabbing some styling spray from the SOS kit, she sprays Polly's upturned head to help maintain body. Jaz smooths back the top front section, and holds it in place with a crystal beaded slide, creating a 1950s-inspired half-up, half-down style.

...polly's day-to-night transformation

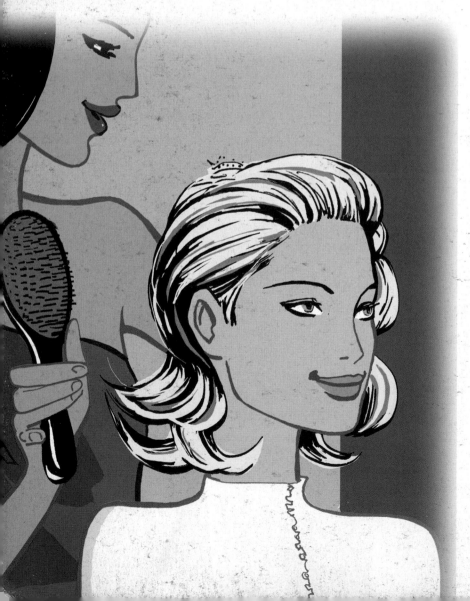

"Don't go too crazy with the gold look," Polly warns Jaz, who had promised to create a spectacular night-time look for her. In moments of pre-wedding anxiety she had imagined leading the first dance with glittery striped cheekbones.
"You lot have such little faith in me," says Jaz, slipping a glitter stick back into her make-up bag. "When have I ever been over the top?" The girls cackle wildly as they remind each other of Jaz's more extreme forays into fashion — her tie-dyed hair, her luminous fishnet tights...Jaz just smiles and begins dusting shimmering gold powder on Polly's cheekbones and hair. After an extra layer of mascara and a touch of eyeliner to enhance Polly's blue eyes, she slicks some clear gloss across her lips, a look that's glamorous without being heavy. "OK, you jokers," she says, standing back to admire her handy work. "It's time to get Mrs Simon back to her party."

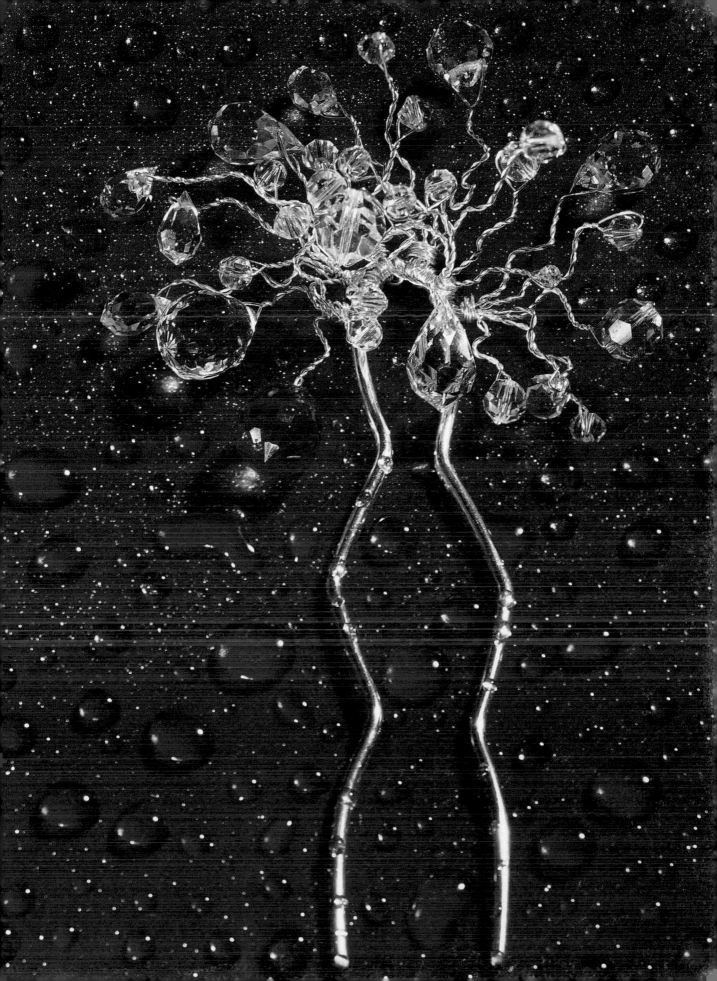

making it last

Whether you are doing your own wedding hair or visiting your stylist, there are certain tricks that will give your hair extra staying power. Make sure your bridesmaids and mother read these tips, too!

1 If you are having an updo, wash your hair the night before the wedding, rather than on the day, since just-washed hair can be harder to tame. Those with bangs may want to part the front section and wash them separately.

2 When you use any styling product, it is very important that most of it is applied at the roots, not the ends. This will stop the hair from being too flat.

3 Silky hair that usually hangs loose in a pretty but stubborn curtain can be tamed by the addition of styling agents. Thickening volumizing spray, wax and mousse will all help the tiara or veil grip onto the hair. Make sure that you do not overcondition fine hair, since this will weigh it down.

4 To put more volume into your style, alternate between hot and cold heat settings when you are blow-drying your hair. Dry the hair first using hot air, then give each section a cold blast — this will set body and bounce as the hair cools down and will help to hold the style in shape for longer.

5 Extra-large rollers create great volume. Work from the top to the bottom of the head, taking sections of hair that are approximately one to two inches wide, depending on its length and health. Roll the hair under in the direction you want the style to lay and ensure that the rollers sit snugly against the scalp for maximum body. Once all the rollers have been inserted, spritz the hair with a styling spray for a long-lasting lift at the roots.

6 Roller-set your hair to make it more manageable and easier to put up on the day.

7 When using hair products, try to choose them all from the same range for the most effective results — they are designed to work together.

8 Backcombing is the backbone of all updos, giving both volume and staying power. It may look bad for your hair, but it is essential.

Having a trial run with your veil and tiara is extremely important. Clear combs are the most effective way of securing a veil discreetly and firmly, and you may need to employ hair pins in a shade similar to your hair color for extra support. Tiaras often come with hooks for clips to be slipped into or with a comb to grip the hair as part of their design. Give your style a serious workout to make sure it has staying power; you will be miserable if you find yourself anxiously trying to balance a slipping tiara all day. Backcombing often helps give the hair texture to which things can grip, as will using product in the hair. Always ask the store from which you buy your veil or tiara to show you how to secure it — they are the experts.

SOS kit

No bride should venture into the elements without her SOS kit. Take whatever you need to feel secure, then nominate your bridesmaid with the biggest handbag to look after it.

Hairspray and shine spray
Bobby pins and hair clips — and plenty of them
Natural-bristle smoothing brush
Tail comb
Hot rollers
Bun ring
Hairpiece

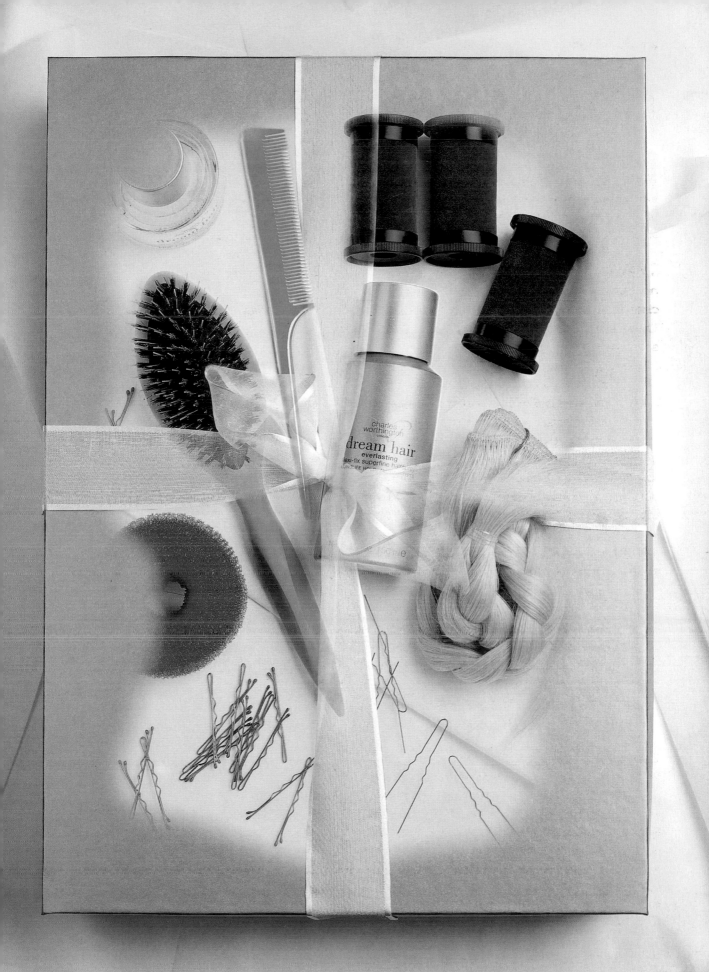

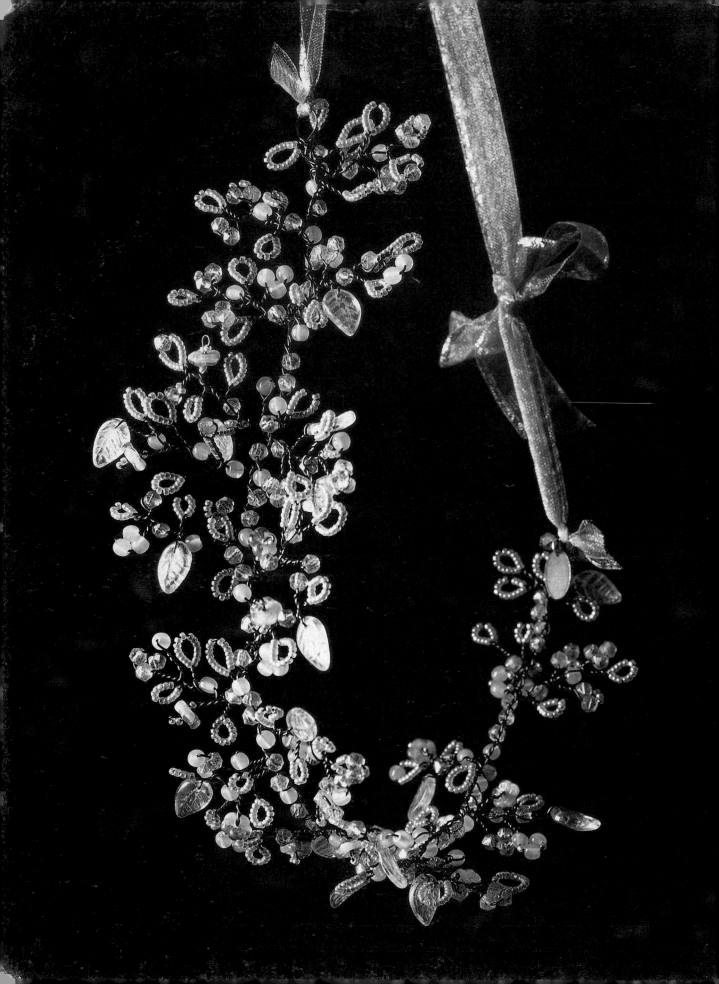

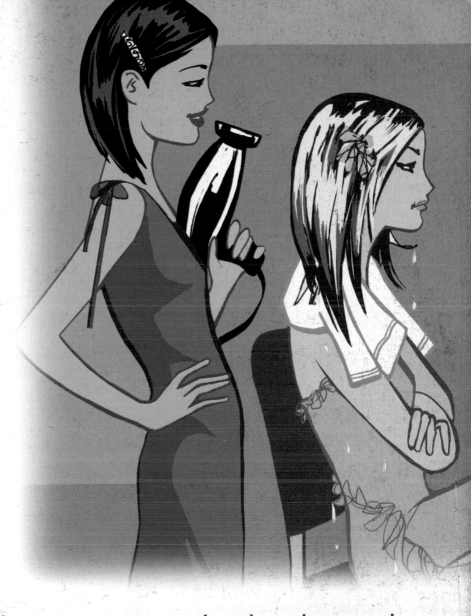

"I can't believe I'm doing this," mutters Chrissie, as she prepares to dash out into the rain to collect Polly's bag from the car. The weather has finally broken, the clear skies turning black with heavy showers. After five minutes in the doorway of the country inn where the reception is being held, she finally accepts that she'll just have to make a run for it.

The 20-second round trip leaves her completely soaked. Her hair is plastered to her head and her lovely dress is glued to her skin. As she slinks through the door, hugging the wall, and starts up the stairs to the suite, she spots Knell Kendrew, the head of Devastation Records arriving at the reception. She could cry on the spot. Never one to indulge in soul-searching, Chrissie's finally realized what

...chrissie gets caught in the rain

has been making her so touchy of late. It seems that everyone else is moving on in their lives, while she's left stuck behind the reception desk at Devastation Records, waiting for the big break that never seems to come.

"There you are! You're soaked and it's completely my fault!" cries Polly, making her way down the stairs towards her, in her freshly made-up perfection.

"Don't panic anyone," says Jaz, rummaging in her bag with one hand and nudging Chrissie into the suite with the other. "Charles left me an SOS kit for exactly this kind of crisis. Get that dress off."

Once inside, Chrissie wriggles out of her wet dress, drapes it on the radiator and slips on one of the fluffy white robes hanging on the door. She takes a seat at the dressing table and begins

removing her melting mascara. Jaz combs some shine spray from Charles's SOS kit through the length of Chrissie's hair. With some deft twisting, she pulls it back into a band, folds the hair over and secures it into a low, loose bun, with a few strands pulled out. The effect is pretty and sexy — the perfect match for her ruffled dress. Maybe she isn't going to have to hide from Knell after all.

post-ceremony

Once the ceremony is over, a grand style may seem slightly extreme, so perform a quick transformation by detaching your veil and leaving your tiara in place.

day to night

For a different evening look, make sure your daytime style can translate easily into night-time glamour. Too much product will leave the hair limp and dull, so use one that will brush out easily, such as hairspray. Take a bridesmaid with you when trying out looks with your hairdresser so that she can see how your style needs to be changed, using your own SOS kit.

LEFT
The hair is divided into one-inch square sections, and each one is bound with thin copper wire which

allows you to sculpt the tendrils into the desired shape. Finish off with a simple accessory.

going away

If you are traveling as soon as the reception is over, you'll want a hairstyle that is tidy and manageable. If you have long hair, try a chic, simple ponytail or scooped-up chignon, while a smudge of pomade is great for tousling or slicking back short hair. Some wedding-day hairstyles are likely to leave your hair kinky and unmanageable when you remove all the clips and paraphernalia. Happily, this means that you can employ the classic going-away style — the Grace Kelly headscarf.

RIGHT
For this glamorous "Jackie O" look, the hair is set on large hot rollers to give volume and wave, and then backcombed at the roots to create big-impact hair. Finish off with a spritz of hairspray to hold.

post-ceremony hair tips

Plan your day-to-night and going-away styles before the day. You may need to buy extra kit.

If your wedding-day hairstyle looks fine with your going-away outfit, don't change if you don't need to.

Keep it simple — by the time you leave the reception, you won't want to fuss over something complicated.

Don't be tempted to add more extra product — it will only make your hair look limp and dull.

Make sure you can travel with your hairstyle — you don't want to have to sit bolt upright on a long flight.

Take your SOS kit with you in your carry-on luggage.

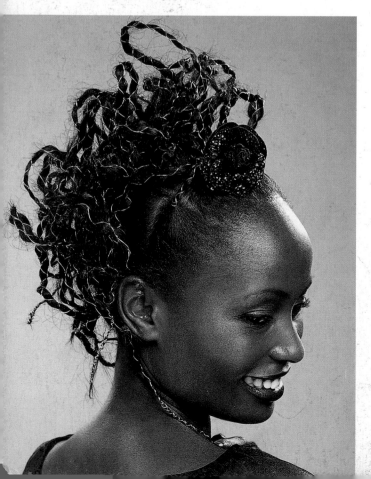

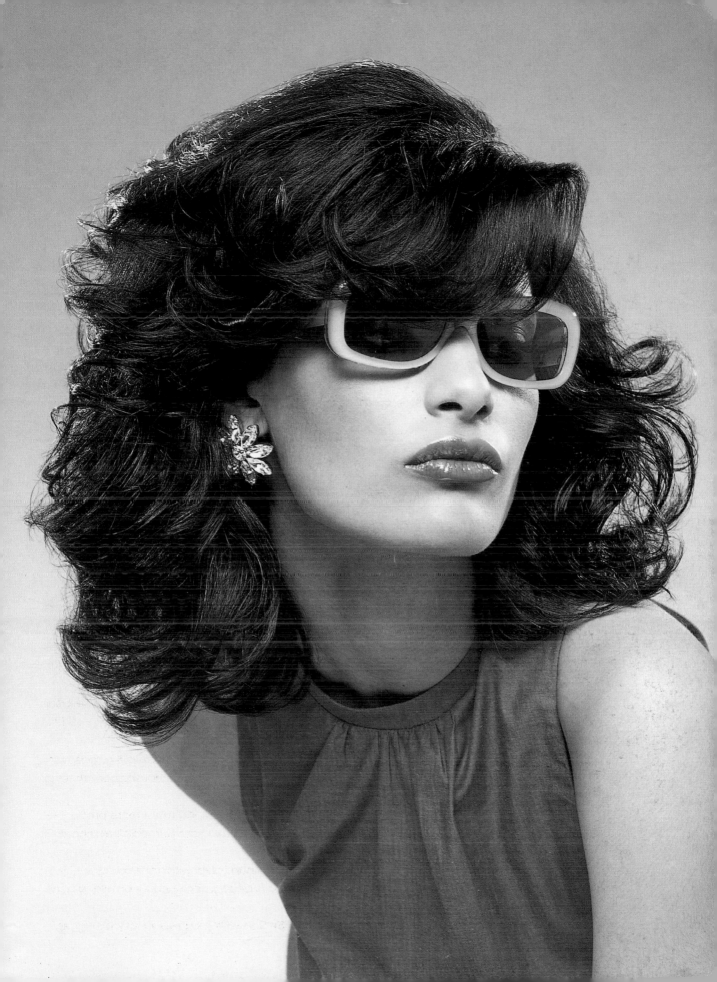

happily ever after...

All of the girls, except Chrissie, were hovering in the doorway of the plush country hotel, waiting for the happy couple to make their exit.

"Well, I think we should move to Upper East Side. That's where everything happens these days; don't you think so, Laura?" said Jaz. Laura mumbled non-committally. She had hoped that maybe she wouldn't be sharing a place anymore — at least, not with her girlfriends. But judging from John's mood this evening, he seemed less likely to want to co-habit than inhabit another country altogether.

"Oh, look!" cried Kate, breaking her train of thought, "Here they come!" Kisses, tears, hugs and more confetti rained down on the wedding party as the couple slowly made their way through the crowd. Jaz looked around frantically, "Where is Chrissie? She's going to miss them!" On cue, Chrissie came bobbing through the crowd. An arm reached out and pulled her out of the throng. It was Knell.

"Chrissie?" she said. Chrissie looked up at Knell, the most powerful woman at Devastation Records, and smiled nervously. She was unsure how to respond to the older woman, knowing that her looks and flirty charms would have no effect.

"Oh, hi Knell, what are you doing here?" she managed to ask.

"Simon's good friends with my son," Knell explained. "They were at college together. Anyway, I'm glad to have bumped into you here, I've seen a different side to you this evening."

"Yeah, I bet you have," thought Chrissie gloomily. Herself wearing a wrinkled dress and her make-up washed off by a torrential downpour was not the kind of lasting impression she wanted to linger with Knell. "I suppose you wondered why you didn't get the gig with Pout," Knell continued, referring to Chrissie's unsuccessful audition for a girl band earlier in the year. "It was because you didn't bring anything new and different. Basically, you were the same as the girls already in the band — all polish and perfection." Chrissie winced internally, reminded of why Knell was regarded as one of the toughest women in the industry. Knell placed an arm around her shoulders, "But seeing you tonight has made me reconsider. Maybe what you need is a change of image... something more natural. People are growing tired of the same old manufactured girl-band line-up. Come and see me on Monday, we'll talk." Knell gently pushed Chrissie back into the crowd, signifying that their meeting was over. Chrissie continued her struggle to get to the girls in a state of shock. Maybe she was going to get her shot at the limelight after all, and, even better, she wasn't going to have to share it!

"Quick, here they come," squealed Kate grabbing handfuls of confetti and throwing them into the air. The girls kissed and hugged the happy couple, tears flowing and giggles erupting — Polly was married, like a real grown-up!

As the car drove off towards the airport, Chrissie turned back to the other three left behind. "OK," she said, "let's go and get some big glasses of Champagne and toast the loss of another single girl."

They started off inside. "Oh, not you, Laura," said Jaz, putting her hand to her mouth apologetically. "You've got to go and see John, he's waiting for you in the rose garden. I forgot to tell you, sorry."

"Why?" asked Laura, nervously.

"I'm not sure," cried Jaz over her shoulder. "He just said he had something to ask you..."

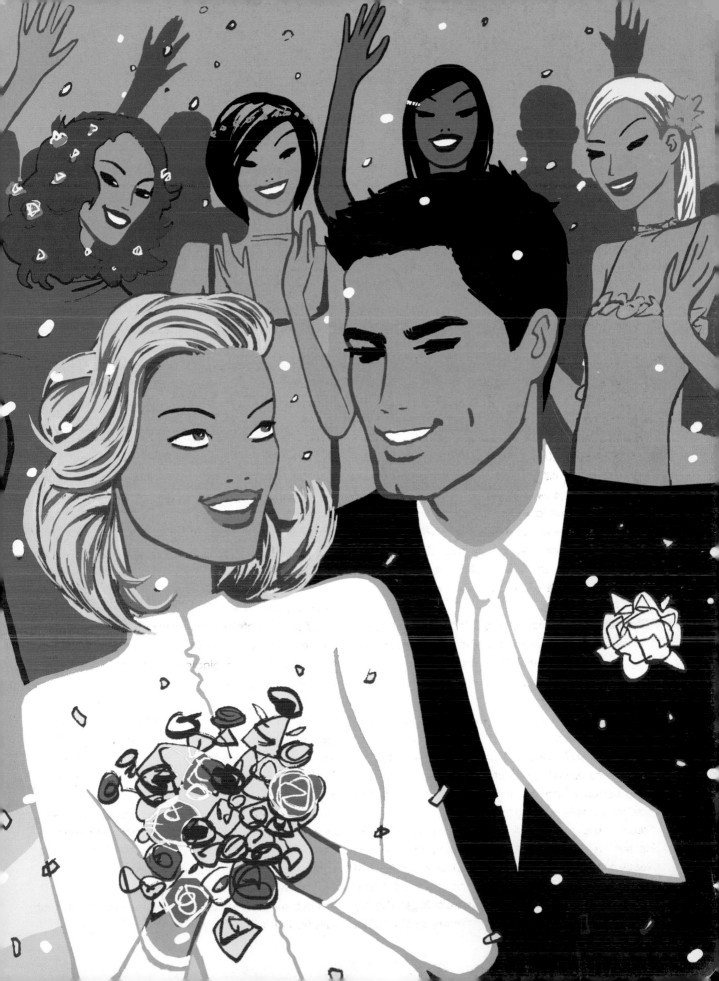

index

acknowledgments

Thank you to Adam Reed and Carolyn Newman
at the Percy Street salon.
With special thanks to Julie Gibson Jarvie, Penny Stock,
and Venetia Penfold, without whom the book wouldn't
have been possible.

The publishers would like to thank the following for fashion loans for the shoot:
Lara Bohinc 107 (0044 20 7405 7744), Elizabeth Emanuel (0044 20 7486 7979),
Nicole Farhi (0044 20 7499 8368), Joelynian (0044 20 7267 4770),
Joseph (0044 20 7225 3335) and Amanda Wakeley (0044 20 7590 9105).

With special thanks to the following:

Bud (by appointment only), tel: 0044 20 8537 0626

Butler & Wilson, 20 South Molton Street, London W1K 5QY, tel: 0044 20 7409 2955

Isabel Kurtenbach Designs (by appointment only), tel: 0044 20 7854 9647,
email: design@isabelkurtenbach.com, website:www.isabelkurtenbach.com

Nicola Pulvertaft (by appointment only), tel: 0044 7747 792 082

Amanda Wakeley, 80 Fulham Road, London SW3 6HR, tel: 0044 20 7590 9105

Basia Zarzycka (by appointment only), 52 Sloane Square, London SW1W 8AX, tel:
0044 20 7730 1660, email: basia@basia.com, website: www.basias.com